589 0109313

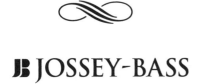

ℬ JOSSEY-BASS

PREVENTION IS PRIMARY

Strategies for Community Well-Being

Larry Cohen, Vivian Chávez,
and Sana Chehimi, Editors

Foreword by Georges C. Benjamin

Copublished by American Public Health Association

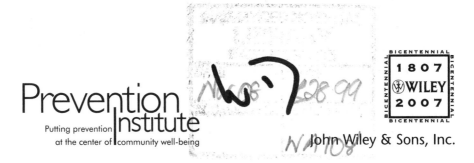

Prevention Institute
Putting prevention
at the center of community well-being

BICENTENNIAL
1807
⊕WILEY
2007
BICENTENNIAL

John Wiley & Sons, Inc.

Copyright © 2007 by Prevention Institute. All rights reserved.

Published by Jossey-Bass
A Wiley Imprint
989 Market Street, San Francisco, CA 94103-1741   www.josseybass.com

No part of this publication may be reproduced, stored in a retrieval system, or transmitted in any form or by any means, electronic, mechanical, photocopying, recording, scanning, or otherwise, except as permitted under Section 107 or 108 of the 1976 United States Copyright Act, without either the prior written permission of the publisher, or authorization through payment of the appropriate per-copy fee to the Copyright Clearance Center, Inc., 222 Rosewood Drive, Danvers, MA 01923, 978-750-8400, fax 978-646-8600, or on the Web at www.copyright.com. Requests to the publisher for permission should be addressed to the Permissions Department, John Wiley & Sons, Inc., 111 River Street, Hoboken, NJ 07030, 201-748-6011, fax 201-748-6008, or online at http://www.wiley.com/go/permissions.

Limit of Liability/Disclaimer of Warranty: While the publisher and author have used their best efforts in preparing this book, they make no representations or warranties with respect to the accuracy or completeness of the contents of this book and specifically disclaim any implied warranties of merchantability or fitness for a particular purpose. No warranty may be created or extended by sales representatives or written sales materials. The advice and strategies contained herein may not be suitable for your situation. You should consult with a professional where appropriate. Neither the publisher nor author shall be liable for any loss of profit or any other commercial damages, including but not limited to special, incidental, consequential, or other damages.

Readers should be aware that Internet Web sites offered as citations and/or sources for further information may have changed or disappeared between the time this was written and when it is read.

Jossey-Bass books and products are available through most bookstores. To contact Jossey-Bass directly call our Customer Care Department within the U.S. at 800-956-7739, outside the U.S. at 317-572-3986, or fax 317-572-4002.

Jossey-Bass also publishes its books in a variety of electronic formats. Some content that appears in print may not be available in electronic books.

Cataloging-in-publication data has been applied for.

ISBN 978-0-7879-8318-5

Printed in the United States of America
FIRST EDITION
PB Printing   10 9 8 7 6 5 4 3 2 1

CONTENTS

LIST OF TABLES, FIGURES, AND EXHIBITS

Tables

Figures

Exhibits

ACKNOWLEDGMENTS

We gratefully acknowledge the following institutions and individuals who made *Prevention Is Primary* a reality:

The Max Factor Family Foundation, for funding of student support to work at Prevention Institute on this text.

The California Endowment, Kaiser Permanente, and The California Wellness Foundation for their overall support of Prevention Institute's work.

The San Francisco State University Department of Health Education, for giving Vivian Chávez the opportunity to teach courses in community organizing, public health, and social justice over the past seven years, as well as encouraging a career grounded in primary prevention.

Kate Pastor and Ashby Wolfe, for their role as student editors, researchers, and writers. Kate wrote most of the sidebars, and Ashby researched and helped write elements of several chapters.

Jeremy Cantor and Jesse Appelman, for providing extensive content and organizational assistance in bringing this work to completion.

Jessica Scully, for her patient and thorough edits on several portions of the text.

Will Courtenay, for his box on men's health and review of the gender chapter.

We also acknowledge Ruth Bosco, Patti Culross, Rachel Davis, Jamila Edwards, Caitlin Merlo, and Greta Tubbesing.

Last but certainly not least, a big thank-you goes to the entire Prevention Institute staff for their enthusiastic support of the project and the extra demands it made on everyone.

Larry Cohen, Vivian Chávez, and Sana Chehimi
Editors

FOREWORD

Georges C. Benjamin

The United States spends $1.7 trillion annually on health care delivery and millions more on alternative treatments. The sum of these expenditures means we spend more per capita than any other industrialized nation. Yet according to the World Health Organization, when compared to these other nations the United States is far from the healthiest (World Health Organization, 2004).

The current U.S. health care delivery system does little to promote health, has significant challenges with delivering consistent quality, and has significant disparities in health outcomes. Over 47 million Americans do not have health insurance, and these people often receive medical care late in the course of their disease, often without the opportunity for preventive care. There are hundreds of thousands of underinsured individuals as well who frequently suffer the same fate.

Having an insurance card is not enough, however, when one considers that even in the nation's near-universal coverage program for seniors, there are still gaps in preventive health services like adult immunizations, screening colonoscopy, and mammography. Basic elements of healthy communities, such as healthy food, access to opportunities for physical activity, and clean air and water, are too often missing in low-income communities and communities of color. These disparities demonstrate the schism between the extraordinary potential of primary prevention and the reality of health policy and practice at the population level. As the nation becomes older, more ethnically diverse, and more deeply plagued by chronic illness, these disparities will become more apparent and widen.

Public health improvement is a continuum from health promotion and disease prevention to timely and appropriate clinical care. It is delivered in a social and economic context that affects health and quality of life. Understanding this context improves our ability to efficiently address our most pressing health concerns.

Good public health practice creates a community benefit. It is science-based and prevention-oriented. A good public health system should reduce morbidity and mortality and improve quality of life. It may even right a wrong. It can save money, but like most things, it usually requires an investment in time, money, and effort.

A 2006 survey by the nonpartisan research advocacy group Research!America and *Parade* magazine found that 86 percent of Americans believe that it is important to prevent their own health problems. Yet getting people to practice prevention continues to be a problem. Whether this is due to a lack of knowledge, lack of belief in preventive measures, or inability to connect the dots from preventive measures to outcomes, this text strives to fill that void. It does so by addressing prevention in its purest form: primary prevention.

The authors of the chapters assembled here are foremost authorities in the field of population health. They represent an important collection of experts in a range of public health and prevention disciplines. Examples include Deborah Prothrow-Stith, who was a trailblazer in defining violence as a public health problem and proposing prevention strategies for its reduction, and Howard Frumkin and Andrew Dannenberg, who have been effective advocates for changing the way we design, build, and rebuild communities and whose work offers clear guidance about the intersection between the built environment and health. The authors from Prevention Institute, led by Larry Cohen, along with his coeditors Vivian Chávez and Sana Chehimi, are an exceptional group who have made it their life's work not only to think about prevention in the academic sense but to go one step further and put their ideas into practice through their direct work with communities.

This book tackles such emerging issues as community resilience and revisits old concerns such as social justice and community organizing as primary prevention tools. The need to invest in strategies to empower communities more effectively was brought into our communal consciousness during Hurricanes Katrina and Rita, which hit the Gulf Coast of the United States in 2005, and the social failures that followed.

Using prevention as one tool in improving health and reducing costs is an increasing topic of discussion and is being touted as a component of the solution to controlling health care costs and improving national health. Primary prevention is about cost avoidance as well. The challenge is to understand its use, practice it, and evaluate its success. This book is designated to help readers understand the complex concepts of primary prevention in their purest form and incorporate them into practice. The old adage that "an ounce of prevention is worth a pound of cure" is the substance of this book; it is also about proving it.

References

Charlton Research Company. (2006). *Taking our pulse: The Parade/Research!America health poll.* Retrieved November 10, 2006, from http://www.researchamerica.org/polldata/2006/ParadePreventionPoll_slides_31906.pdf

World Health Organization. (2004). *The world health report 2004—Changing history.* Retrieved November 14, 2006, from http://www.who.int/whr/2004/en/index.html

To past, current, and future leaders in prevention,
for their continuous dedication to achieving community well-being
and linking it to social justice

THE CONTRIBUTORS

Bonnie Benard, M.S.W, has brought the concept of resilience to the attention of national and international audiences for more than two decades. She is currently a senior program associate in WestEd's Health and Human Development Program in Oakland, California. She writes widely, leads professional development, and makes presentations in the field of prevention and resilience and youth development theory, policy, and practice. Her book *Fostering Resiliency in Kids: Protective Factors in the Family, School, and Community* is credited with introducing resilience theory and application to the fields of prevention and education. Her most recent book, *Resiliency: What We Have Learned,* synthesizes the latest developments in resilience research and describes how it has been applied in the most successful efforts to support young people. Benard's work in resilience has also led to the development of the Resilience and Youth Development Module of the California Department of Education's Healthy Kids Survey, which polls students throughout California and elsewhere on their perceptions of supports and opportunities in their schools, homes, communities, and peer groups.

Georges C. Benjamin, M.D., F.A.C.P., is well known in the world of public health as a leader, practitioner, and administrator. Benjamin has been the executive director of the American Public Health Association (APHA), the nation's oldest and largest organization of public health professionals, since December 2002. He came to that post from his position as secretary of the Maryland Department of Health and Mental Hygiene, where he played a key role in developing Maryland's bioterrorism plan. Prior to becoming the state's chief health executive, Benjamin served four years as its deputy secretary for public health services.

An established administrator, author, and orator, Benjamin managed a 72,000 patient-visit ambulatory care service as chief of the Acute Illness Clinic at the Madigan Army Medical Center in Tacoma, Washington. Later, in Washington, D.C., he served as chief of emergency medicine at the Walter Reed Army Medical Center. As chairman of the department of community health and ambulatory care at the District of Columbia General Hospital, he managed a $7 million budget and 175 employees. Benjamin directed one of the busiest ambulance services in the nation as interim director of the Emergency Ambulatory Bureau of the District of Columbia Fire Department and worked as a health policy consultant. He also served as acting health commissioner for the District of Columbia.

Benjamin serves on several federal advisory committees, including the advisory committee for the director of the Centers for Disease Control and Prevention. He also serves on the boards of Research!America, Partnership for Prevention, and Advocates for Highway and Auto Safety. He is a member of the Institute of Medicine of the National Academies of Science.

Vivian Chávez, Dr.P.H., is an associate professor in the Department of Health Education at San Francisco State University. Her research interests include community-based participatory research, youth empowerment, global health, community organizing, and violence prevention. Her scholarship is informed in part by her standpoint as a woman of color and concerns the mind-body divide characteristic of higher education. Chávez has extensive media experience and over the past decade has worked to integrate the study of media literacy with policy advocacy. She codeveloped and practices a concept known as the "pedagogy of collegiality," a teaching approach that builds critical consciousness in learners. At SFSU, she teaches courses in public health, community organizing, multicultural women's health, and planning programs for adult learners. Chávez is a faculty member of the International Honors Program (IHP) on health and community. IHP's culturally competent approach to curriculum development combines traditional in-class lectures with independent study, hands-on field exploration, case studies, and group projects in Asia and Africa.

Sana Chehimi, M.P.H., is a program manager at Prevention Institute, a national nonprofit dedicated to advancing community well-being through primary prevention. Chehimi focuses her efforts on developing tools and strategies to advance primary prevention practice, with a particular emphasis on promoting environments that promote healthy eating and physical activity. She leads the development of the Environmental Nutrition and Activity Community Tool (ENACT), a Web-based resource designed to improve local nutrition and physical activity environments and oversees the institute's media advocacy efforts through the Rapid Response Media Network. Chehimi has written numerous reports and publications for Prevention Institute, including an assessment of the impact of the neighborhood food environment. Prior to joining Prevention Institute, she worked on basic science research in HIV and as a community treatment advocate for individuals living with the virus. She received her master's degree in public health from the University of California-Berkeley, with an emphasis on health and social behavior.

Molly Chidsey, B.A., a pollution prevention specialist for Multnomah County, Oregon's Sustainability Initiative, is enthusiastic about truly sustainable communities. Originally from Cleveland, Ohio, she received a bachelor's degree in English from Baldwin-Wallace College, with minors in sociology and environmental science. Chidsey has worked with national and local sustainability efforts, including organizing midwestern colleges to participate in Campus Ecology with the National Wildlife Federation, organizing the National "Mercury-Free Medicine" campaign of the international Health Care Without Harm coalition, and local air pollution efforts in Cleveland and Detroit.

Chidsey joined the Multnomah County Sustainability Initiative in 2002 to develop a new pollution prevention program and so far has worked to raise the average recycling rate for county facilities and developed a resolution for Multnomah County and the city of Portland that directs both agencies to form a toxics reduction strategy using the precautionary principle. She also helps staff the sustainable procurement strategy and the Sustainable Development Commission, a citizen's advisory board to the city of Portland and Multnomah County.

Though she believes there is not enough art or humor in the environmental movement, she is serious about sustainability and welcomes creativity as a tool to solve ecological problems.

Larry Cohen, M.S.W., is the founder and executive director of Prevention Institute, a nonprofit national center dedicated to improving community health and well-being by building momentum for effective primary prevention. Prevention Institute was developed to be a national focal point for advancing primary prevention with strategies and tools to help communities, governments, foundations, academics, and individuals. Cohen developed the *Spectrum of Prevention,* a tool that enables groups to devise a comprehensive approach to effective prevention, and several tools on coalition building, including *Eight Steps to Effective Coalition Building,* as well as materials on turf and interdisciplinary collaboration. He provides national training, consultation, and facilitation related to strategy, policy development, and coalition building in areas of health disparities, community health, physical activity and nutrition, mental health, health promotion, and injury and violence prevention. Cohen has written for numerous publications and has played a key role in establishing effective prevention policy, including the development of the nation's first multicity tobacco laws. He also played a significant role in strengthening California's bicycle, motorcycle, and auto safety efforts, as well as contributing to the development of the nation's food-labeling regulations. Cohen also developed and taught one of the nation's first youth violence prevention courses at the University of California-Berkeley's School of Public Health. He has received several awards for his work in public health, including the U.S. Department of Health and Human Services Secretary's Award for Community Health Promotion for broad work in primary prevention, the American Cancer Society Award for his work on no-smoking ordinances, and the Outstanding Preceptor Award at the UC-Berkeley School of Public Health. He received his master's degree in social welfare and his bachelor's degree in economics from the State University of New York, Stony Brook.

Andrew L. Dannenberg, M.D., M.P.H., is the associate director for science in the Division of Emergency and Environmental Health Services at the National Center for Environmental Health (NCEH), part of the Centers for Disease Control and Prevention in Atlanta. He oversees activities in NCEH focused on the health aspects of community design, such as land use, transportation, urban planning, and other issues related to the built environment. His current research projects include exploring the use of a health impact assessment as a tool to inform community planners and the use of model zoning codes to promote health. Dannenberg is also an adjunct professor of epidemiology and of environmental and occupational health at the Emory University Rollins School of Public Health. Prior to 2001, he served as director of CDC's Division of Applied Public Health Training with oversight responsibility for the Epidemic Intelligence Service and other training programs, as preventive medicine residency director and injury prevention epidemiologist at the Johns Hopkins School of Public Health, and as a cardiovascular epidemiologist at the National Institutes of Health. Dannenberg received a medical degree from Stanford University and a master of public health degree from Johns Hopkins University, and he completed a family medicine residency at the Medical University of South Carolina.

Lori Dorfman, Dr.P.H., directs the Berkeley Media Studies Group, a project of the Public Health Institute, where she oversees BMSG's research on the news, media advocacy training for advocates, and professional education for journalists.

She earned her doctorate in 1994 from the University of California-Berkeley's School of Public Health, where, using participant observation and content analysis, she studied how television news frames health. Her recent research examines how local television news and newspapers portray a variety of public health issues, including racial discrimination, children's health, nutrition and agriculture, paid family leave, youth and violence, intimate-partner violence, and alcohol, tobacco, and other drugs. Dorfman cowrote the major texts on media advocacy, *Public Health and Media Advocacy: Power for Prevention* and *News for a Change: An Advocates' Guide to Working with the Media,* and teaches a course for master's students on mass communication and public health at UC-Berkeley's School of Public Health. She conducts media advocacy training for grassroots organizations and public health leaders, consults for government agencies and community programs across the United States and internationally, and publishes articles on public health and mass communication. Dorfman's publications are available from http://www.bmsg.org.

Jonathan M. Ellen, M.D., is professor and vice chair of the Department of Pediatrics at the Johns Hopkins University's School of Medicine. He is also director of the Johns Hopkins Pediatrics Outcomes and Policy Research Center. His research has focused on prevention of sexually transmitted diseases, including HIV, among adolescents. He has investigated factors associated with the acquisition of STIs and factors associated with STI screening, treatment, and care. In addition, Ellen has studied the effectiveness of two innovative community-based strategies for controlling STIs—the Syphilis Elimination Program and UJIMA Mobile STI/HIV clinic. He has cochaired the Community Prevention Leadership Group for Adolescent HIV Prevention Trials Network; he leads five multisite research protocols focused on HIV prevention, including Connect to Protect; he has provided scientific consultation to STI investigators in England, the Caribbean, and South Africa; he has been invited to deliver lectures at international meetings; and he advises the Centers for Disease Control and Prevention in the United States and the Ministry of Health in Jamaica on STI prevention and control.

Catherine S. Erickson, B.A., M.P.H., earned her bachelor's degree in political science at Duke University and her M.P.H. in public health nutrition at the University of California-Berkeley. She has participated in research related to fresh-food access in low-income neighborhoods and links between the sustainable agriculture and health care communities.

Stephanie Ann Farquhar, Ph.D., is associate professor of community health at Portland State University in Portland, Oregon, and clinical assistant professor at Oregon Health and Sciences University. She draws primarily from the principles of community-based participatory research to address issues of social and environmental equity as they relate to health. In partnership with the Multnomah County Health Department and several community organizations, Farquhar recently completed a three-year Centers for Disease Control and Prevention grant to examine the role of community health workers and popular education in Latino and African American communities in Portland. She is currently investigating on a four-year National Institute for Occupational Safety and Health grant that seeks to reduce pesticide exposure among indigenous farmworkers in Oregon. Farquhar is on the board of directors of the Oregon Center for Environmental Health and served as a commissioner on the city-county Sustainable Development Commission.

Prior to arriving at the School of Community Health, Farquhar completed a one-year W. K. Kellogg Foundation Community Health Scholars postdoctoral fellowship and worked with residents of rural North Carolina to change discriminatory state-level natural disaster recovery policies. She earned her doctorate at the University of Michigan School of Public Health.

Howard Frumkin, M.D., Dr.P.H., is director of the National Center for Environmental Health/Agency for Toxic Substances and Disease Registry (NCEH/ATSDR) at the Centers for Disease Control and Prevention in Atlanta. NCEH/ATSDR works to maintain and improve the health of the American people by promoting a healthy environment and by preventing premature death and avoidable illness and disability caused by toxic substances and other environmental hazards.

Frumkin is an internist, environmental and occupational medicine specialist, and epidemiologist. His research interests include public health aspects of urban sprawl and the built environment; air pollution; metal and PCB toxicity; climate change; health benefits of contact with nature; and environmental and occupational health policy, especially regarding minority workers and communities, and those in developing nations. Before joining the CDC in 2005, he was professor and chair of the Department of Environmental and Occupational Health at the Rollins School of Public Health of Emory University and professor of medicine at Emory Medical School in Atlanta. He is the author or coauthor of over one hundred scientific journal articles and chapters, and his books include *Urban Sprawl and Public Health, Emerging Illness and Society, Environmental Health: From Global to Local,* and *Safe and Healthy School Environments.*

Wayne H. Giles, M.D., M.S., joined the Centers for Disease Control and Prevention in July 1992; he is currently the acting director for the Division of Adult and Community Health at the CDC's National Center for Chronic Disease Prevention and Health Promotion. He holds a bachelor's degree in biology from Washington University, a master of science degree in epidemiology from the University of

Maryland, and a doctor of medicine degree from Washington University, and he has completed residencies in both internal medicine (at the University of Alabama at Birmingham) and preventive medicine (at the University of Maryland).

His past work experience has included studies examining the prevalence of hypertension in Africa, clinical trials evaluating the effectiveness of cholesterol-lowering agents, and studies examining racial differences in the incidence of stroke. Giles currently oversees programmatic and research activities in cardio-vascular diseases, arthritis, aging, health care utilization, and racial and ethnic disparities in health within the Division of Adult and Community Health at the CDC. He has published more than one hundred articles in peer-reviewed journals and has written several book chapters.

Ongoing research includes the surveillance of cardiovascular disease, secondary prevention activities related to cardiovascular disease, racial and socio-economic determinants of end-state renal disease, and the evaluation of genetic and environmental risk factors for cardiovascular disease. Giles has been honored with numerous awards, including the Distinguished Researcher Award bestowed by the International Society on Hypertension in Blacks and the Jeffrey P. Koplan Award granted by the CDC.

Leandris C. Liburd, Ph.D., M.P.H., serves as chief of the Community Health and Program Services Branch at the Centers for Disease Control and Prevention in Atlanta, where she directs public health programs addressing community health promotion and the elimination of health disparities. Her principal research is focused on understanding the intersection of race, class, and gender in chronic disease risks, management, and prevention. She spent twelve years as a community interventionist in the CDC's Division of Diabetes Translation, where her work was focused on developing community models for diabetes prevention and control programs in racial and ethnic communities in the continental United States, around the Pacific Rim, along the U.S. border with Mexico, and among Native American tribes in the Southwest. She has written extensively on community-based public health approaches to chronic disease prevention and control, the influence of culture and gender on health beliefs and behaviors, and the elimination of health disparities. Liburd holds a bachelor of arts degree from the University of Michigan at Ann Arbor, a master of public health degree in health education from the University of North Carolina at Chapel Hill, and a doctor of philosophy degree in medical anthropology from Emory University.

Siobhan Maty, Ph.D., M.P.H., is an assistant professor in the School of Community Health at Portland State University in Portland, Oregon. She is a social epidemiologist who uses a community-based participatory research approach in addition to traditional epidemiologic methods to study the social determinants of health, health disparities, the epidemiology of diabetes and obesity, and the translation of research into action to achieve social change. She is currently teaching undergraduate and graduate students, in addition to working on several community-based participatory epidemiologic research projects with ethnically and socioeconomically diverse communities in the greater Portland region.

Leslie McBride, Ph.D., is an associate professor in the School of Community Health at Portland State University in Portland, Oregon, where she teaches graduate and undergraduate courses in integrative health and qualitative research. Since 1977, she has conducted research into and taught courses on various aspects of women's health.

Leslie Mikkelsen, M.P.H., R.D., is managing director of Prevention Institute. A key emphasis of her work is on systems approaches to promoting healthy eating and physical activity. She provides training and facilitation for local and state coalitions and has written research papers for the California Endowment and the Robert Wood Johnson Foundation outlining strategies for shifting community environments to support healthier behaviors. She coordinates the Strategic Alliance for Healthy Food and Activity Environments, a network advocating to make healthy eating and physical activity options more accessible in California. Before joining Prevention Institute, Mikkelsen worked for the Alameda County (California) and New York City food banks, where she directed programs designed to address hunger and mobilize community advocacy to support antihunger policies.

Meredith Minkler, Dr.P.H., is professor of health and social behavior and director of the Dr.P.H. program at the School of Public Health, University of California-Berkeley. She has three decades of experience in community building and organizing and community-based participatory research activities in underserved communities. Her current research includes documenting the impacts of community-based participatory research on public policy, empowerment intervention studies with youth and the elderly, and national studies of health disparities in older Americans. Minkler has written more than one hundred articles and book chapters and has written, cowritten, or edited seven books, including *Community Organizing and Community Building for Health, Community-Based Participatory Research for Health* (with Nina Wallerstein), *Grandmothers as Caregivers* (with Kathleen Roe), and *Critical Perspectives on Aging* (with Carroll L. Estes).

Marion Nestle, Ph.D., M.P.H., is Paulette Goddard Professor in the Department of Nutrition, Food Studies, and Public Health at New York University, a department she chaired for fifteen years (1988–2003). She received her Ph.D. in molecular biology and her M.P.H. in public health nutrition from the University of California-Berkeley. She has held faculty positions in the Department of Biology at Brandeis University and at the University of California San Francisco School of Medicine, where she was associate dean for human biology programs. From 1986 to 1988, she was senior nutrition policy adviser in the U.S. Department of Health and Human Services and managing editor of the 1988 *Surgeon General's Report on Nutrition and Health*. She is the author of *Food Politics: How the Food Industry Influences Nutrition and Health; Safe Food: Bacteria, Biotechnology, and Bioterrorism;* and *What to Eat.*

Neha Patel, M.S., obtained her degree in environmental health management from Oregon State University in 2003. She is the program director for the Oregon Center for Environmental Health, which works to protect public health and the environment through community action to eliminate environmental pollutants. Over the past six years, Patel has coordinated the center's award-winning Health Care Without Harm campaign for environmentally responsible health care. In 2006, she accepted the national Pioneers of Precaution award on behalf of the center for the creation of a toxics reduction strategy adopted by local government operations using the precautionary principle.

Daniel Perales was born in Brownsville, Texas. He received his B.A. degree from the University of California-Berkeley and his M.P.H. and Dr.P.H. degrees from the University of Texas School of Public Health in Houston. Perales is an associate professor of public health in the Department of Health Science at San Jose State University. He teaches a course in health promotion planning and evaluation in the university's M.P.H. program and courses in social marketing and epidemiology in the undergraduate program. Over the past fifteen years, he has conducted research that includes observational studies of bicycle safety helmet use in two California counties and a needle exchange HIV/AIDS harm reduction program. He has also conducted evaluations of programs related to tobacco control, adolescent pregnancy prevention, nutrition education and food security, child immunization, and coalition development and maintenance. In 1995 and 1996, he served on the American Public Health Association's Strategic Planning Committee. Perales is treasurer and a former vice president of the Society for Public Health Education. He is also a past member of the editorial board of *Health Education and Behavior,* the editorial advisory board of the journal *Health Promotion Practice,* and the editorial board of the *Californian Journal of Health Promotion* and serves on Prevention Institute's board of directors.

Deborah Prothrow-Stith, M.D., is a nationally recognized public health leader, known for her efforts to have youth violence defined as a public health problem. She created a social movement to prevent violence in Boston that has had repercussions for the entire nation. In 1987, she was appointed the first woman commissioner of public health for the Commonwealth of Massachusetts, where she established the first Office of Violence.

Prothrow-Stith developed and wrote *The Violence Prevention Curriculum for Adolescents*. She is also the author of *Deadly Consequences* and cowrote two books with Howard Spivak, M.D.: *Murder Is No Accident* and *Sugar and Spice and No Longer Nice*. She has written or cowritten more than eighty articles on medical and public health issues.

Prothrow-Stith is the associate dean for faculty development and professor of public health practice at the Harvard School of Public Health, where she created and served as founding director of the Division of Public Health Practice. A Spelman College and Harvard Medical School graduate, she has received ten honorary doctorates, the 1993 World Health Day Award, the 1989 Secretary of Health and Human Services Award, and a presidential appointment to the National Commission on Crime Control and Prevention.

Michelle Ramirez, Ph.D., is a medical anthropologist at Kaiser Permanente's Center for Health Research in Portland, Oregon. She has conducted women's health research in Nayarit, Yucatán, and Oaxaca, Mexico. She has completed postdoctoral training at Oregon Health and Science University in public health and preventive medicine and is currently researching health issues among long-term colorectal cancer survivors.

Michael S. Spencer, Ph.D., M.S.W., is an associate professor at the University of Michigan School of Social Work and faculty affiliate of the Program on American Cultures and the National Poverty Center. His research focuses on the health and mental health of populations of color. His current research examines the causes and consequences of disparities in the health, mental health, and service use of people of color. Spencer is one of the principal investigators for the REACH Detroit Partnership, a community-based participatory research partnership. The goal of REACH Detroit is to reduce health disparities, particularly diabetes, among African American and Latino Eastside and Southwest Detroit residents through the promotion of a healthy lifestyle and self-management of health. Spencer is also the principal investigator of the Family Development Project, a University of Michigan–Detroit Head Start community-based research partnership whose goal is to improve mental health service use and delivery among families enrolled in the Detroit Head Start programs. Spencer teaches courses in contemporary cultures in the United States, multicultural and multilingual organizing, facilitation training for dialogues in diversity and social justice, social work practice in communities and social systems, community development, and human behavior in the social environment.

Makani Themba-Nixon is executive director of the Praxis Project, a nonprofit organization dedicated to helping communities use media and policy advocacy to advance health equity and justice. She was previously director of the Grass Roots Innovative Policy Program (GRIPP), a national project to build capacity among local organizing groups to engage policy advocacy to address institutional racism in welfare and public education. She served as staff for the California state legislature, was media director for the Southern Christian Leadership Conference in Los Angeles, and worked five years for the Marin Institute for the Prevention of Alcohol and Other Drug Problems, including three years as director of its Center for Media and Policy Analysis.

Themba-Nixon has published numerous articles and case studies on race, media, policy advocacy, and public health. She is coauthor of *Media Advocacy and Public Health: Power for Prevention*, a contributor to the volumes *We the Media, State of the Race: Creating Our 21st Century*, along with many other edited book projects. She is also the author of *Making Policy, Making Change*, which examines media and policy advocacy for public health through case studies and practical information. Her latest book, cowritten with Hunter Cutting, is *Talking the Walk: Communications Guide for Racial Justice*.

Lawrence Wallack, Dr.P.H., is dean of the College of Urban and Public Affairs at Portland State University and emeritus professor of public health at the University of California-Berkeley. He is one of the primary architects of media advocacy, an innovative approach to working with mass media to advance public health. He has published extensively and lectures frequently on topics related to the news media and public health and social issues. He is the principal author of *News for a Change: An Advocate's Guide to Working with the Media* and *Media Advocacy and Public Health: Power for Prevention*. He is also coeditor of *Mass Media and Public Health: Complexities and Conflicts*.

Wallack has been the recipient of several awards, including the Robert Wood Johnson Foundation Innovator Award (2000–2005); Distinguished Wellness Lecturer, University of California-Berkeley (1997); the Alfred W. Childs Distinguished Award for Faculty Service, School of Public Health, University of California-Berkeley (1996–1997); and University of California Health Net Wellness Award Lecturer (1994).

Wallack has appeared on *Nightline, Good Morning America*, the *CBS Evening News*, the *Today Show*, Cable Network News, *Oprah*, and numerous local news and public affairs programs to discuss his research and comment on policy issues regarding public health problems.

Nina Wallerstein, Dr.P.H., is professor and director of the master's in public health program in the University of New Mexico's Department of Family and Community Medicine. She has worked in empowerment and popular education and community-based participatory research since the mid-1970s. Recent books include *Community-Based Participatory Research in Health* (with Meredith Minkler) and *Problem-Posing at Work: A Popular Educator's Guide* (with Elsa Auerbach).

Dan Wohlfeiler, M.J., M.P.H., is chief of the Office of Policy and Communications of the Sexually Transmitted Disease Control branch of the California Department of Health Services. From 1990 to 1998, he served as education director of San Francisco's STOP AIDS Project, a leading HIV-prevention organization run by and for gay and bisexual men in San Francisco. He is a nationally recognized expert on structural interventions for HIV prevention and offers training through the California STD/HIV Prevention Training Center. His current interests focus on structural and network-level interventions for STD/HIV prevention.

Ashby Wolfe, M.D., joined Prevention Institute in 2005 as a contributing editor for the text *Prevention Is Primary*. She has worked on a number of recent public health projects, including an investigation of access to care among low-wage workers in New York and California. She also assisted Prevention Institute in preparing a paper on violence prevention for the Robert Wood Johnson Foundation. Her current policy interests include health care access, reproductive health, and primary prevention. She is currently beginning an analysis of federal policy and prevention initiatives targeted at California's Medicare and Medicaid populations. She received her doctor of medicine degree from the Stony Brook University School of Medicine in New York and is currently pursuing a dual master's degree in public policy and public health at the University of California-Berkeley.

Katie Woodruff, M.P.H., believes that the news media have tremendous power in shaping how the public and policymakers perceive social issues. Her research and training activities help groups harness that power to work for social change. Woodruff is program director for the Berkeley Media Studies Group, which studies the process of news gathering and analyzes media content to support media advocacy training for community and public health leadership groups. She provides strategic consultation and media advocacy training to community groups and public health professionals working on a range of public health and public interest issues, including violence prevention, alcohol control, tobacco control, injury control, children's health, child care, and affirmative action. She also conducts research on news content and has published case studies and articles on applying media advocacy to public health and social justice issues. She earned a master's degree in public health, with a focus on community health education, at the University of California-Berkeley and a bachelor's degree in creative writing at Brown University. Woodruff is a coauthor of *News for a Change: An Advocate's Guide to Working with the Media.*

INTRODUCTION

Larry Cohen, Vivian Chávez, Sana Chehimi

Prevention works. From mandatory seat belt use to unleaded paint and gasoline, from fluoridated water to childhood immunizations, our daily lives are filled with reminders that prevention saves lives and reduces unnecessary suffering. An estimated 50 percent of annual deaths in the United States are preventable (McGinnis & Foege, 1993; Mokdad, Marks, Stroup, & Gerberding, 2004). As George W. Albee, one of the foremost leaders of the prevention movement, noted, "No mass disorder afflicting mankind is ever brought under control or eliminated by attempts at treating the affected individual," explaining that prevention efforts targeting whole populations are needed instead (1983, p. 24). However, despite a demonstrated track record of positive health impacts, prevention efforts in practice are increasingly deprioritized and marginalized in favor of action after the fact.

The purpose of *Prevention Is Primary: Strategies for Community Well-Being* is to inspire a new generation of community leaders with the power of primary prevention in *practice*. We focus in particular on *primary prevention*—taking action to prevent health and social problems *before* their onset—a proven strategy for improving health and well-being for all segments of society. Primary prevention emphasizes the particular value of fostering health-supporting community environments and of making the healthy choice the easy choice.

Primary prevention is a skill; you "cannot assume that just anyone can do prevention. A person who is skilled and knowledgeable about prevention . . . is more likely to have the resources to resist being drawn into intervention, crisis management, and service provision at the expense of prevention, proactive planning, and capacity building" (MacDonald & Green, 2001, p. 763). *Prevention Is Primary* defines a coherent set of principles and approaches to develop the skills and guide the practice of prevention in a wide range of contemporary health and social problems.

We draw our inspiration from the leadership of all the advocates who, across decades, disciplines, and issue areas, have made every effort to move prevention from the margins to the center of community health. One notable standout on this list is Henrik Blum, who exemplifies the kind of academic for whom this text was created. Blum did not limit himself to the theoretical aspects of academia. His efforts to develop the "determinants of health" to identify the underlying causes of health problems revealed the prominence of the social, cultural, and physical environment as a key health determinant (Blum, 1981). Rather than "lurching from crisis to crisis," Blum was committed to the power of participatory community health planning, feeding into a cycle of policy development and implementation to develop profound solutions to health and social problems.

Prevention Is Primary aims to change the ways in which a new generation of community and public health leaders approach health by making a strong case for primary prevention. Rather than focus on a single discipline or preventable condition, we have deliberately chosen to build on the cross-disciplinary wisdom and experiences of a variety of practitioners.

We have organized the text into three parts: "Defining the Issues," "Key Elements of Effective Prevention Efforts," and "Prevention in Context." The parts are arranged in sequence, and we suggest that readers move through them sequentially. Each part includes its own introduction, providing the context and analysis for each of the included chapters. A number of chapters are complemented by sidebars, written by or on behalf of the editors, which further contextualize primary prevention from a variety of disciplines and perspectives. These sidebars represent the perspectives of the editors, not necessarily the chapter authors.

Part One, "Defining the Issues," begins with a thorough definition of what primary prevention is and, equally important, what it is not. The part continues by describing the overarching framework and principles guiding *quality* prevention efforts, including a focus on social justice and health equity, gender, and community resilience.

Part Two, "Key Elements of Effective Prevention Efforts," describes the transition from prevention theory to implementation and practice—from interdisciplinary collaboration to the evaluation of primary prevention efforts.

Part Three, "Prevention in Context," explores the application of prevention efforts to a wide range of contemporary health and social issues and demonstrates both current successes and the potential inherent in prevention practice.

As editors with a passion for prevention, we realize that although we have tried our best, no one text can fully represent the comprehensive nature of primary prevention. To that end, we have set up a Web site, http://www.prevention institute.org/prevention_text.html, where we will continue to post prevention case studies, tools and resources, and profiles of prevention leaders. We hope that you will not only turn to this Web site as your careers progress but will also contribute to its content.

Although we recognize that we are members of a global community with transnational connections and implications, we focus predominantly in this book on the United States. We also recognize that whereas primary prevention efforts will not resolve every health and social problem, they are nonetheless a much needed complement to care and treatment.

As much as this book is about health, it is equally about social justice. As the civil rights leader Fannie Lou Hamer of the Student Nonviolent Coordinating Committee stated, "I'm sick and tired of being sick and tired" (DeMuth, 1964, p. 549), and she translated her despair at U.S. injustice into voter registration leadership. For the new generation of leaders, the readers this book is intended for, health and justice must be inseparable. As César Chávez explained, "We can choose to use our lives for others to bring about a better and more just world for our children" (National Farm Worker Ministry, 2005, p. 1). "Our movement," Chávez stated, referring to the United Farm Workers, "is spreading like flames across a dry plain" (1966, p. 14). Our hope, in universities across the country and the world, is that this book becomes a small spark in the movement for good health for all.

References

Albee, G. W. (1983). Psychopathology, prevention, and the just society. *Journal of Primary Prevention, 4,* 5–40.

Blum, H. L. (1981). Social perspective on risk reduction. *Family and Community Health, 3,* 41–50.

Chávez, C. E. (1966, March 17). The plan of Delano. *El Malcriado,* pp. 11–14.

DeMuth, J. (1964, June 1). Tired of being sick and tired. *The Nation,* pp. 548–551.

MacDonald, M. A., & Green, L. W. (2001). Reconciling concept and context: The dilemma of implementation in school-based health promotion. *Health Education & Behavior, 28,* 749–768.

McGinnis, J. M., & Foege, W. H. (1993). Actual causes of death in the United States. *Journal of the American Medical Association, 270,* 2207–2212.

Mokdad, A. H., Marks, J. S., Stroup, D. F., & Gerberding, J. L. (2004). Actual causes of death in the United States, 2000. *Journal of the American Medical Association, 291,* 1238–1245.

National Farm Worker Ministry. (2005, November 22). Litany of Christian hope. Retrieved October 7, 2006, from http://www.nfwm.org/worshipresources/litanies.shtml

PART ONE

DEFINING THE ISSUES

Typically, medical approaches treat people after they get sick and look at one individual at a time. But a better option for societal health and well-being would be to create quality prevention techniques to keep people from getting sick in the first place. What is *quality* prevention? It is far more than a message in a brochure or information received during a medical visit. The four chapters in Part One explain the fundamental concepts needed to complement medical treatment with quality prevention efforts and to improve and maintain societal health.

Chapter One, "Beyond Brochures: The Imperative for Primary Prevention," by Larry Cohen and Sana Chehimi, establishes the need to address the factors that cause unnecessary illness, injury, and death. The authors show that primary prevention provides an important solution to an overburdened health care system where, as health care services weaken, everyone is increasingly at risk and marginalized populations are most vulnerable. A prevention-oriented approach to health and well-being is needed to help eliminate the injustice of the greatest impact of illness and injury falling on disfranchised populations. The authors note that primary prevention is far from a new idea and highlight its long and proven record of success. The chapter emphasizes the importance of a comprehensive approach and presents the "spectrum of prevention," a framework for putting primary prevention into practice.

Health disparities—gaps between health outcomes by race and ethnicity and other factors—are often stark for people of color. In Chapter Two, "Achieving

Health Equity and Social Justice," Wayne Giles and Leandris Liburd reveal that health disparities are primarily the result of social structures and processes rather than individual genetic factors. While inequities in and access to quality medical services for people of color are well documented and contribute to disparities, addressing medical care inequities is just one part of a larger solution. Modifying key elements of the community environment can decrease the number of people who become ill or injured to begin with. Thus the adoption of a primary prevention-oriented framework, including comprehensive efforts directed at the broader social and policy environments that promote health and prevent disease, offers the opportunity for improving both health and equity.

Michelle Ramirez, Siobhan Maty, and Leslie McBride, the authors of Chapter Three, "Gender, Health, and Prevention," focus on another distinction that affects health outcomes: gender. They argue for incorporating a gender orientation into primary prevention efforts. The authors note that gender is a social construct, a set of cultural expectations of behavior and identity separate from biological sex. For any given condition, some similar but also some very different social and cultural processes affect levels of prevalence for men and women. From the editors' perspective, it is critical to consider gender because it is one of the important and often ignored explanations behind the aggregated statistics of ill health. The dominant cultural paradigm for a "real man" includes heterosexuality, risk taking, prodigious appetite, high levels of control and power, and physical indestructibility. For "real women," it includes heterosexuality, caretaking, attractiveness, seamless juggling of family and career, emotional responsiveness, and physical restraint. The authors look at four vital health issues—intimate partner violence, traffic injuries, cardiovascular disease, and depression—and lay out the differential ways in which social definitions such as gender create expectations of behavior and conditions that give rise to these health issues. The authors end by offering examples of effective initiatives.

In Chapter Four, "The Hope of Prevention: Individual, Family, and Community Resilience," Bonnie Benard describes resilience, the ability of individuals, families, and communities to face and overcome challenges and obstacles, as a key building block of prevention. Focusing primarily on risk factors, the more traditional approach to community health, can have the effect of stigmatizing and demoralizing individuals and communities. Protective factors, such as strong social networks and partnerships, caring relationships between community members, and education and literacy, help people grow stronger. These factors also give communities the ability to build their own capacity to effect change and prevent illness and injury.

CHAPTER ONE

BEYOND BROCHURES

The Imperative for Primary Prevention

Larry Cohen, Sana Chehimi

Some years ago, a prominent individual suffered a major heart attack right across the street from the local county hospital. Although the initial prognosis was poor, the care provided by the hospital resulted in a quick and near-complete recovery. The county board of supervisors proudly emphasized the hospital's success during its next meeting. In the presence of the media, the supervisors congratulated key health officials on the outstanding care and treatment provided, noting in particular the high quality of the hospital staff, medical equipment, and training. As the proceedings were winding down, one supervisor asked, "But what about prevention? Do we have quality prevention?" Without missing a beat, the health director answered, "Yes." Pointing to a pile of brochures titled *Staying Heart Healthy*, he proclaimed, "We have these!"

This isn't an isolated case. Many aspects of health in the United States, from how resources are allocated to who has access to care, suffer from a lack of focus on prevention. Far too often, prevention is an afterthought (Cowen, 1987). The predominant approach to health and well-being in this country focuses on medical treatment and services—*after the fact*—for the many Americans who are sick and injured each year. Unfortunately, there is a lack of corresponding emphasis on quality community and large-scale prevention efforts in order to avoid those same illnesses and injuries *in the first place*. Furthermore, prevention is often relegated to a message in a brochure or to a few moments during a medical visit. Yet these approaches are not quality prevention efforts—human behavior is complicated, and awareness of a health risk does not automatically lead to taking protective action (Ghez, 2000).

Effectively addressing the range of health and social problems of the twenty-first century requires a fundamental paradigm shift that generates equity for the most vulnerable members of society and maximizes limited resources: moving from medical treatment *after the fact* to prevention *in the first place* and from targeting *individuals* to a comprehensive *community* focus. The imperative for this shift in thinking is best described by the psychologist and noted prevention advocate George Albee (1983), who noted that ". . . no mass disorder afflicting mankind is ever brought under control or eliminated by attempts at treating the affected individual . . ." (p. 24).

This chapter moves prevention *beyond brochures* by presenting an alternative to the dominant individual-based prevention and treatment model. We begin by defining primary prevention and offering recent and historical examples of prevention successes, demonstrating that prevention is the basis of public health and that prevention works. We then make the case for primary prevention, emphasizing that prevention supports health care infrastructure, is an effective use of health care resources, and assists those most in need by decreasing disparities in health. Finally, we describe the six complementary levels of the *spectrum of prevention*, which provide a multifaceted and sustainable framework for achieving community change.

Primary Prevention: Moving Upstream

In a 2002 speech to the Commonwealth Club in San Francisco, Gloria Steinem observed, "We are still standing on the bank of the river, rescuing people who are drowning. We have not gone to the head of the river to keep them from falling in. That is the 21st century task." Steinem's remark refers to a popular analogy, "moving upstream," that is used to highlight the importance and relevance of primary prevention (Ardell, 1977/1986).

Moving Upstream

While walking along the banks of a river, a passerby notices that someone in the water is drowning. After pulling the person ashore, the rescuer notices another person in the river in need of help. Before long, the river is filled with drowning people, and more rescuers are required to assist the initial rescuer. Unfortunately, some people are not saved, and some victims fall back into the river after they have been pulled ashore. At this time, one of the rescuers starts walking upstream. "Where are you going?" the other rescuers ask, disconcerted. The upstream rescuer replies, "I'm going upstream to see why so many people keep falling into the river." As it turns out, the bridge leading across the river upstream has a hole through which people are falling. The upstream rescuer realizes that fixing the hole in the bridge will prevent many people from ever falling into the river in the first place.

The act of "moving upstream" and taking action *before* a problem arises in order to avoid it entirely, rather than treating or alleviating its consequences, is called primary prevention. The term *primary prevention* was coined in the late 1940s by Hugh Leavell and E. Guerney Clark from the Harvard and Columbia University Schools of Public Health, respectively. Leavell and Clark described primary prevention as "measures applicable to a particular disease or group of diseases in order to intercept the causes of disease before they involve man . . . [in the form of] specific immunizations, attention to personal hygiene, use of environmental sanitation, protection against occupational hazards, protection from accidents, use of specific nutrients, protection from carcinogens, and avoidance of allergens" (Goldston, 1987, p. 3). Although Leavell and Clark's *definition* is mostly disease-oriented, the applications of primary prevention extend beyond medical problems and include the prevention of other societal concerns, ranging from violence to environmental degradation, that also affect health and well-being. Primary prevention efforts are, by definition, proactive and should generally be aimed at populations, not just individuals. Returning to the upstream analogy, fixing the hole in the bridge will benefit not only those at greatest risk for falling in but everyone who crosses it, the rescuers on the riverbank, and everyone who helps pay for rescue costs.

Leavell and Clark further identified two other degrees of prevention, termed *secondary* and *tertiary prevention*. Secondary prevention consists of a set of measures used for early detection and prompt intervention to control a problem or disease and minimize the consequences, while tertiary prevention focuses on the reduction of further complications of an existing disease or problem, through treatment and rehabilitation (Spasoff, Harris, & Thuriaux, 2001).

Leavell and Clark's "overarching concept of prevention," described in Table 1.1 through the example of childhood lead poisoning, actually refers to three distinctive activities that might be better termed "prevention, treatment, and rehabilitation" (Goldston, 1987, p. 3). As noted by Albee (1987, p. 12), "All three forms of preventive intervention are useful and defensible." However, whereas primary prevention *alone* is not enough to address pervasive health and social problems, it remains the foremost method that we can employ in order to *eliminate* future health and social problems. Albee goes on to note that "any *reduction in incidence* must rely heavily on proactive efforts with large groups, and such actions involve primary prevention approaches" (p. 12).

Prevention Works: The History of Prevention Efforts

In practice, primary prevention involves policies and actions that fix the metaphorical holes in the bridge that lead to sickness and injury. Primary prevention works to reduce the ailments that would otherwise be treated.

One well-known and very successful modern example of primary prevention is the National Minimum Age Drinking Act of 1984, which required all states to raise the minimum age to purchase alcohol to twenty-one or risk losing major transportation funding. The National Highway Traffic Safety Administration

TABLE 1.1. RECOGNIZING THE DIFFERENCES BETWEEN PRIMARY, SECONDARY, AND TERTIARY PREVENTION: CHILDHOOD LEAD POISONING.

Primary prevention

Dramatic reductions in the blood lead levels of U.S. children from 1970 to 1990 were attributed to population-based environmental policies that banned the use of lead in gasoline, paint, drinking-water pipes, food and beverage containers, and other products that created widespread exposure to lead (Centers for Disease Control and Prevention, 2004).

Primary prevention is the only way to reduce the neurocognitive effects of lead poisoning (Lee & Hurwitz, 2002).

Secondary prevention

Lead-level screening programs for at-risk children followed by the treatment of children with high levels and removal of lead paint from households. Screening can prevent recurrent exposures and the exposure of other children to lead by triggering the identification and remediation of sources of lead in children's environments (New York State Department of Health, 2004).

Tertiary prevention

The treatment, support, and rehabilitation of children with lead poisoning who manifest complications of the disease. Lead chelation of the blood and soft tissues of exposed individuals can reduce morbidity associated with lead poisoning. Chelation can reduce the immediate toxicity associated with acute ingestion of lead but has limited ability to reverse the neurocognitive effects of chronic exposure (Lee & Hurwitz, 2002).

(NHTSA) estimates that as a result of minimum-drinking-age laws, 18,220 lives were saved between 1975 and 1999 (U.S. Department of Transportation, 1999).

This law is far from the first example of primary prevention. In fact, public health has always been founded on prevention. The first public health measures were vast environmental improvements aimed at keeping entire populations healthy. *The Sanitary Conditions of the Labouring Population of Great Britain*, a seminal report published in 1842 by the English civil servant Edwin Chadwick, noted that widespread preventive measures were necessary to preserve the health of England's workforce (Duffy, 1990). Initial public health efforts focused primarily on improving water supplies, refuse and sewage disposal, housing, ventilation, disinfection, and general cleanliness in a community (Vetter & Matthews, 1999). Labor, housing standards, and other health regulations were also developed during this period in an effort to curtail disease and premature death (Duffy, 1990).

What many experts recognize as the seminal event of the prevention movement was a simple but exceptionally effective action taken by John Snow, a physician, during England's 1854 cholera outbreak. Cholera spreads rapidly, causing diarrhea, vomiting, and if untreated, eventual death from dehydration. During the 1854 outbreak, five hundred people from an impoverished section of South London died within a ten-day period as a result of the disease. Many people needed treatment. However, instead of just treating his patients individually, Snow, who is credited with some of the initial investigative work in epidemiology for his work during an earlier cholera outbreak, also decided to "move upstream" and locate the source of the problem (Summers, 1989).

By studying the trends of the particular outbreak, Snow mapped the origin to a specific water pump on Broad Street. He used the information he had collected about the source of cholera to prevent its spread. Instead of warning locals not to drink water from the contaminated pump or attempting to treat the water for drinking, Snow took his initial efforts a step further and had the pump's handle removed to prevent new cases of cholera from the pump (Summers, 1989).

Snow's story illustrates the importance of taking environmental factors into account when diseases or other problems occur in a community, as well as displaying the grace and common sense associated with prevention.

Primary Prevention: Recent Examples and Future Challenges

Actions like Snow's are behind many public health successes. Many injuries have been averted and lives saved by such primary prevention measures. In addition to the minimum-drinking-age law, recent examples of primary prevention include the following:

- *Antismoking legislation.* California's aggressive antitobacco effort under Proposition 99 resulted in thirty-three thousand fewer deaths from cardiovascular disease in the first three years (Kuiper, Nelson, & Schooley, 2005).
- *Routine immunizations.* Combined with disease control programs, routine immunizations have contributed significantly to child survival, averting more than two million deaths a year worldwide as well as countless episodes of illness and disability (UNICEF, 2005).
- *Water fluoridation.* Water fluoridation is effective in reducing dental decay by 20 to 40 percent (American Dental Association, 2005).
- *Motorcycle helmet laws.* Motorcycle helmet laws, enacted in six states (California, Maryland, Nebraska, Oregon, Texas, and Washington) since 1989, have successfully reduced motorcycle fatalities by an average of 27 percent in the first year (NHTSA, 2004).

These examples provide compelling evidence that primary prevention is effective. But despite this evidence, there is resistance to primary prevention. Unfortunately, primary prevention is often treated as if it were a *distraction* from the real and urgent pressure to meet the needs of those who are presently ill.

Why is this the case? One reason is that until prevention efforts succeed, it is generally difficult to conceptualize what prevention "looks like." Meanwhile, the need to provide treatment services to affected individuals is clear. Thus it is easy to understand that someone who experiences domestic violence may need counseling and other supportive services but harder to understand how to change whole populations to prevent occurrences of domestic violence before they begin.

We can learn how to overcome obstacles and to create effective prevention initiatives by studying previous successes. Nearly every prevention effort, including those mentioned in this chapter, was at its initiation viewed as "impossible." The first antismoking advocates routinely heard "You're crazy!" and "That will never work!" as they attempted to pass no-smoking laws for restaurants and public places. Indeed, in light of the powerful tobacco industry and the skepticism of the general public, the passage of no-smoking laws seemed ambitious at best. Today, however, we often take for granted what once seemed impossible. Many (but certainly not all) public spaces are smoke-free, from airplanes to hospitals and increasingly bars and restaurants. (Loftus, 2002).

Another common but unfounded criticism is that the impact of primary prevention is invisible; how can we know if an illness or injury has been *prevented* or simply did not occur? Although prevention is often difficult to quantify on an individual level, when viewed in aggregate at the population level, the significant impact of prevention becomes immediately quantifiable. Consider the impact mandatory use of seat belts and infant and child safety seats has had in the primary prevention of death and injury from automobile crashes. Between 1978 and 1985, every state, beginning with Tennessee, passed laws requiring safety seats for child passengers (Harvard Injury Control Research Center, 2003–2006). Between 1975 and 2003, mandatory car seat use resulted in the prevention of close to six thousand deaths and injuries in the United States (NHTSA, 2003). Clearly, prevention on the community level has a substantial impact.

The Case for Primary Prevention

Primary prevention offers the hope of eliminating unnecessary illness, injury, and even death. Nearly 50 percent of annual deaths in the United States—and the impaired quality of life that frequently precedes them—are preventable in part because they are attributable to external environmental or behavioral factors (McGinnis & Foege, 1993; Mokdad, Marks, Stroup, & Gerberding, 2004).

A focus on primary prevention can reverse this current trend by converting some of the resources used to treat injuries and illnesses into efforts that effectively prevent them in the first place.

According to the noted public health expert Henrik Blum (1981), medical care and interventions "play key restorative or ameliorating roles. But they are predominantly applied only after disease occurs and therefore are often too late and at a great price" (p. 43). Despite the widely held belief in the United States that the state of being healthy is derived primarily from health care, Blum notes that in reality, there are four major determinants of health: environment, heredity, lifestyle, and health care services. Of these four, Blum found that "by far the most potent and omnipresent set of forces is the one labeled 'environmental,' while behavior and lifestyle are the second most powerful force" (p. 43).

Health Care Needs Prevention

"America's health care system is in crisis precisely because we systematically neglect wellness and prevention," noted U.S. Senator Tom Harkin (2005). Although they are often viewed as an after-the-fact add-on to treatment, primary prevention strategies are a natural complement to medical care and treatment. As the capacity of the U.S. health care system approaches a breaking point (Cooper, Getzen, McKee, & Prakash, 2002; see Exhibit 1.1), prevention becomes even more critical. A systematic investment in prevention lessens the burden on the health care system, translating into higher-quality care and treatment services for those truly in need.

EXHIBIT 1.1. A SNAPSHOT OF THE U.S. HEALTH CARE SYSTEM.

High costs, poor access to health care services, and fundamental inadequacies in the provision of services contribute to poorer health outcomes for the nation.

High Costs for Health Care

- In the United States, per capita spending for health care in 2002 was $5,267— a full 53 percent more than in any other country (Anderson, Hussey, Frogner, & Waters, 2005).

- In 2003, the United States spent 15.3 percent of its gross domestic product (GDP) on health care. Projected spending may reach 18.7 percent of GDP by 2013 and 32 percent of GDP by 2030 (Borger et al., 2006).

- In 2004, employer health insurance premiums increased by 11.2 percent—nearly four times the rate of inflation (Kaiser Family Foundation & Health Research and Educational Trust, 2004).

- Only 2 percent of annual health care spending in the United States goes toward the prevention of chronic diseases (Centers for Disease Control and Prevention, 2003).

Poor Access to Health Care Services

- In 2005, some 41.2 million persons (14.2 percent of the U.S. population) were uninsured, and 51.3 million persons (17.6 percent) had been uninsured for at least part of that year (Cohen & Martinez, 2005).

- Individuals with little or no health insurance coverage are more likely to visit emergency rooms and to use emergency rooms as their usual source of health care (McCaig & Burt, 2005). As the number of emergency room visits has increased, the number of emergency departments has decreased dramatically (Barlett & Steele, 2004).

- Poor access to services is likely to worsen as the population ages, rates of chronic disease increase, corporations continue to reduce their contributions to health care (Abelson, 2005), and the number of primary care health professionals dwindles.

Inadequate Quality of Care

- Among thirteen developed nations, the United States ranks second to last on sixteen health indicators and last in infant mortality (Starfield, 2000).

- Patients in the United States receive the recommended care for health conditions only about half the time (McGlynn et al., 2003).

- Two-thirds of emergency department directors in the United States report shortages of on-call specialists. In addition, thirty states are experiencing nursing shortages, with the number expected to increase to forty-four states by 2020 (American College of Emergency Physicians, 2004).

- Medical errors and hospital-acquired infections cause more deaths than AIDS, breast cancer, firearms, diabetes, and auto accidents combined; recent estimates place the number of annual deaths attributable to medical error at 195,000 and the number attributable to hospital infections at 103,000 (American College of Emergency Physicians, 2004).

Primary Prevention Helps Those Most at Risk

"All members of a community are affected by the health status of its least healthy members" (Institute of Medicine, 2002, p. 37). The burden of illness and lack of access to care in the United States is not borne equally across the population. Both frequency of illness and quality of care are often a reflection of socioeconomic status, ethnicity, and race (Agency for Healthcare Research and Quality, 2000). According to the Centers for Disease Control and Prevention (CDC), "The demographic changes that are anticipated over the next decade magnify the importance of addressing disparities in health status" (2006). Groups currently experiencing poorer health status are expected to grow as a proportion of the total U.S. population; therefore, the future health of America as a whole will be influenced substantially by our success in improving the health of these groups, since we are all cared for by the same system and so share limited resources. A national focus on disparities in health status is particularly important as major changes unfold in the way in which health care is delivered and financed.

African Americans, Hispanics, Native Americans, Alaska Natives, and Pacific Islanders consistently face higher rates of morbidity and mortality, and compelling evidence indicates that race and ethnicity correlate with persistent and often increasing health disparities compared to the U.S. population as a whole. Research has now shown that after adjusting for individual risk factors, differences remain in health outcomes among various communities (PolicyLink, 2002). Primary prevention can serve to eliminate underlying health disparities through its upstream population focus; as Albee (1996) notes, "Logically, prevention programs should include efforts at achieving social equality for all" (p. 1131). For example, improving access to healthy foods in order to prevent the onset of diabetes due to poor nutrition for at-risk individuals in a community would result in positive health benefits for other community members as well.

Primary Prevention Is a Good Investment

The CDC has pointed out, "If we are serious about improving the health and quality of life of Americans *and* keeping our health care budget under control . . . we cannot afford to ignore the power of prevention" (2003, p. 6).

Health care is among the most expensive commitments of government, businesses, and individuals combined. A targeted investment in prevention not only decreases the financial burden on the health care system but also staves off unnecessary and rising medical costs. According to the U.S. Preventive Services Task Forces' *Guide to Clinical Preventive Services* (1996), primary prevention is generally considered the most cost-effective way to provide effective health care, due to its role in alleviating the unnecessary suffering and high costs of specialized care associated with disease. A primary prevention approach also helps defer the social costs associated with illness and injury that arise from lost productivity and expenditures for disability, workers' compensation, and public benefit programs (see Exhibit 1.2).

Putting Primary Prevention into Practice

Communities are addressing increasingly complex social and health problems, from HIV to violence to diabetes. Practitioners face the challenge of devising new services and programs *in response* to these issues, yet the commitment to preventing them in the first place lags. Prevention initiatives and efforts often focus on

EXHIBIT 1.2. PRIMARY PREVENTION: A LESSON IN RESPONSIBLE SPENDING.

The cost of after-the-fact treatment and services is generally far greater than the cost of prevention for a number of social and physical ailments (U.S. Department of Health and Human Services, 2003):

- Between 1990 and 1998, the California Tobacco Control Program saved an estimated $8.4 billion in overall smoking-related costs and more than $3.0 billion in smoking-related health care costs (Lindblom, 2005).
- Removing the lead from all pre-1950 homes today would yield $48 billion in net benefits (Messonnier, Corso, Teutsch, Haddix, & Harris, 1999).
- Fortifying cereals with folic acid reduces neural tube defects by 50 percent and saves $4 million a year (Messonnier et al., 1999).
- Every dollar spent on the measles-mumps-rubella vaccine saves $16.34 in direct medical costs (Messonnier et al., 1999).
- Every dollar spent on the chickenpox vaccine saves $5.40 in direct medical costs (Messonnier et al., 1999).
- Every dollar spent on the Women, Infants and Children (WIC) Program reduces the costs associated with low-birthweight babies by $2.91 (Messonnier et al., 1999).
- For each dollar spent on the Safer Choice Program (a school-based program focused on the prevention of HIV, other STDs, and teen pregnancy), about $2.65 is saved on medical and social costs (Messonnier et al., 1999).
- For every dollar spent on preconception care programs for women with diabetes, $1.86 can be saved by preventing birth defects among their offspring (Messonnier et al., 1999).
- Each dollar spent on optimal water fluoridation results in up to $80 in reduced dental expenses (Messonnier et al., 1999).

changing individual behaviors alone while ignoring the societal context surrounding them. An effective prevention strategy to respond to these challenges
must target not just individual behaviors but also the environment in which they
occur. Primary prevention requires a shift from a focus on programs to a focus on
more far-reaching prevention initiatives and from a focus on the individual to a
focus on the environment.

Far more than simply air, water, and soil, the term *environment* refers to the
broad social and environmental context in which everyday life takes place. As Lori
Dorfman, Lawrence Wallack, and Katie Woodruff point out in Chapter Six, "Personal choices are always made in the context of a larger environment. Prevention
can address both ends of the spectrum. In fact, many health and social problems
are related to conditions outside the immediate individual's control. A focus limited to personal behavior change ultimately fails us as a society because it narrows
the possible solutions inappropriately."

The importance of an integrated, multifaceted approach to prevention is also
recognized by the Institute of Medicine, which concluded in its 2000 report *Promoting Health,* "It is unreasonable to expect that people will change their behavior
easily when so many forces in the social, cultural, and physical environment conspire against such change (Institute of Medicine, 2001, p. 4). In recognizing this
fact, it is essential that a successful prevention initiative be comprehensive. That
is to say that it must address the environmental as well as individual factors that
influence health in a community.

How do we craft comprehensive solutions? The Spectrum of Prevention[1] offers
a systematic framework for developing effective and sustainable primary prevention
programs (see Figure 1.1). The six levels of the spectrum allow practitioners to
move beyond the common "brochures as prevention" approach by defining a variety of areas in which prevention can be implemented. The levels of the spectrum
are complementary. When used together, each level reinforces the others, leading to
greater effectiveness. According to Ottoson and Green (2005), "One of the lessons
of successful efforts in community-based health information has been that activities must be coordinated and mutually supportive across levels and channels of influence, from individual to family to institutions to whole communities. This is the
lesson of an ecological understanding of complex, interacting, community program components and the causal chains by which they affect outcomes" (p. 53).

To illustrate, let's use the example of breastfeeding. Breastfeeding is beneficial for boosting an infant's immune system and is also considered one of the best
forms of nutrition for infants (Reynolds, 2001).

A century ago, nearly 100 percent of babies were breastfed. Despite slight increases in recent years, today only 17 percent of women adhere to the recommended guidelines of breastfeeding a child for a full six months after birth (Wolf,
2003). Rates have declined dramatically over the past century for a number of

FIGURE 1.1. THE SPECTRUM OF PREVENTION.

Influencing policy and legislation
Changing organizational practices
Fostering coalitions and networks
Educating providers
Promoting community education
Strengthening individual knowledge and skills

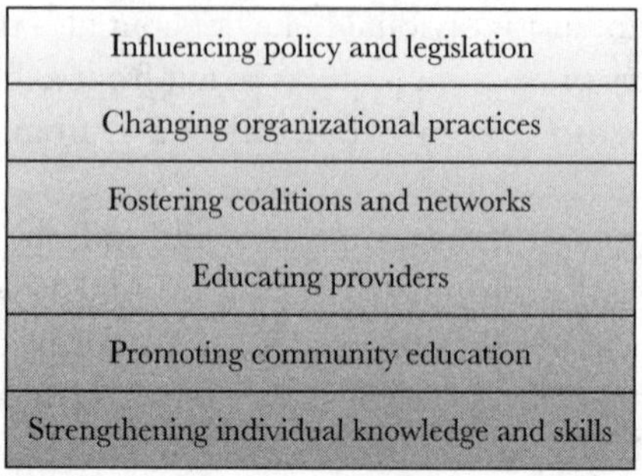

reasons, including lack of accommodations for working mothers who are breast-feeding, social mores about the acceptability of breastfeeding in public, and the development and marketing of baby formulas as a primary source of infant nutrition (Wolf, 2003). Recently, however, as more evidence becomes available to clinicians, breastfeeding is again being promoted in order to improve the public's health.

The cultural context surrounding breastfeeding, however, is still a significant barrier in the United States. As sociologist Joan Retsinas noted, "While it is known that breastfeeding is better, our society is not structured to facilitate that choice" (quoted in Wright, 2001, p. 1). Groups like the Women, Infants and Children's (WIC) Program funded by the U.S. Department of Agriculture to improve birth outcomes and early childhood health have prioritized breastfeeding for low-income women and children through nutritional support programs (Ahluwalia & Tessaro, 2000).

Making progress requires more than simply helping mothers with the skills to successfully breastfeed. Creating and maintaining widespread social norms for breastfeeding is critical. This requires activities along each level of the spectrum of prevention.

The first level of the spectrum, *strengthening individual knowledge and skills*, emphasizes enhancing individual skills that are essential in healthy behaviors. Clinical services are one common opportunity for delivering these skills, though there are many avenues of importance. Individual skill building is essential to the success of breastfeeding for new mothers. Women need support both before and after their child is born in order to successfully initiate and maintain breastfeeding. Often an ob-gyn, presenting expectant parents with information on the benefits of breastfeeding for themselves and their infants, can be an early influencer on the decision to breastfeed. In-hospital support, round-the-clock hotlines, and lactation counselors help troubleshoot the challenges a mother encounters and motivate her to continue in her breastfeeding commitment.

The second level of the spectrum, *promoting community education*, entails reaching people with information and resources in order to promote their health and safety. Typically, many health education initiatives focus on developing brochures, holding health fairs, and conducting community forums and events. Such one-time exposures can be a valuable element of a broader campaign but often don't have a big impact. We need to understand that nowadays, the mass media are the primary sources of education for almost everyone. Although there have been creative efforts to use the media to improve health, the massive expenditures of corporations far overshadow public health efforts in the mass media. As Ivan Juzang (2002) of MEE Productions points out, word of mouth can be a powerful and effective tool. It's the best advertising money can't buy. Creating positive word of mouth allows your prevention message to live on, even after a formal campaign is over, as community members take ownership of the message and begin to initiate their own activities that support it.

Educating a larger community about the benefits of breastfeeding is a step toward creating community environments in which breastfeeding is both encouraged and viewed as normal. Posters have been used in health care settings to signal the value of breastfeeding. One example of a large-scale community media campaign is the one coordinated by the U.S. Department of Health and Human Services and the Ad Council (U.S. Department of Health and Human Services, Office of Women's Health, 2001).

Locally, the news media can provide rich—and free—opportunities to emphasize public health. A great example was the Berkeley, California, Public Health Department's event to enter the *Guinness Book of World Records* by bringing together the largest number of breastfeeding mothers in history (BBC News, 2002).

Advocates also cite corporate advertising as one of the roadblocks in encouraging social change toward increased breastfeeding. Manufacturers often idealize the use of formula for infant nutrition by touting convenience; Derrick Jellife coined the term *commerciogenic malnutrition* to describe the impact of industry marketing practices on infant health (Baby Milk Action, n.d.). A resulting boycott, and the media attention it engendered, created large-scale awareness that the decline in breastfeeding was not simply a matter of unfettered individual choice.

The third level of the spectrum is *educating providers*. Because health care providers are a trusted source of health-related information, they are a key group to reach with strategies for prevention. Similarly, teachers and public safety officials are often identified as key groups to reach with new information and methods. The notion of who is a provider should be approached more broadly, however, and extends beyond the "usual suspects" to include faith leaders; postal workers and other public servants; business, union, and community leaders; and cashiers—anyone who is in a position to share information or influence the opinions of others.

Because of their prominence with expectant mothers, a first place to start is with ob-gyn and pediatric staff. Maternity staff have been trained that a good practice is to encourage breastfeeding within a half hour of birth. In California, Riverside County's nutrition services department has created a "marketing team" modeled on pharmaceutical company representatives that visit prenatal and pediatric care providers to supply them with educational materials, displays, take-away cards, and training to ensure that they have the resources necessary to help their patients choose to breastfeed their babies and continue to do so. An additional approach is the involvement of business leaders, who can assist mothers in transitioning back into the workplace. Training includes helping business leaders understand their role when mothers return to work and how to set up facilities that allow breastfeeding in the workplace. Another innovative model of provider education, developed in some African American communities, involves sharing information about the benefits of breastfeeding between beauty shop employees and their clients, who in turn share it with their neighbors (Best Start Social Marketing, 2003).

Level four of the spectrum, *fostering coalitions and networks*, focuses on collaboration and community organizing. Fostering collaborative approaches brings together the participants necessary to ensure an initiative's success and increase the "critical mass" behind a community effort. Coalitions and expanded partnerships are vital in successful public health movements including breastfeeding promotion. The metaphor of a jigsaw puzzle is appropriate, with each piece having value but taking on a greater significance when all the pieces are put together in the right way. Collaboration is not an outcome per se, like the other levels of the spectrum, but rather a tool used to achieve an objective. Often the best way to ensure a comprehensive strategy is to build a diverse coalition.

Collaborations may take place at several levels: at the community level—including grassroots partners working together such as in community organizing; at the organizational level—including nonprofits working together to coordinate the efforts of business, faith, or other interest groups; and at the governmental level, with different sectors of government linking with one another. Typical partnerships include elements of all three. In health fields, interdisciplinary and intergovernmental partnerships are probably less common than community-based organizations and grassroots efforts, which hold enormous promise for advancing the work of primary prevention (Cohen, Baer, & Satterwhite, 2002). Often the best way to ensure a comprehensive strategy is to build a diverse coalition. Eight Steps to Effective Coalition Building (Cohen et al., 2002) is a framework that guides advocates and practitioners through the process of coalition building, from deciding whether or not a coalition is appropriate to selecting the best membership and conducting ongoing evaluation.

An important objective of coalition building is to identify and work toward goals that can have greater impact on the community overall than any coalition participant might achieve alone. A key part of leadership, then, is finding an interest common to most or all groups and facilitating work toward achieving vital shared goals.

Returning to our example, collaboration between organizations and the fostering of coalitions are vital in the promotion of breastfeeding. To effect not only individual behavior change but social norm change as well, leadership is needed from health experts, grassroots advocates, social service workers, politicians, business groups, and the media. On the international level, a broad collaboration of community members around the world led to the effective challenge of corporations promoting infant formula ("Challenging Corporate Abuses," 1993). At the local level, building on public knowledge of the importance of breastfeeding and engaging the business and medical community led to changes in the organizational practices of businesses and hospitals.

The fifth level of the spectrum, *changing organizational practices*, deals with organizational change from a systems perspective. Reshaping the general practices of key organizations can affect both health and norms. Such change reaches the members, clients, and employees of the company as well as the surrounding community and serves as a model for all. Changing organizational practices is more easily achievable in many cases than policy change and can become the testing ground for policy. Government and health institutions are key places to make change because of their role as standard setters. Other critical arenas include media, business, sports, faith organizations, and schools. Nearly everyone belongs to or works in an organization, so this approach gives collaborators an immediate place to initiate change surrounding a particular issue.

Two key areas for organizational practice change that support breastfeeding are the Baby-Friendly Hospital Initiative and workplace policies around maternity leave and lactation support. As part of the Baby-Friendly Hospital Initiative, participating hospitals provide an optimal environment for the mother to learn the skills of breastfeeding, including allowing mothers to keep their newborns in the same room rather than in the hospital nursery, and encourage initiating breastfeeding within a half hour after birth. These hospitals stop the standard practice of sending mothers home with discharge packs that include artificial baby formula. This initiative has resulted in significant increases in breastfeeding initiation rates (Phillip et al., 2001).

For mothers who work, breastfeeding can be difficult unless their employers adopt policies that facilitate breastfeeding. Such organizational policies include allowing enough maternity leave to solidly establish breastfeeding and designing environments that make it easier for mothers to pump and store breast milk while at work. Media portrayals of breastfeeding as normal, as opposed to portraying breasts as almost entirely sexualized, could also facilitate breastfeeding.

The sixth level of the spectrum has the potential for achieving the broadest impact across a community: *influencing policy and legislation.* Policy is the set of rules that guide the activities of government or quasi-governmental organizations. Policy thus sets the foundation or framework for action. By mandating what is expected and required, sound policies can lead to widespread behavior change on a communitywide scale that may ultimately become the social norm. Over the course of the past several years, major health improvements have occurred as a result of policy change, including a reduction in diseases associated with cigarette smoking, a decrease in workplace and roadway accidents due to dramatically greater use of safety equipment, and reductions in lead poisoning.

Although policy is frequently thought of as either state or federal, evidence indicates that highly effective prevention policy can be developed on the community level and that local policy development is integral to the success of prevention programs (Holder et al., 1997). As a result, sound policies can lead to widespread behavior change on a communitywide scale. As noted by the Municipal Research and Services Center of Washington (2000), "Policy making is often undervalued and misunderstood, yet it is the central role of the city, town, and county legislative bodies."

Using our breastfeeding example, policies that support breastfeeding mothers include laws mandating maternity leave and requiring workplaces to make accommodations for employees who breastfeed. Additional legislation at the state level can help modify the existing structure of a system in order to promote the healthier choice for a mother and her newborn infant. A California policy proposed in 2004 would have provided comprehensive education about infant feeding options to new mothers and would have banned the marketing of infant formulas in California hospitals. However, despite widespread support, the bill failed to receive adequate votes for passage.

Local, state, and federal policies are still needed to protect a woman's right to breastfeed in public and to encourage and achieve adequate nutrition for our society's children in their earliest years of life. Although many barriers exist, the sixth level of the spectrum is an essential piece to achieving such social change.

One reason the spectrum can be a powerful tool for prevention is that it is helpful in designing efforts that change norms. Norms shape behavior and are key determinants of whether our behaviors will be healthy or not. More than habits, often based in culture and tradition, norms are regularities in behavior to which people generally conform (Ullmann-Margalit, 1990).

Typically, the tipping factor for normative change requires efforts at the broadest levels of the spectrum, *changing organizational practices* or policies, because such actions change the community environment. (The other elements of the spectrum are usually important also, contributing to and building on this momentum for change.) As Schlegel (1997) points out, policy change can trigger norm change by altering what is considered acceptable behavior, encouraging people to think actively about their own behavior, and providing relevant information and a supportive environment to promote change. The emergence of new social norms occurs when enough individuals have made the choice to change their current behavior.

Norm change regarding smoking behaviors is probably the most frequently cited example of this tipping factor and makes the importance of interplay between elements of the spectrum visible. After the surgeon general's report in 1964 that smoking harms health and numerous reports of research implying that secondhand smoke was risky (*promoting community education*), local communities formed coalitions to shape policy in restaurants, public places, and workplaces (*influencing policy*). The ensuing policy controversy received media attention (not only explaining the law but also why smoking is risky) (*promoting community education*), and the newfound attention led to more requests for training for health and civic leaders (*educating providers*). Doctors started to change their practices—more offered stop-smoking clinics and warned patients about the dangers of smoking (*strengthening individual knowledge and skills*). Once passed, the implementation of the policy required *changing organizational practices* to comply with the policy. This led to training, conducted by coalition partners, of government employees, restaurateurs, and business owners. This spurred an increase in people wanting to quit, and quit-smoking clinics became busier. As the number and extent of policies grew, momentum built for further changes. "What's next?" asked policymakers and enterprising reporters. And the process started again—banning vending machines, boosting tobacco taxes, and forbidding smoking in bars and public recreation areas. Individual choice still exists, and people still behave according to their own personal preferences. What has changed is society's perception about what is acceptable smoking behavior. This shift in the social norms changes the preference and improves the health of millions.

A well-designed strategy, while seizing opportunities that may arise, always considers a variety of levels of the spectrum. Also, data and evaluation are key. They are not levels of the spectrum because they are not outcome-related activities per se, but they are critical in informing and enhancing the spectrum strategy.

Building a Prevention Movement

Former U.S. Surgeon General David Satcher (2006) once explained, "There is still a big gap between what we know and what we do, and that gap is lethal. When it comes to the health of our communities, we must never be guilty of low aim." We cannot afford to aim low because our own well-being and that of our friends, families, and communities is at stake. We are getting seriously injured and ill unnecessarily far too often. When seeking care to address these ills, we are not served optimally by the health care system. This is especially the case for those most in need, but increasingly for all of us, the system does not perform adequately.

Prevention is necessary to address this situation. Through high-quality prevention, we can create community environments that foster good health. Prevention is our best hope for reducing unnecessary demand on the health care system. Healthy environments also provide optimal support for people who are injured or ill to heal and recover their health. Chronic disease among members of the American population is on the rise, new communicable disease threats have appeared, and Surgeon General Richard Carmona has predicted that due to chronic diseases related to poor eating habits and physical inactivity, this may be the first generation of children whose life expectancies will be lower than those of their parents (U.S. Department of Health and Human Services, 2004). Effective prevention strategies are needed to reverse these alarming trends.

Some people say that the easy problems have been solved. In fact, until they were solved, none of them were easy. But in retrospect, we can understand the key elements that made past problems solvable. The problems we face today are in fact made easier by what we have learned through earlier prevention efforts. Applying these lessons to emerging health concerns is vital as public health leaders help communities flourish in the current century.

Note

1. The Spectrum of Prevention was originally developed by Larry Cohen in 1983 while working as director of prevention programs at the Contra Costa County Health Department. It is based on the work of Marshall Swift (1975) in preventing developmental disabilities.

References

Abelson, R. (2005, May 6). States and employers duel over health care. *New York Times*, p. C1.

Agency for Healthcare Research and Quality. (2000, February). *Fact sheet: Addressing racial and ethnic disparities in health care* (AHRQ Publication No. 00-PO41). Rockville, MD: Author. Retrieved July 27, 2006, from http://www.ahrq.gov/research/disparit.htm

Ahluwalia, I. B., & Tessaro, L. M. (2000). Georgia's breastfeeding promotion program for low-income women. *Pediatrics, 105*, E85. Retrieved July 27, 2006, from http://www.pediatrics.org/cgi/content/full/105/6/e85

Albee, G. W. (1983). Psychopathology, prevention, and the just society. *Journal of Primary Prevention, 4*, 5–40.

Albee, G. W. (1987). The rationale and need for primary prevention. In S. E. Goldston & California Department of Mental Health (Eds.), *Concepts of primary prevention: A framework for program development*. Sacramento: California Department of Mental Health, Office of Prevention.

Albee, G. W. (1996). Revolutions and counterrevolutions in prevention. *American Psychologist, 51*, 1130–1133.

American College of Emergency Physicians. (2004, September). *On-call specialist coverage in U.S. emergency departments: ACEP survey of emergency department directors*. Irving, TX: Author.

American Dental Association. (2005). *Fluoridation facts*. Chicago: Author. Retrieved July 11, 2006, from http://64.233.187.104/search?q=cache:gGT-gOwjmqgJ:www.ada.org/public/topics/fluoride/facts/+fluoridation+facts&hl=en&gl=us&ct=clnk&cd=1

Anderson, G. F., Hussey, P. S., Frogner, B. C., & Waters, H. R. (2005, July). Health spending in the United States and the rest of the industrialized world. *Health Affairs, 24*, 903–914.

Ardell, D. B. (1986). *High level wellness: An alternative to doctors, drugs, and disease* (10th anniv. ed.). Berkeley, CA: Ten Speed Press. (Original work published 1977)

Baby Milk Action. (n.d.) *Briefing paper: History of the campaign*. Retrieved July 28, 2006, from http://www.babymilkaction.org/pages/history.html

Barlett, D. L., & Steele, J. B. (2004). *Critical condition: How health care in America became big business—and bad medicine*. New York: Doubleday.

BBC News, World Edition. (2002, August 4). U.S. Breaks breastfeeding record. Retrieved July 28, 2006, from http://news.bbc.co.uk/2/hi/americas/2171092.stm

Best Start Social Marketing. (2003, December). *Using loving support to build a breastfeeding-friendly community: Follow-up report to Indiana WIC Program*. Retrieved July 29, 2006, from http://www.indianaperinatal.org/files/education/EMPR1003.pdf

Blum, H. L. (1981). Social perspective on risk reduction. *Family and Community Health, 3*, 41–50.

Borger, C., Smith, S., Truffer, C., Keehan, S., Sisko, A., Poisal, J., & Clemens, M. K. (2006). Health spending projections through 2015: Changes on the horizon. *Health Affairs, 25*, W61–W73.

Centers for Disease Control and Prevention. (2003). *The power of prevention: Reducing the health and economic burden of chronic disease*. Atlanta, GA: Author. Retrieved from http://www.cdc.gov/nccdphp/publications/PowerOfPrevention/pdfs/power_of_prevention.pdf

Centers for Disease Control and Prevention. (2004). Preventing lead exposure in young children: A housing-based approach to primary prevention of lead poisoning. Atlanta, GA: Author.

Centers for Disease Control and Prevention, Office of Minority Health. (2006). *Eliminating racial and ethnic health disparities*. Atlanta, GA: Author. Retrieved July 11, 2006, from http://www.cdc.gov/omh/AboutUs/disparities.htm

Challenging corporate abuses: An interview with Elaine Lamy. *Multinational Monitor*, 15(7–8). (1993, August). Retrieved July 28, 2006, from http://multinationalmonitor.org/hyper/issues/1993/08/mm0893_08.html

Cohen, L., Baer, N., & Satterwhite, P. (2002). Eight steps to effective coalition building. In M. E. Wurzbach (Ed.), *Community health education and promotion: A guide to program design and evaluation* (2nd ed., pp. 144–161). Gaithersburg, MD: Aspen.

Cohen, R. A., & Martinez, M. E. (2005). *Health insurance coverage: Estimates from the National Health Interview Survey*. Retrieved June 1, 2006, from http://www.cdc.gov/nchs/nhis.htm

Cooper, R. A., Getzen, T. E., McKee, H. J., & Prakash, L. (2002). Economic and demographic trends signal an impending physician shortage. *Health Affairs, 21*, 140–154.

Cowen, E. L. (1987). Research on primary prevention interventions: Programs and applications. In S. E. Goldston (Eds.), *Concepts of primary prevention: A framework for program development* (pp. 33–50). Sacramento: California Department of Mental Health.

Duffy, J. (1990). *The sanitarians: A history of American public health.* Champaign: University of Illinois Press.

Ghez, M. (2000). Getting the message out: Using media to change social norms on abuse. In C. M. Renzetti, J. L. Edleson, & R. K. Bergen (Eds.), *Sourcebook on violence against women* (pp. 417–438). Thousand Oaks, CA: Sage.

Goldston, S. E. (Ed.). (1987). *Concepts of primary prevention: A framework for program development.* Sacramento: California Department of Mental Health.

Harkin, T. (2005, February 17). Remarks at the annual conference of the American College of Preventive Medicine, Washington, DC.

Harvard Injury Control Research Center. (2003–2006). Child safety seats. In *Success stories in injury prevention.* Boston: Author. Retrieved July 11, 2006, from http://www.hsph.harvard.edu/hicrc/success.html

Holder, H. D., Saltz, R. F., Grube, J. W., Treno, A. J., Reynolds, R. I., Voas, R. B., et al. (1997). Summing up: Lessons from a comprehensive community prevention trial. *Addiction, 92,* 293–302.

Institute of Medicine. (2001). *Promoting health: Intervention strategies from social and behavioral research* (B. D. Smedley & L. S. Syme, Eds.). Washington, DC: National Academies Press.

Institute of Medicine. (2002). *Unequal treatment: Confronting racial and ethnic disparities in health care* (B. D. Smedley, A. Y. Stith, & A. R. Nelson, Eds.). Washington, DC: National Academies Press.

Juzang, I. (2002, November 20–22). Presentation at the Preventing Obesity in the Hip-Hop Generation Workshop sponsored by the California Adolescent Nutrition and Fitness Program (CANFit) and Motivational Educational Entertainment (MEE) Productions, San Diego, CA.

Kaiser Family Foundation & Health Research and Educational Trust. (2004, September 9). *Employer health benefits: 2004 annual survey.* Menlo Park, CA: Author. Retrieved July 29, 2006, from www.kff.org/insurance/7148/upload/2004-Employer-Health-Benefits-Survey-Full-Report.pdf

Kuiper, N. M., Nelson, D. E., & Schooley, M. (2005). *Evidence of effectiveness: A summary of state tobacco control program evaluation literature.* Atlanta, GA: Centers for Disease Control and Prevention, Office on Smoking and Health. Retrieved July 11, 2006, from http://www.cdc.gov/tobacco/sustainingstates/pdf/lit_Review.pdf

Lee, D. A., & Hurwitz, R. L. (2002). Childhood lead poisoning: Exposure and prevention. In B. D. Rose (Ed.), *UpToDate* [CD-ROM]. Wellesley, MA: UpToDate.

Lindblom, E. (2005, February 24). *Comprehensive statewide tobacco prevention programs save money.* Washington, DC: Campaign for Tobacco-Free Kids.

Loftus, M. J. (2002, Spring). Making smoking history. *Public Health.* Retrieved November 13, 2006, from http://www.whsc.emory.edu/_pubs/ph/spring02/smoking.html

McCaig, L. F., & Burt, C. W. (2005, May). *National hospital ambulatory medical care survey: 2003 emergency department summary.* Hyattsville, MD: National Center for Health Statistics.

McGinnis, J. M., & Foege, W. H. (1993). Actual causes of death in the United States. *Journal of the American Medical Association, 270,* 2207–2212.

McGlynn, E. A., Asch, S. M., Adams, J., Keesey, J., Hicks, J., DeCristofaro, J., et al. (2003). The quality of health care delivered to adults in the United States. *New England Journal of Medicine, 348,* 2635–2645.

Messonnier, M. L., Corso, P. S., Teutsch, S. M., Haddix, A. C., & Harris, J. R. (1999, April). An ounce of prevention:. What are the returns?—A handbook. *American Journal of Preventive Medicine, 16,* 248–263.

Mokdad, A. H., Marks, J. S., Stroup, D. F., & Gerberding, J. L. (2004, March 10). Actual causes of death in the United States, 2000. *Journal of the American Medical Association, 291,* 1238–1245.

Municipal Research and Services Center of Washington. (2000, September). *Policy making introduction.* Retrieved July 27, 2006, from http://www.mrsc.org/Subjects/Governance/legislative/intro.aspx

National Highway Traffic Safety Administration. (2003). *Traffic safety facts, 2003* (DOT HS 809 775). Washington, DC: Author. Retrieved July 11, 2006, from http://www.nrd.nhtsa.dot.gov/pdf/nrd-30/NCSA/TSFAnn/2003HTMLTSF/TSF2003.htm

National Highway Traffic Safety Administration. (2004, January). *State legislative fact sheet: Motorcycle helmet use laws.* Washington, DC: Author. Retrieved July 11, 2006, from http://www.nhtsa.dot.gov/people/injury/new-fact-sheet03/MotorcycleHelmet.pdf

New York State Department of Health. (2004, June). *Eliminating childhood lead poisoning in New York State by 2010.* Albany: Author.

Ottoson, J., & Green, L. (2005). Community outreach: From measuring the difference to making a difference with health information. *Journal of the Medical Library Association, 93,* S49–S56.

Phillip, B. L., Merewood, A., Miller, L. W., Chawla, N., Murphy-Smith, M. M., Gomes, J. S., et al. (2001). Baby-Friendly Hospital Initiative improves breastfeeding initiation rates in a U.S. hospital setting. *Pediatrics, 108,* 677–681.

PolicyLink. (2002). *Reducing health disparities through a focus on communities.* Oakland, CA: Author. Retrieved July 29, 2006, from http://www.policylink.org/Research/HealthDisparities

Reynolds, A. (2001). Breastfeeding and brain development. *Pediatric Clinics of North America, 28,* 159–171.

Satcher, D. (2006, April 7). Keynote address at the opening of the California Endowment's Center for Healthy Communities, Los Angeles.

Schlegel, A. (1997). Response to Ensminger & Knight. *Current Anthropology, 38,* 18–19.

Spasoff, J. M., Harris, S. S., & Thuriaux, M. C. (Eds.). (2001). *A dictionary of epidemiology* (4th ed.). New York: Oxford University Press.

Starfield, B. (2000, July 26). Is U.S. health really the best in the world? *Journal of the American Medical Association, 284,* 483–485.

Steinem, G. (2002, February 13). *A 21st century feminism.* Paper presented at the Commonwealth Club of California. Retrieved July 29, 2006, from http://www.commonwealthclub.org/archive/02/02-02steinem-intro.html

Summers, J. (1989). Broad Street pump outbreak. In *Soho: A history of London's most colourful neighborhood* (pp. 113–117). London: Bloomsbury.

Swift, M. S. (1975). *Alternative teaching strategies, helping behaviorally troubled children achieve: A guide for teachers and psychologists.* Champaign, IL: Research Press.

U.S. Department of Health and Human Services, Office of Women's Health. (2001). *Health and Human Services blueprint for action on breastfeeding.* Washington, DC: Author.

U.S. Department of Health and Human Services. (2003). *Prevention makes common "cents."* Washington, DC: Author.

U.S. Department of Health and Human Services, Office of the Surgeon General. (March 2, 2004). Testimony on the growing epidemic of childhood obesity. Retrieved on July 28, 2006, from http://www.surgeongeneral.gov/news/testimony/childobesity03022004.htm

U.S. Department of Transportation. (1999, December). Fact sheet: Minimum drinking age laws. In *Community how-to guide on . . . public policy* (app. 7). Washington, DC: Author. Retrieved July 29, 2006, from http://www.nhtsa.dot.gov/people/injury/alcohol/ Community Guides HTML/PDFs/Public_App7.pdf

U.S. Preventive Task Force. (1996). *Guide to clinical preventive services* (2nd ed.). Rockville, MD: Author.

Ullmann-Margalit, E. (1990). Revision of norms. *Ethics, 100,* 756–767.

UNICEF. (2005, September). A report card on immunization, number 3. In *Progress for children.* New York: Author. Retrieved June 18, 2006, from http://www.unicef.org/ progressforchildren/2005n3/PFC3_English2005.pdf

Vetter, N., & Matthews, I. (1999). *Epidemiology and public health medicine.* London: Harcourt.

Wolf, J. H. (2003). Low breastfeeding rates and public health in the United States. *American Journal of Public Health, 93,* 2000–2010.

Wright, A. L. (2001). The rise of breastfeeding in the United States. *Pediatric Clinics of North America, 48,* 1–12.

CHAPTER TWO

ACHIEVING HEALTH EQUITY AND SOCIAL JUSTICE

Wayne H. Giles, Leandris C. Liburd

The Institute of Medicine recently concluded that "disparities in health care are among the nation's most pressing health problems. Research has extensively documented the pervasiveness of racial and ethnic disparities in health" (2002, p. 3). Different social groups, whether defined by gender, race or ethnicity, income, education, or region, experience dramatically different levels of health. There is a substantial and growing literature on the relationship between social conditions, broadly understood, and health status, including population and subgroup susceptibility to selected conditions, severity of the clinical manifestation of certain diseases, and survival rates (Dressler, 1993; Feinstein, 1993; Geronimus, 2000; Liburd, Jack, Williams, & Tucker, 2005; Rose, 1985; Wallace & Wallace, 1997). For example, African American men can expect to live an average of sixty-nine years, while Caucasian women can expect to live an average of eighty years (National Center for Health Statistics, 2005). This eleven-year difference suggests that some social groups have very different experiences with respect to health than others.

In addition to racial and ethnic disparities, there are stark disparities in health by gender and socioeconomic status. For example, persons with lower educational

The views and opinions in this chapter are those of the authors and do not necessarily reflect the views of the Centers for Disease Control and Prevention or the Department of Health and Human Services.

attainment have higher mortality than those with advanced education, and men have higher mortality than women (see Figure 2.1). In statistical terms, we observe among women with greater than twelve years of education a mortality rate of 171 per 100,000 population, while men with less than twelve years of education have a mortality rate of 826 per 100,000 population—a fivefold difference! There are also marked disparities in health by region, with the East South Central portion of the United States, which includes Alabama, Kentucky, Mississippi, and Tennessee having the highest mortality and the West North Central region, which includes Iowa, Kansas, Minnesota, Missouri, North Dakota, and South Dakota, having the lowest mortality (see Figure 2.2). The growing sentiment among health practitioners and policymakers across the country and the world is that such disparities in health status and outcomes are unacceptable.

In this chapter, we argue that health disparities are largely socially constructed on the basis of race and ethnicity, gender, education, income, and region and not the result of a poor genetic endowment. In addition to access to quality health care, we describe in this chapter the role of stress, employment, race, and socioeconomic status in achieving health equity. We conclude that health disparities can be not just reduced but eliminated through comprehensive, coordinated, and sustained public health efforts directed at the behaviors, systems, and broader social and policy environments that promote health and prevent disease.

FIGURE 2.1. AGE-ADJUSTED MORTALITY FROM ALL CAUSES, UNITED STATES, 2003, BY EDUCATIONAL ATTAINMENT AND GENDER.

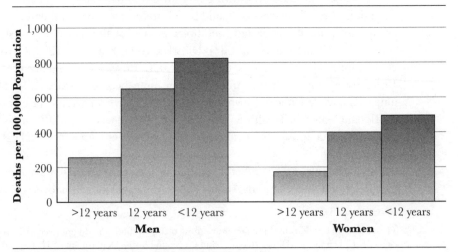

Source: National Center for Health Statistics (2005).

FIGURE 2.2. AGE-ADJUSTED MORTALITY, UNITED STATES, 2003, BY REGION.

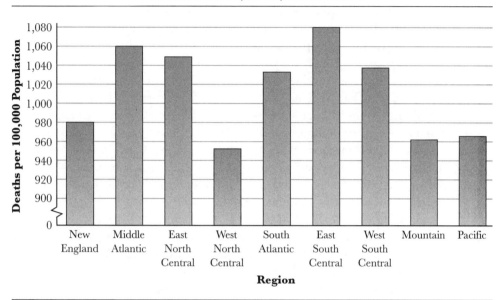

Source: National Center for Health Statistics (2005).

What Is Health Equity?

The terms *health disparities* and *health equity*, while clearly not household expressions, are fairly common to many health practitioners, program managers, policymakers, and researchers (Braveman, 2006). The terms *health disparities* or *health inequities* are generally used in the United States, while *health equity* is more common in Europe. The definitions for these terms have evolved over time, but there is little consensus on usage or meaning. One of the best definitions was developed by Margaret Whitehead in the early 1990s. Whitehead defined health disparities as "differences in health that are not only avoidable and unnecessary but in addition unjust and unfair." Health equity is defined as "providing all people with fair opportunities to attain their full health potential to the extent possible" (Braveman, 2006, p. 167). The central implication for primary prevention in this definition is that disparities in health reflect conditions that are avoidable, unjust, and unfair.

Paula Braveman and her colleagues at the World Health Organization provide yet another definition of health equity as when individuals' "needs rather than their social privileges guide the distribution of opportunities and well-being.

In virtually every society in the world, social privilege is reflected in differences in socioeconomic status, gender, geographic location, ethnic/religious differences and age. Pursuing equity means trying to reduce avoidable gaps in health status and services between groups with different levels of social privilege" (Braveman, Krieger, & Lynch, 2000, p. 232). A key aspect to this definition is social privilege. Disparities are not merely differences in health between groups but differences between groups with varying levels of social privilege. Social privilege can be defined as one's relative position in a hierarchy determined by prestige, power, or wealth. In the United States, for instance, high socioeconomic position tends to result in better health (Braveman et al., 2000).

When health inequities are described as "avoidable," what is implicit is that they are socially constructed and not fundamentally the result of genetic differences. Although certain conditions, such as sickle cell anemia, are strongly correlated with genetics, the majority of inequities result from social context, behavioral and environmental factors, and disparities in access to treatment and medical services.

As one conceptualizes health equity, it is important to realize that there are at least two types of equity, horizontal and vertical (Krieger, Williams, & Moss, 1997). *Horizontal equity*, which means equal treatment for equal needs, would ensure that all persons with an equally severe heart attack, for example, would be treated in the same way. In many instances however, this is not the case. Specifically, those without health insurance, the poor, and racial and ethnic minorities may receive less aggressive treatments than their more socially privileged counterparts. One survey found that African American women who suffer a heart attack were 75 percent less likely to receive invasive care then Caucasian men (Giles, Anda, Casper, Escobedo, & Taylor, 1995).

Vertical equity refers to different levels of treatment for different needs. That is, one would expect a greater expenditure of resources to treat the people most in need. Here again, research has shown that this is frequently not the case. We find, for example, that poorer individuals, who have many more chronic conditions (are more in need), are less likely to receive preventive health care than wealthier individuals, who often have fewer chronic conditions (National Center for Health Statistics, 2005).

Vertical equity may be related to the health care financing schemes characterized by O'Rourke and Iammarino (2006) as "progressive" and "regressive." A progressive approach takes a rising percentage of payments as income increases, while a regressive approach takes a falling percentage as income increases. The primary financing system employed in the United States is a regressive approach that according to O'Rourke and Iammarino "guarantees and perpetuates inequities" (p. 59). In other words, persons with the highest income pay a smaller percentage of their total income for health insurance, while low-income families pay a higher percentage, thereby reducing their disposable income, which in turn "exacerbates the effects of poverty" (p. 59). This cycle can contribute to the observed patterning of health disparities.

Determinants of Health Disparities

Typically, when policymakers and public health professionals attempt to address health disparities, they focus on the elimination of inequities in health care, that is, within the organized health care system. We agree that all persons are entitled to receive high-quality health care without regard to gender, race, socioeconomic status, or other social variables that have historically driven unequal treatment. However, the elimination of health disparities requires attention to the physical, mental, and dental health of all communities, as well as the social and political context in which health occurs or is threatened. The prevention of health disparities requires interventions that are holistic and address the allocation of public health and medical resources, quality of care, and the environments in which people live. In addition, public health interventions intending to eliminate health disparities need to systematically address their underlying determinants. Only by addressing the full continuum of health can one expect to effectively eliminate disparities.

Access to Care

Although medical care plays an important role in health, its contribution is weaker than usually assumed. According to Blum (1981), there are four major determinants of health: environment, heredity, lifestyle, and health care services. Of these four, "by far the most potent and omnipresent set of forces is the one labeled 'environmental,' while behavior and lifestyle are the second most powerful force" (p. 43). Clinical care has played a small role in improving population health over the past two hundred years; better nutrition, sanitation, and living conditions have played a much greater role. Nevertheless, timely and appropriate preventive medical services and effective therapies to manage acute and chronic illnesses can improve health, enhance quality of life, and reduce disparities (Williams, 2003). Yet access to health care in this country is severely limited, and people with access fall into three categories: the insured, the underinsured, and the uninsured.

Socially disadvantaged groups have lower levels of health insurance coverage and hence less access to health care (National Center for Health Statistics, 2005). O'Rourke and Iammarino (2006) argue, for example, that *underinsured* is merely a "euphemism meaning that you are insured only as long as nothing serious happens" (p. 59). Furthermore, socially disadvantaged groups differ greatly in their utilization of health care. There are multiple barriers both at the institutional and the personal level that can lead to lower utilization of care, such as organizational characteristics of the health care system that make it easier for socioeconomically advantaged individuals to receive care (more accessible office hours, the availability of transportation, and so on), language and cultural barriers, and prior experiences.

Differences in the way health care providers and their institutions respond to social groups may also lead to variations of care. For example, there is compelling evidence that white women and minorities receive less intensive and poorer-quality care than their white male counterparts (Giles, Anda, et al., 2005; Institute of Medicine, 2002).

Stress

Exposure to stress is a risk factor for a number of health problems, and coping responses can ameliorate at least some of the negative effects associated with stress (Politzer et al., 2001). Politzer and colleagues have noted that compared to their economically and socially advantaged counterparts, disadvantaged minorities, individuals of low socioeconomic status, and those living in rural areas have higher levels of stress and fewer resources to cope. The types of stressors to which individuals are exposed, the availability of resources to cope with stress, and the patterned nature of responses to environmental challenges are shaped by the larger social and economic environments in which people live. For example, if someone lives in an environment where there is a liquor store on every corner and that individual is under increasing amounts of stress, the method used to cope with stress may include increased consumption of alcohol. By contrast, another individual who lives in an environment with walking and biking paths, might deal with the same level of stress by becoming increasingly physically active.

The Role of Employment

Men and women, low- and high-socioeconomic-status individuals, and socially privileged and disadvantaged minorities are differentially exposed to economic marginalization and separation from the labor force. Because of historical and continuing individual and institutional discrimination, lower levels of preparation for the labor market, and the mass movement of jobs from areas of concentrated minorities and low-income populations, racial and ethnic minorities and other persons of low socioeconomic status have markedly higher rates of unemployment and job instability than their socially advantaged counterparts (Cutler, Glaser, & Vigdor, 1997). Moreover, individuals of low socioeconomic status and members of disadvantaged minority groups are more likely to be employed in occupational settings and job categories characterized by high levels of psychosocial stress, physical demands, and exposure to toxic substances (Williams, 2003). All of these factors can lead to increasing levels of disease morbidity and mortality.

Health Disparities: Trajectory and Factors

The trajectory of health disparities in Figure 2.3 depicts three elements that contribute to inequitable health outcomes for low-income populations and people of color. First, individuals are born into a society that neither treats people nor distributes opportunity equally; these are known as *root factors*. These root factors, such as discrimination, poverty, and other forms of oppression, play out at the community level, affecting the community environment (*environmental factors*). People experiencing health disparities more frequently live in environments with toxic contamination and greater exposure to high rates of joblessness; inadequate access to nutritious food and exercise; less effective transportation systems; and targeted marketing of unhealthy products. These kinds of environmental factors shape behaviors (*behavioral factors*), such as eating and activity patterns, tobacco and alcohol use, and violence. The combination of environmental and behavioral factors contributes to an increased number of people in need of screening, diagnosis, and treatment (*medical services*). Inequities in medical services for people of color are well documented and contribute to even greater health disparities.

FIGURE 2.3. TRAJECTORY OF HEALTH DISPARITIES.

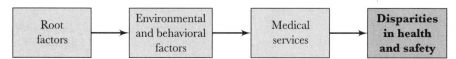

This diagram should not be read as a linear causal model. Placing all resources into medical services could improve care after an illness or injury but would not substantially improve overall health outcomes. This is because it would not address the number of people becoming disproportionately sick or injured in the first place. In fact, extensive research has indicated that the first two elements have a more significant impact on population health. As was mentioned previously, Blum (1981) found that the major determinants of health are the environment, heredity, lifestyle, and health care services. Of these, "by far the most potent and omnipresent set of forces is the one labeled 'environmental,' while behavior and lifestyle are the second most powerful force" (p. 43).

Another way to think about reducing health disparities is to think backward from a given condition. The first step back is from the injury or illness to what McGinnis and Foege (1993) called the "actual causes or death." For instance, lung cancer can be traced back to smoking. This could lead to strategies to abate an individual's smoking behavior. However, as the Institute of Medicine has stated, "It is unreasonable to expect that people will change their behavior so easily when so many forces in the social, cultural, and physical environment conspire against change" (2001, p. 4). The second step back is to consider the environmental factors that directly affect health or influence behavior. In the

(Continued)

case of lung cancer and smoking, we can step back to factors such as availability of tobacco and cultural norms that reinforce smoking as desirable.

Taking the second step back to address the environmental factors depicted in the trajectory presents a key opportunity for prevention. Prevention Institute conducted a re-view of the research and literature and delineated thirteen environmental factors that ei-ther directly influence health outcomes (such as air and water quality) or directly influence behaviors that in turn affect health outcomes (for example, the availability of healthy food affects nutrition). They fall into three interrelated clusters:

- *Opportunity:* racial justice and intergroup relations; jobs and local ownership; education
- *People:* social networks and trust; community engagement and efficacy; acceptable behaviors and attitudes
- *Place:* what's sold and how it is promoted; look, feel, and safety; parks and open space; getting around; housing; air, water, and soil; arts and culture

More information about the clusters and factors can be found at http://preventioninstitute. org/healthdis.html.

Issues in Addressing Racial Disparities

The conditions that structure health disparities are complex and too often en-during. Strategies to effectively eliminate health disparities must also confront and grapple with these complex issues until we realize positive change.

Race and Socioeconomic Status

Many people have argued that much of the racial and ethnic disparities in health can be explained by differences in socioeconomic resources. Consistent with other research, racial differences in life expectancy become smaller when comparing blacks and whites with similar levels of income (Cho & Hummer, 2000). How-ever, within each level of socioeconomic status, racial differences in life expectancy still persist (Lin, Rogot, Johnson, Sorlie, & Arias, 2003). The persistence of racial and ethnic differences in health after taking income into account could reflect the role of other measures of socioeconomic resources in health disparities, the non-comparability of income indicators across race, the residual effects of early life adversity, or the contribution of risk factors linked to discrimination and racism (or some combination of these).

Racial and Ethnic Subgroups

It is important when examining racial and ethnic disparities to examine the health status of racial and ethnic subgroups whenever possible. For example, the life experiences of Puerto Ricans in New York may be very different from those of Mexican Americans in Texas. In the United States, combining subgroups may mask groups with a higher level of risk. For example, when examining the health status of Asians, their overall health status can be classified as good; however, when the groups are disaggregated into Laotians, Cambodians, Hmong, and Vietnamese, we find poorer health status than when simply comparing all Asian groups combined against the overall white population (Giles, Kittner, Hebel, Losoconzy, & Sherwin, 1995). Combining Asian, Pacific Islander, Hispanic, American Indian, and even African American groups into one large group masks differences and obscures understanding the causal factors that are at the root of disparities.

Strategies to Reduce Disparities

Given that specific health risks are embedded in the larger social and political contexts in which people live, effective interventions to eliminate disparities must take account of the historical and cultural factors that shape experiences and the living conditions of various groups. Interventions are needed that alter features of the environment to maximize health and buffer negative exposures. Potential policies to reduce social disadvantage include improving employment opportunities, neighborhood and housing quality, and transportation services. In addition, new taxes, income support policies, and employment initiatives that assist the most vulnerable and reduce long-term poverty may be effective strategies. One example of a program that has proved effective in changing environmental factors is the Moving to Opportunity program, which provided assistance to randomly selected families in high-poverty neighborhoods to help them move to better neighborhoods. The program showed that three years after moving, the mental health of both parents and offspring had improved (Leventhal & Brooks, 2003).

The Task Force on Community Preventive Services has identified more than two hundred community-based interventions that can be used to improve social environments and health (ZaZa, Briss, & Harris, 2005). These include strategies to improve neighborhood living conditions; opportunities for learning and capacity development; community development and employment opportunities; prevailing norms, customs, and processes; social cohesion and civic engagement; and collective efficacy and health promotion, disease prevention, and health care opportunities.

The Centers for Disease Control and Prevention's Racial and Ethnic Approaches to Community Health (REACH 2010) program has demonstrated that national vision when coupled with local interventions can be an extremely effective strategy in reducing long-standing disparities in health. Through this national program, local communities have demonstrated dramatic improvements in disparities in cholesterol screening, hypertension, diabetes, and lifestyle behaviors such as cigarette smoking (Bachar et al., 2006; Giles & Liburd, 2006; Nguyen et al., 2006). For example, in South Carolina, coordinated by the Medical University of South Carolina and implemented in African American communities in Georgetown and Charleston, the REACH 2010 project has improved outcomes for persons with type-2 diabetes. The community coalitions work to improve diabetes care and control for more than twelve thousand African Americans. Some of their strategies include "walk and talk" groups, providing diabetes medicines and supplies, and creating learning environments where health professionals and people with diabetes learn together.

The impact of four hundred years of slavery and social inequality has not been erased from African American communities in the South. The programs sponsored by the REACH 2010 program in South Carolina not only build skills in diabetes self-management but also teach adults a process of learning that is transferable to other areas of their life. In other words, the health education programs have become a source of continuing education for adults who have historically not had access to the same health information as their white counterparts. Furthermore, having opportunities to interact with physicians and other health care providers outside of the hierarchical structure of the clinical setting has been instrumental in demystifying the position of power held by physicians and is teaching adults with type-2 diabetes their entitlements to a particular quality of health care that has historically been withheld from them (Airhihenbuwa & Liburd, 2006).

African Americans served by the REACH 2010 program are learning that despite what they have observed and construed to be inevitable outcomes of type-2 diabetes, such as end-stage renal disease and lower-extremity amputations, there are proven strategies to prevent these devastating outcomes, and these strategies are available and accessible to them.

Just two years after the program began, African Americans in Charleston and Georgetown, South Carolina, are more physically active, they're being offered healthier foods at group activities, and they're getting better diabetes care and control. In addition, what's been particularly noteworthy about this program is that African Americans are now receiving the recommended preventive care such as testing for hemoglobin A1C levels or blood sugar levels, lipid profiles, and kidney function, as well as getting dilated eye exams annually. Participants are also having their blood pressure monitored regularly. It is now documented that the initial 21 percent disparity in hemoglobin A1C testing between African Americans and whites has been virtually eliminated in these two communities.

To highlight a few additional REACH community demonstration projects that focus their intervention work beyond the clinical care setting, the Fulton County, Georgia, Department of Health and Wellness's REACH for Wellness project addresses the psychosocial health of African American women through a comprehensive personal empowerment program known as the Sisters Action Team. In addition to teaching stress management techniques, the Sisters Action Team is working to establish safer communities, walking clubs, bike trails, and more green space. It is also educating state legislators about the necessity of living wages and affordable housing as a requisite for better health outcomes.

Bronx Health REACH, a coalition of diverse community and organizational partners led by the Institute for Urban Family Health, has forged a "broad-based advocacy movement to eliminate racial disparities in health and health care . . . focused on increasing the number of eligible individuals enrolled in health insurance programs, ensuring non-discriminatory health care, increasing the representation of people of color in the health professions, and ensuring culturally competent health education and treatment" (Bronx Health REACH, 2004, p. 4). Through a combination of faith-based partnerships, a legal and regulatory committee, a training curriculum for health care providers, and community-based health education, the Bronx Health REACH initiative is working to eliminate the disparity in diabetes prevalence among African Americans and Latinos living in the Bronx, New York.

One final example of an intervention addressing the social determinants of cardiovascular disease and diabetes is the establishment of a neighborhood farmer's market by the Charlotte, North Carolina, REACH project. REACH simultaneously increases the availability and financial accessibility of fresh fruits and vegetables in an African American community and creates new markets for local farmers to sell their produce (Liburd et al., 2005). There is evidence from Charlotte and other urban communities that when fresh fruits and vegetables are available, consumption of these healthier foods increases (Zenk et al., 2005).

Conceptual Framework

Figure 2.4 provides a conceptual framework for a comprehensive public health strategy to eliminate disparities in health. The current reality with regard to disparities is noted in the middle panel: Unfavorable social, political, and environmental conditions exist in many communities, and these may be due to historical injustices, discrimination, racism, and sexism. They result in unhealthy environments for many

Americans, experienced through poor housing conditions, lack of transportation, few opportunities for employment, and lack of access to healthy foods and physical activity. These unfavorable environments then lead to adverse behaviors that promote disparities, including unhealthy eating, lack of physical activity, and an increasing likelihood of sexually transmitted diseases. These adverse behaviors then lead to the development of major risk factors, including high blood pressure, high cholesterol, diabetes, and obesity and overweight. The risk factors favor the development of diseases, including HIV/AIDS, tuberculosis, cancer, heart disease, and stroke. These higher rates of disease lead to increased disability and recurrence of disease, which may be reflected in reduced health status and health-related quality of life. The final result is higher mortality and a shorter life span among the affected groups.

While the middle pattern depicts the current reality, the top panel depicts the vision of the future, whereby all social groups live in communities where the social, political, and environmental conditions are favorable to the promotion of health and the elimination of disparities. Including increased opportunities for employment, education, and wealth, this favors the development of behavior patterns among the population that promote health and eliminate disparities—lower rates of tobacco use, increased physical activity, healthy eating—which in turn lead to low population risks for disease, lower disease outcomes, and full functional capacity and low risk of recurrent disease, all of which results in an improved overall quality of life.

To move from the present reality to the vision of the future requires policy and environmental changes that promote social, political, and environmental conditions favorable to disparity elimination. This might entail policies that promote equal access to employment and education and policies and environments that ensure that communities have access to safe places to engage in physical activity and access to healthy nutrition. In addition, these policies and practices may increase community awareness related to health and should lead to increased risk factor detection and control, permitting better emergency and acute care as persons develop conditions, improved rehabilitation and long-term care, and improved end-of-life care.

The bottom panel illustrates the size of the population that is targeted by each type of intervention. Policy and environmental strategies will target the entire population, while those related to the health care system will each address smaller and smaller subsets of the population. Thus the greater impact occurs with strategies that focus on the primary prevention of diseases at the policy and environmental-change levels. However, when addressing health disparities, it is imperative to engage in the full continuum of intervention activities, including the prevention of

FIGURE 2.4. FRAMEWORK FOR A COMPREHENSIVE PUBLIC HEALTH STRATEGY TO ELIMINATE HEALTH DISPARITIES.

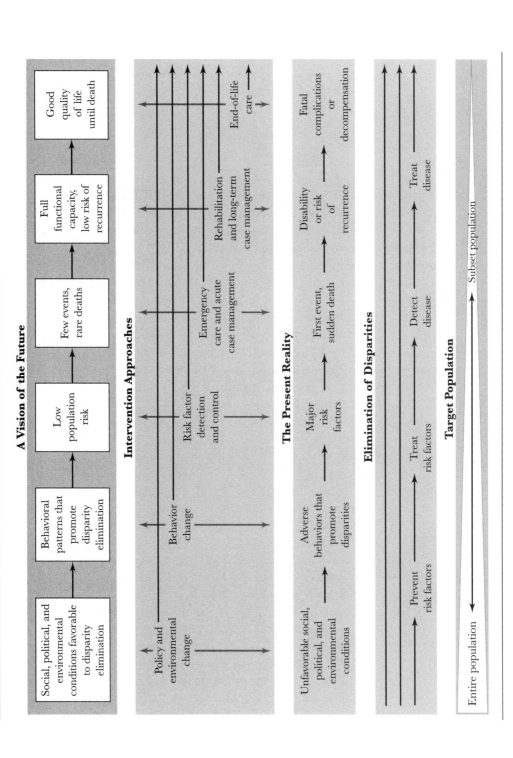

risk factors, treatment of risk factors, detection of disease, and treatment of disease. It is through policy and environmental-policies changes, behavior changes, risk factor detection and treatment, emergency care, and rehabilitation that this full continuum is addressed.

Conclusion

Taking the necessary steps toward eliminating health disparities across vulnerable populations challenges traditional public health sensibilities. Relying solely on public health programs that encourage individuals to adopt healthy behaviors is inadequate; emphasis on setting up social conditions that promote health must occur at the same time. Reducing disparities in health requires national leadership that provides direction and financial resources, government action at the regional and local levels, and active support and commitment from community organizations and individuals. This combination of national vision and resources with local action allows for flexibility in planning and implementation at the local level. Interventions aimed at improving health that are not coupled with interventions that seek to reduce social disadvantage are unlikely to substantially reduce disparities.

A deeper understanding of the context in which health disparities occur is needed as a first step to developing interventions that effectively eliminate conditions that are avoidable, unjust, and unfair. The public health community must move toward more innovative, broadly focused strategies for prevention. In training the next generation of public health workers, we must include "intervention research on the social determinants of health, break down the silos that perpetuate 'design superiority and paradigm elitism,' and have a willingness to learn from academic disciplines that have not previously informed public health practice" (Liburd et al., 2005, p. 23). Public health workers must also support and work with community institutions dedicated to achieving social equality for disfranchised communities, as well as challenge unjust policies that perpetuate health inequalities. Historically black colleges and universities, Hispanic colleges and universities, tribal colleges, the business sector, and national and regional minority organizations with state and local chapters are all possible collaborators.

Taken together, a sustained focus on achieving favorable social, political, and environmental conditions that promote good health coupled with access to affordable and high-quality health care and communities informed about how to prevent disease and injuries will set this nation on the path to the elimination of health disparities.

References

Airhihenbuwa, C. O., & Liburd, L. C. (2006, August). Eliminating health disparities in the African American population: The interface of culture, gender, and power. *Health Education and Behavior, 33,* 488–501.

Bachar, J. J., Lefler, L. J., Reed, L., McCoy, T., Bailey, R., & Bell, R. (2006, July 5). Cherokee Choices: A diabetes prevention program for American Indians. *Preventing Chronic Disease, 3.* Retrieved October 8, 2006, from http://www.cdc.gov/pcd/issues/2006/jul/05–0221.htm

Blum, H. L. (1981). Social perspective on risk reduction. *Family and Community Health, 3,* 41–50.

Braveman, P. A. (2006). Health disparities and health equality: Concepts and measurement. *Annual Review of Public Health, 27,* 167–194.

Braveman, P. A., & Gruskin, S. (2003). Defining equity in health. *Journal of Epidemiology and Community Health, 57,* 254–258.

Braveman, P. A., Krieger, N., & Lynch, J. (2000). Health inequities and social inequalities in health. *Bulletin of the World Health Organization, 78,* 232–233.

Bronx Health REACH. (2004, April). Health disparities destroy lives and dreams. *End Health Disparities Now,* p. 4.

Cho, Y., & Hummer, R. A. (2000). Disability status differential across fifteen Asian and Pacific Islander groups and the effects of nativity and duration of residence in the U.S. *Social Biology, 48,* 171–195.

Cutler, D. M., Glaser, E. L., & Vigdor, J. L. (1997). Are ghettos good or bad? *Quarterly Journal of Economics, 112,* 827–872.

Dressler, W. W. (1993). Health in the African American community: Accounting for health inequalities. *Medical Anthropology Quarterly, 7,* 325–345.

Feinstein, J. S. (1993). The relationship between socioeconomic status and health: A review of the literature. *Milbank Quarterly, 71,* 279–322.

Geronimus, A. T. (2000). To mitigate, resist, or undo: Addressing structural influences on the health of urban populations. *American Journal of Public Health, 90,* 867–872.

Giles, W. H., Anda, R. F., Casper, M. L., Escobedo, L. G., & Taylor, H. A. (1995). Race and sex differences in the rate of invasive cardiac procedures in U.S. hospitals: Data from the National Hospital Discharge Survey. *Archives of Internal Medicine, 155,* 318–324.

Giles, W. H., Kittner, S. J., Hebel, J. R., Losoconzy, K. G., & Sherwin, R. W. (1995). Determinants of black-white differences in the risk of cerebral infarction: The National Health and Nutrition Examination Survey Epidemiologic Follow-Up Study. *Archives of Internal Medicine, 155,* 1319–1324.

Giles, W. H., & Liburd, L. C. (2006). Reflections on the past, reaching for the future: REACH 2010—the first seven years. *Health Promotion Practice, 7,* S179–S180.

Institute of Medicine. (2001). *Promoting health: Intervention strategies from social and behavioral research* (B. D. Smedley & S. L. Syme, Eds.). Washington, DC: National Academies Press.

Institute of Medicine. (2002). *Unequal treatment: Confronting racial and ethnic disparities in health care* (B. D. Smedley, A. Y. Stith, & A. R. Nelson, Eds.). Washington, DC: National Academies Press.

Krieger, N., Williams, D. R., & Moss, N. E. (1997). Measuring social class in U.S. public health research: Concepts, methodologies, and guidelines. *Annual Review of Public Health, 18,* 341–378.

Leventhal, T., & Brooks, G. J. (2003). Moving to opportunity: An experimental study of neighborhood effects on mental health. *American Journal of Public Health, 93,* 1576–1582.

Liburd, L. C., Jack, L., Williams, S., & Tucker, P. (2005). Intervening on the social determinants of health. *American Journal of Preventive Medicine, 29*(5 Suppl. 1), 18–24.

Lin, C. Y., Rogot, E., Johnson, N. J., Sorlie, P., & Arias, E. (2003). A further study of life expectancy by socioeconomic factors in the National Longitudinal Mortality Study. *Ethnicity and Disease, 13,* 240–247.

McGinnis, J. M., & Foege, W. H. (1993). Actual causes of death in the United States. *Journal of the American Medical Association, 270,* 2207–2212.

National Center for Health Statistics. (2005). *Health, United States, 2005, with chartbook on trends in health of all Americans.* Hyattsville, MD: Author.

Nguyen, T. T., McPhee, S. J., Gildengorin, G., Nguyen, T., Wong, C., Lai, K. Q., et al. (2006). Papanicolaou testing among Vietnamese Americans: Results of a multifaceted intervention. *American Journal of Preventive Medicine, 31,* 1–9.

O'Rourke, T., & Iammarino, N. (2006). The American mirage of equity: Is social justice myth or reality? *American Journal of Health Education, 37,* 58–62.

Politzer, R., Yoon, J., Shi, L., Hughes, R., Regan, J., & Gaston, M. (2001). Inequity in America: The contribution of health centers in reducing and eliminating disparities in access to care. *Medical Care Research and Review, 58,* 234–278.

Rose, G. (1985). Sick individuals and sick populations. *International Journal of Epidemiology, 14,* 32–38.

Wallace, R., & Wallace, D. (1997). Socioeconomic determinants of health: Community marginalization and the diffusion of disease and disorder in the United States. *British Medical Journal, 314,* 1341–1345.

Williams, D. R. (2003). The health of men: Structured inequities and opportunities. *American Journal of Public Health, 93,* 724–731.

ZaZa, S., Briss, P. A., & Harris, K. W. (2005). *The guide to community preventive services.* New York: Oxford University Press.

Zenk, S. N., Schulz, A. J., Israel, B. A., James, S. A., Bao, S., & Wilson, M. L. (2005). Neighborhood racial composition, neighborhood poverty, and the spatial accessibility of supermarkets in metropolitan Detroit. *American Journal of Public Health, 95,* 660–667.

CHAPTER THREE

GENDER, HEALTH, AND PREVENTION

Michelle Ramirez, Siobhan Maty, Leslie McBride

Many researchers and public health practitioners have come to accept the important role that gender plays in influencing health outcomes. Gender roles vary cross-culturally, although all cultures produce particular systems of gender relations that affect life-cycle roles, choices, and often inequalities in health (Lane & Cibula, 1999). In this chapter, we examine the influence of gender on particular health outcomes from both a social science and a public health perspective and the importance of considering gender in the context of prevention. Rather than provide an exhaustive account of differences in morbidity and mortality between men and women, we elucidate how socially constructed gender roles influence individual behavior and social institutions and interact with other social determinants. Information, research, and examples regarding primary prevention and gender are minimal. We hope that this chapter contributes to the exploration of how gender can be integrated into the design and implementation of initiatives intended to improve the public's health. As public health practitioners interested in prevention, it is imperative that we consider individuals as nested within a larger social context, of which gender is a fundamental construct.

What Is Gender?

The social scientific practice of distinguishing biological sex from social gender has begun to percolate into the language of prevention, etiology, and causation within health research (Krieger, 2003; Phillips, 2005). The terms *sex* and *gender* are often used interchangeably, but the two concepts have fundamentally different meanings. *Sex* refers to the biological differences between men and women—chromosomes, internal and external sex organs, hormonal makeup, and secondary sex characteristics (Östlin, George, & Sen, 2001). *Gender,* by contrast, refers to the ways in which biological differences between men and women are culturally elaborated into notions of masculinity and femininity that are attributed to and expected of people within a given cultural system (Whitehead, 1997). This distinction has tremendous relevance for public health prevention efforts because culturally constructed gender roles and expectations influence behaviors that can either put men and women at risk or have a protective effect for particular health outcomes.

For example, men are less likely than women to seek professional help for health conditions such as substance abuse, depression, loss of physical function, and stressful life events (Galdas, Cheater, & Marshall, 2005). For many men, social norms maintain that they should not need to seek help and can handle problems on their own (Addis & Mahalick, 2003). Further, men's reluctance to seek help for themselves but willingness to do so for others is a trait thought to be associated with masculinity (O'Brien, Hunt, & Hart, 2005). Women are more likely to attend to minor symptoms and see health care providers more often than men due to their socialization as gatekeepers of their own and their family's health (Hemard, Monroe, Atkinson, & Blalock, 1998; Lorber, 1997; Waldron, 1995). However, women's greater health care–seeking behavior has been proposed as one of the reasons that women live longer but report greater morbidity than men (Doyal, 1995; Lorber, 1997).

Not only does gender influence the behavior of individual men and women, but it is also embedded in the major social organizations of society, including the family, the economy, politics, and the medical and legal systems, and its influence can result in unequal access to resources, biased public representation, and discriminatory institutional policies (Lorber, 1997; Östlin et al., 2001). The biomedical treatment of women and their bodies provides ample evidence of gender-based institutional discrimination. Much of the activism and research related to women's health that we see today was spawned by the women's health movement in the 1960s, which, in addition to providing alternative services and promoting health advocacy, developed a political analysis of gender inequality within the health care system. During this time, scholars, activists, and practitioners documented the medical mistreatment of women by physicians and health care institutions, the medicalization of women's lives, and the subjugation of women by the predominantly white, male medical establishment (Morgen, 2006).

One of the central tenets of feminist scholarship asserts that patriarchy privileges men by taking the male body as the "standard" universal body, while female bodies are found to be lacking and deficient by comparison (Annadale & Clark, 1996; Martin, 1992). For example, a natural life-cycle event such as menopause was considered for many years to be a "hormone deficiency disease" that required hormone medication regimens to keep women youthful and attractive (Lock, 1993; Wilson, 1966). Some medical anthropologists assert that the construction of menopause as a disease, rather than a normal biological event, illustrates the North American cultural tendency to devalue aging women's bodies because youthful, reproductive bodies are the culturally sanctioned ideal. Indeed, women's experience of menopause varies cross-culturally and is directly linked to how a given society regards women (Beyene, 1989; Lock, 1993). The example of menopause demonstrates how the experiences of health and illness are socially constructed rather than biologically determined. In other words, the experience of menopause is not a fixed universal biological reality but is influenced by active, cooperative social interchange (Gergen, 1985), which demonstrates that biomedicine is not a purely objective scientific enterprise but rather reflects the gender biases of the larger culture.

Gender continuously interacts with other social factors such as social class, race, and sexual orientation. These and other social factors work together to determine the development of social and health inequalities between and within different groups of women and men (Östlin et al., 2001). Gender, race, ethnicity, sexuality, and social class intersect in the lived experiences of people who occupy different social locations and negotiate power within the health care system and society at large (Morgen, 2006). For example, in the United States, men generally have a lower life expectancy than women, but African American and Native American men have the lowest life expectancy of all racial and ethnic groups (Staples, 1995). Staples argues that institutional racism combined with the "masculine mystique," which indoctrinates men into ignoring an illness until it becomes disabling, threaten to institutionally decimate much of the black male population. Thus gender interacts with other forms of social and institutional inequalities to produce detrimental health outcomes not only for African American men but for other socially marginalized groups.

In sum, gender is a construct that individually and in conjunction with other social factors creates social norms that affect the behavior of men and women, provide various protections and risks related to health, and shape institutional policies and practices that privilege one gender over another (generally men over women). It is crucial to consider gender, because it is one of the important differentiators hidden within aggregated health statistics.

We now look at how gender interacts with four different public health issues—intimate partner violence, traffic injuries, cardiovascular disease, and depression. We will examine the epidemiological data—and lay out rates and variations between women and men, the differential ways in which gender and social norms create conditions that influence incidence, and examples of promising initiatives that have been developed using a primary prevention-focused understanding of the impact of gender on health.

Intimate Partner Violence

Intimate partner violence (IPV) is part of a larger pattern of violence, and different types of violence affect different victims. Violence is one of the leading causes of early death for people aged fifteen to forty-four years worldwide (World Health Organization, 2002a). Nearly 5.3 million incidents of IPV occur each year among U.S. women aged eighteen and older, and 3.2 million occur among men. Approximately 1.5 million women and 835,000 men are raped or physically assaulted annually by an intimate partner (Tjaden & Thoennes, 2000b). However, national data indicate that the majority of violent injuries result from male violence against women (Gerlock, 1999). Several U.S. national surveys found that women were twice as likely to be injured in domestic violence incidents and were more likely than men to report being IPV victims (Tjaden & Thoennes, 2000a).

The United Nations' 1993 Declaration on the Elimination of Violence Against Women defines violence against women as ". . . any act of gender-based violence that results in, or is likely to result in, physical, sexual or psychological harm or suffering to women" (UN Doc. A/48/49). According to Heise, Ellsberg, and Gottmoeller (2002), violence against women is "the most pervasive yet least recognized human rights violation in the world" (p. S5) and is both a consequence and a cause of gender inequality. Studies conducted in various cultural settings have found that violence against women is most common where gender roles are rigidly defined and enforced and where masculinity is linked to toughness, male honor, or dominance (UN Doc. A/48/49). Other cultural norms associated with abuse include tolerance of physical punishment of both women and children, acceptance of violence as a means to resolve interpersonal conflicts, and the perception that men have ownership of women (Heise, 1998).

Documenting the magnitude of violence against women and producing reliable, comparative data to guide policy have been exceedingly difficult because women are reluctant to declare incidents of violence out of fear of reprisals and feelings of shame (World Health Organization, 2005). The WHO Multi-Country Study on Women's Health and Domestic Violence Against Women (2005) responded by collecting survey data from twenty-four thousand households in ten geographically diverse countries. According to this study, women who had ever experienced physical or sexual partner violence, or both, were significantly more likely to report poor or very poor health than women who had never experienced partner violence. IPV not only causes physical damage but also involves psychological distress and trauma. Depression and posttraumatic stress disorder are the most prevalent mental health sequelae of IPV (Golding, 1999). Also noteworthy is that recent experiences of illness were associated with lifetime experiences of violence. This suggests that the physical effects of violence may last long after the actual violence has ended and that cumulative abuse affects health most strongly. The WHO study also confirms that violence against women is a global problem and that violence by intimate partners rather than by other perpetrators is the dominant form of violence in women's lives.

Implications for Prevention. Several studies indicate that 11 to 30 percent of injured women who present in accident and emergency departments have been abused by a male partner (Campbell, 2002). Therefore, Campbell suggests a need for universal rather than incident-based screening for IPV in emergency care settings. However, screening for IPV is not primary prevention. If a woman reports violence, she is already experiencing abuse, so this type of intervention should be considered secondary or tertiary prevention. Efforts aimed at raising consciousness about IPV by reducing the stigma, shame, and denial associated with partner violence, and strengthening informal support networks by encouraging family and community members to support women living with violence may not be sufficient to radically alter gender roles and norms to an extent that would allow greater equity between men and women.

Amy Ernst (2006), a physician, asserts that to prevent the incidence of violence, public health efforts must focus on the perpetrators of violence. Intervention programs can use media to encourage men to speak out against violence and challenge its social acceptability. These actions will counter notions that all men condone violence and will provide alternative models of masculinity (WHO, 2005).

Cohen and colleagues (2006) also propose a multitiered approach to the primary prevention of IPV to change social norms regarding violence. The authors suggest that applying the spectrum of prevention (see Figure 1.1. in Chapter One), which involves strengthening individual knowledge and skills, promoting community education, educating providers, fostering coalitions and networks, changing organizational practices, and influencing policy and legislation, could lead to a change in gender-related attitudes, beliefs, values, and practices at the individual, institutional, and societal levels.

An example of a primary prevention program aimed at reducing IPV is the Men Can Stop Rape (MCRS) project. MCRS is a program in the District of Columbia and California that empowers young males and the institutions that serve them to work with women as allies in the primary prevention of rape and other forms of violence. The program uses awareness-to-action education and community organizing to promote gender equity and counter the attitudes, beliefs, and values that condone partner violence. The program is organized around the theme "My strength is not for hurting" and builds the capacity of young men to be strong without being violent (Men Can Stop Rape, n.d.-b). Another MCRS program, the Men of Strength (MOST) Club, provides safe and supportive environments for high school males to associate with male peers while exploring healthy, nonviolent models of masculinity (Men Can Stop Rape, n.d.-a).

Traffic Injuries

"[Lance] Armstrong was piloting his black BMW M5 at roughly twice the speed limit down a rural highway while devouring a teriyaki beef wrap from the take-out window at Roscoe's. . . . The business of eating the wrap while dipping chips into a small container of salsa forced him to take both hands off the wheel periodically and steer with his left knee. When his passenger offered to take the wheel [Armstrong directed], 'You do the interview. . . . I'll drive the car and eat my lunch'" (Murphy, 2006, p. 60).

This quote, from the opening paragraph of a recent *Sports Illustrated* cover story, highlights how gender may express itself in how we drive, the risks we take while on the road, the crashes we may experience, and even the injuries we may suffer. Readers might argue that Lance Armstrong is so highly trained and his reactions so finely tuned that even when taking risks, he may be one of the safest drivers on the road. That misses the point. Here we have a popular magazine, read mostly by men, opening its featured article on an elite athlete, a sports legend, even arguably a national hero, with a detailed account of his risky behavior behind the wheel. Not only that, but Armstrong responds to an offer of help with a command that is wholly emblematic of the male stereotype: *Mind your own business;* I'm *in control.* That this article is about Lance Armstrong does not render its support of gender norms unusual or isolated; we send and receive messages of this sort on a continual basis. Before pursuing further their impact on our behavior, let us examine traffic-related mortality and morbidity statistics as they break down by gender.

Gender is a consistent and significant predictor of involvement in traffic crashes both in the United States and internationally. In 2004, the rate of men's involvement in fatal traffic crashes was more than twice that of women, and a woman's chance of getting hurt in a traffic crash was 25 percent lower than a man's (Insurance Institute for Highway Safety, 2004). However, almost 50 percent of women who died in crashes were passengers, compared with approximately 25 percent of the men. The WHO (2002b) reported that worldwide, men are 2.7

times as likely to die from road traffic injuries as women are. A study in Barcelona, Spain, found that males constituted seven out of every ten road traffic injury cases above the age of fourteen years, and the overall death rate for men was more than three times that for women. In Australia, the Department of Transport and Regional Services reported that male drivers were involved in 75 percent of fatal motor vehicle crashes in 1999 and 2000; young male drivers between seventeen and twenty-five years of age were involved in one in every five fatal motor vehicle crashes in 2000, and females in the same age group were the drivers in only 7 percent of such crashes (Turner & McClure, 2003, p. 123).

What explains these striking differences? One reason males are at greater risk of experiencing injuries and fatalities from traffic crashes is their greater exposure to driving. Worldwide, on average, men spend more time inside moving vehicles than women and are more likely to own cars. Gender norms often dictate that men are much more likely than women to work as automotive mechanics and drivers, including driving long-haul vehicles. These jobs result in males' having greater exposure to the risk of traffic injuries. Cultural traditions may also place restrictions on women's mobility (WHO, 2002b).

While exposure is a key factor, other factors must be considered to explain why, for example, male pedestrians experience injuries and fatalities at much higher rates than females, irrespective of time spent walking on the road (WHO, 2002b). In the United States, males constitute 70 percent of pedestrian fatalities, so factors influenced by prevalent gender expectations such as risk taking, attitudes toward traffic laws and violations, and alcohol use patterns are important to consider.

Studies consistently find that men take more risks when driving and participate in more illegal driving behavior than women. Reviewing findings from several studies, Dana Yagil (1998) concluded that gender and age have an interactive effect on driving behavior, noting that young male drivers are considered a high-risk group in terms of crash involvement, risky driving, aggressive driving, and traffic violations. Similarly, one review of research on gender differences in adolescent driving behavior revealed that ". . . men (particularly young men) engaged in more illegal and risky driving behavior than women, no matter what was measured" (Harre, Field, & Kirkwood, 1996, p. 163).

It may be that men take more risks when driving because they tend to underestimate the hazards involved in various driving activities and overestimate their driving ability (Dejoy, 1992). Overestimating driving ability may encourage what Yagil (1998) refers to as conditional compliance with traffic laws: depending on the situation, men are more likely than women to judge for themselves whether a traffic law is relevant. Women, by contrast, evaluate the content of traffic laws more positively and indicate a stronger sense of obligation to comply with them. Compared to women and older drivers, men and younger drivers expect fewer negative outcomes and more social approval as a result of committing traffic violations (Yagil, 1998). Alcohol use is also implicated in higher crash fatalities among teenagers in the United States (WHO, 2002b). A national sample of 1,725 adolescent males found that males were twice as likely to drive under the influence of alcohol or drugs as females (Elliot, 1987). In Canada, a national youth survey found that of teens who reported drinking at parties, males were three to five times more likely to drive after drinking than females (WHO, 2002b, p. 3).

Implications for Prevention. The differences in attitudes and behaviors we have described reflect gendered ideas about masculinity and femininity. Harre and colleagues (1996) concluded that being able to drive skillfully is perceived as "part of being a man." However, the authors make the important distinction that for many men, driving skillfully is more often defined as driving fast and overtaking other drivers than it is about safety. "Drinking and driving, trying out maneuvers beyond their skills, and speeding may help young men create their gender identities in a culture where seeking risks is part of the construction of manliness" (p. 164). The World Health Organization (2002b) has observed that "gender role socialization and the association of masculinity with risk-taking behavior, acceptance of risk and a disregard of pain and injury may be factors leading to hazardous actions on the part of men. These include, for example, excessive consumption of alcohol, drug use, aggressive behavior to be in control of situations, and risky driving" (p. 3). Young men experience the majority of injuries and fatalities, but young women face significant risks from male behavior as well—as passengers, pedestrians, and drivers of other vehicles on the road.

The WHO (2002b) has called for the design and testing of interventions that both challenge gender-role stereotyping of males as high risk takers and foster safe driving behavior. The WHO recommends targeting children and adolescents of both sexes and suggests involving older men and women to help create an environment conducive to males adopting safer, non-risk-taking behavior and concludes that "positive behavioral changes may be best achieved through community-based approaches, which allow injury prevention messages to be repeated in different forms and contexts" (p. 4). Harre and colleagues (1996) suggest, "As young men tend to begin driving earlier than young women, there is perhaps a greater urgency with regard to early timing of intervention programs aimed at adolescent males" (p. 172).

An example of a program that adopts a primary prevention approach is Friday Night Live (FNL), a teen support program directed toward changing norms about alcohol use and driving and protecting youth in risky situations (California Friday Night Live, 2006). FNL clubs have been formed in high schools across the country. Participants create materials and activities that challenge unhealthy norms around drinking (with a focus on drinking and driving) and also provide free rides home on weekend nights to students who fear that their only way home is with someone who has been drinking. Furthermore, when used by young women as an alternate form of transportation, the FNL groups have a role to play in reducing the incidents of dating violence given that alcohol is often involved in this type of violence (O'Keefe, 1997).

Cardiovascular Disease

The term *cardiovascular disease* (CVD) refers to a group of pathophysiological disorders that occur in the heart or blood vessels. Coronary artery disease, coronary heart disease, pericardial disease, and congenital heart disease are a few of the cardiovascular diseases that affect the heart. Several other cardiovascular disorders affect blood vessels, such as atherosclerosis, high blood pressure, aneurysm, and stroke (Mayo Clinic, 2005).

Cardiovascular diseases are a major source of mortality and morbidity globally. In the United States, more than seventy million adults suffer from cardiovascular disorders, resulting in over six million hospitalizations annually. Over 40 percent of the deaths in the United States each year can be attributed to CVD (Centers for Disease Control and Prevention [CDC], 2005).

Patterns of CVD Risks and Outcomes

In the United States, heart disease and stroke are the first and third leading causes of death, respectively, for both men and women (CDC, 2005). Although CVD is a major cause of death for both genders, women are more likely to die from CVD than men. In fact, female CVD mortality rates have exceeded male CVD mortality rates each year since 1984 (Bell & Nappi, 2000).

The treatment and prognosis of CVD also interact with gender. For example, compared to men, women are more likely to suffer a second heart attack after an initial myocardial infarction (Frasure-Smith, Lesperance, Juneau, Talajic, & Bourassa, 1999) and are twice as likely to die within a year of the event (Vaccarino, Krumholz, Yarzebski, Gore, & Goldberg, 2001). Men suffer more severe chronic illness and die younger than women, whereas women live longer but have more nonfatal morbidity and disability (Rieker & Bird, 2005).

Why Do CVD Risks and Outcomes Differ by Gender?

Evidence suggests that biological systems, behaviors, and social processes underlie the patterns of CVD risk and outcomes (Rieker & Bird, 2005). Viewing CVD risk, outcomes and intervention methods with consideration of sex and gender differences is a relatively recent endeavor. In fact, it was not until 1993 that the Food and Drug Administration (FDA) revised clinical research guidelines to mandate the participation of women of childbearing potential in clinical trials (Schiebinger, 2003). Inclusion of women in subsequent studies has led to improved knowledge of CVD risk, presentation, and prognosis. As a result of this significant policy intervention, future health research studies will improve understanding of the multiple determinants of CVD and identify the best actions to prevent their occurrence in both women and men.

Differences in cardiovascular disease rates may be partly attributable to inherent biological differences between men and women. Recent research assigns the most severe CVD risk disparities to diabetes mellitus, where the risk of CVD is 1.5 to 2.3 times more likely in women with diabetes than in men with the disease (Mosca, 2002). Another example of how biological processes can influence CVD rates is through differential concentration of estrogen, since low levels of estrogen (such as those found in men and postmenopausal women) are known to reduce the uptake of LDL into the cells (Abbey, Owen, Suzakawa, Roach, & Nestel, 1999).

Also, known behavioral CVD risk factors, such as smoking and physical inactivity, are patterned by gender (Eastwood & Doering, 2005). Physical activity and low-fat, high-fiber diets are considered to be protective against the development of cardiovascular disease and other chronic illnesses, such as diabetes, for both women and men. However, given the compounded demands of work and family, many women are limited in the amount of time they have available for physical activity or healthy meal preparation and instead may engage in stress-related behaviors, such as smoking and eating nonnutritious, quick meals (Mosca et al., 2000). Despite these behavioral patterns, studies show that women are more likely than men to engage in health-promoting behaviors (Schoenborn, Adams, Barnes, Vickerie, & Schiller, 2004). For example, the use of alcohol, tobacco, and other drugs or substances is significantly less common among women than among men, and men are more likely to begin using tobacco, alcohol, and other drugs at younger ages than women (Courtenay, 2000a). Furthermore, men who adopt stereotypical beliefs about masculinity have greater health risks, in terms of physical inactivity, alcohol use, and smoking, than their peers with less traditional beliefs (Courtenay, 2000d).

Social determinants of gender disparities in CVD include the types and expectations of gendered social roles and social positions, as well as differential access to resources (such as income, healthy food, social supports, health care services, and safe areas in which to exercise) and opportunities (including education and occupation) available to women and men for health promotion purposes (Mosca, McGillen, & Rubenfire, 1998; Rieker & Bird, 2005). The sociocultural context and institutions of our society, including schools, government, workplaces, and health systems, often perpetuate the gender norms that create and sustain an unequal balance of power between women and men (Wingood & DiClemente, 2000). For example, women's lack of material, personal, and social resources and opportunities relative to men may make them more vulnerable to life stressors and consequently more susceptible to health effects due to psychosocial and physiological stress (McDonough & Walters, 2001).

Although socioeconomic and psychosocial risk factors—such as education, occupation, and stress—have been associated with increased rates of CVD, their effects often differ between women and men. For example, low socioeconomic position in both childhood and adulthood is a stronger risk factor in women than in men for various forms of adult CVD (Brunner, Shipley, Blane, Davey Smith, & Marmot, 1999; Dalstra et al., 2005; Galobardes, Davey Smith, & Lynch, 2006). The division of labor, whether domestic or economic, can lead to differential exposure and vulnerability to illness among women and men. For example, men may be more dependent on their occupational status for self-efficacy or self-esteem, whereas women may change or combine their occupational and other roles more frequently and therefore draw on several sources of self-efficacy and esteem (Siegrist, 2002).

Gender influences other social factors, such as social interaction. Men and women customarily differ in their ability to share feelings, which may lead to anger, anxiety, or social isolation. Each of these negative effects may have biological repercussions in terms of altered hormonal release or immunological response, possible CVD promoters (Hawkley, Masi, Berry, & Cacioppo, 2006; Williams et al., 2000). Moreover, social isolation removes access to education and awareness of preventive factors for cardiovascular health. While social supports have been hypothesized to protect against cardiovascular events (Berkman & Syme, 1979), the degree and type of social supports are thought to differ between men and women. Men tend to draw on fewer individuals or groups for support in comparison to women, which may result from different social needs or skills (Barrett-Connor, 1997).

Making Health Manly: Norms, Peers, and Men's Health

"Health matters are women's matters." "Only women pamper their bodies." There is substantial evidence, at least in the United States, that asking for help and caring for one's health are widely considered to be the province of women (Courtenay, 2000c). Collective beliefs and assumptions such as these are what social scientists refer to as *social norms* (Berkowitz, 2003) or *subjective norms* (Ajzen, 2001).

Given the existence of these norms, it is not surprising that in most Western industrialized countries, women are the greatest consumers of health-related products and

---

(Continued)

services. Women are often first to take responsibility, not only for the health and well-being of themselves and their offspring, but also for the health of men. This helps explain why single men have the greatest health risks—and why the benefits of marriage are consistently found to be greater for men than for women (who can suffer substantial stress in caring for their spouses) (Courtenay, 2000a).

Ultimately, men need to take greater responsibility for their own health. But here is the problem: men receive strong social prohibitions against doing *anything* that women do (Courtenay, 2000c).

Men and boys who engage in behaviors representing feminine gender norms risk being perceived as "wimps" or "sissies." Consequently, men often seek to prove their manhood by *actively rejecting* doing anything that women do—and this includes caring for their health (Courtenay, 2000b). Not surprisingly, there is solid evidence that masculinity is associated with health behavior and even predicts mortality (Courtenay, 2003).

Of course, many men *are* concerned about their health. But as long as men believe that their peers are unconcerned about *their* health, they will be less likely to attend to their own health needs. What this means is that for men to change, social norms will have to change.

Results of a recent survey of more than five hundred men on one U.S. college campus indicated that these men believed that most (55 percent) of their peers were either not at all concerned or only a little concerned about their health. In reality, only 35 percent of the men were unconcerned about their health; most (65 percent) reported being either somewhat or very concerned (Courtenay, 2004). Dissemination of these data could promote the more accurate norm that men at this particular college are indeed concerned about their health.

A similarly effective way to change social norms is with the use of accounts by prominent members of a particular group about how they became involved in their health. Research shows that people can be persuaded to behave in ways that they believe credible, influential colleagues or peers want them to behave (Petty, Wegener, & Fabrigar, 1997). Perhaps then men will begin to see health and well-being as *human* concerns and recognize that following good health habits can be manly as well as lifesaving.

Source: Courtesy of Will Courtenay.

Implications for Prevention. Although cardiovascular disease places a significant burden on society, the problem is largely preventable. Increased awareness of disease risk and prevention is one step toward reducing this burden. For example, in response to the pervasive misperceptions about women and CVD, the American Heart Association launched the Go Red for Women national movement in February 2004. This awareness campaign attempts to empower women "with knowledge and tools so they can take positive action to reduce their risks of heart disease and stroke and protect their health." By utilizing multiple media outlets (Internet, newspapers, billboards, and newsletters) the program provides women with information about how to prevent CVD through healthy eating and exercise, smoking cessation, weight maintenance, and improved blood pressure and blood cholesterol management (American Heart Association, 2006).

A way to address gender differences in help-seeking behaviors would be to create programs that focus on socialization. For example, the Men as Navigators for Health project in North Carolina is using a male lay health adviser model to weaken patterns of male gender socialization that promote high-risk attitudes and behaviors, to develop skills and strategies for lifestyle change, and to enhance men's motivation to access disease prevention and health care services (CDC, 2004).

However, as has been discussed throughout this chapter, information campaigns and behavior modification programs rarely have a sustained impact and should therefore not be considered primary prevention. To achieve sustainable CVD prevention, efforts must be aimed at changing the environment (physical and social) and getting to the root causes of disease. Research has shown significant associations between the level of neighborhood deprivation and cardiovascular risk profiles (smoking, obesity, physical inactivity) of community residents (Cubbin et al., 2006). Many prevention-focused community-level and policy interventions have the potential to improve health outcomes for everyone, while others target exclusively either men or women.

A successful example of an environmental response to these unhealthy risk patterns is found in the Evergreen Cemetery Jogging Path Project. This project was initiated in Boyle Heights, a predominantly Latino area of East Los Angeles. Residents partnered with the Latino Urban Forum to create a 1.5-mile walking and jogging path where they previously had no access to open space. The residents can now safely engage in physical activity. Moreover, the Evergreen Jogging Path has become a catalyst for further community improvement projects (Aboelata et al., 2004).

Another mode of prevention includes the development of policies that affect gender norms, such as Title IX legislation. In 1972, after years of pressure from the burgeoning women's movement, the federal government passed Title IX outlawing sex-based restrictions on any educational activity funded by the federal government. The legislation had an immediate impact on university admissions policies, particularly to professional schools of law and medicine. The highest-profile and most controversial changes were made in athletic programs. Initial claims that "girls aren't as interested in sports" and that schools would lose alumni backing if men's athletics received cuts proved largely baseless (National Women's Law Center, n.d.). This legislation has had a profound impact on female participation in intercollegiate sports. Between 1972 and 2002, female participation increased 400 percent and high school sports participation increased 800 percent (National Women's Law Center, n.d.). Such dramatic changes are likely to have

direct health impacts resulting from exercise such as improved cardiac and respiratory health, reduced risk of depression, and, reduced participation in high-risk
behaviors. In addition, early participation in athletics is predictive of participation in exercise in later life (Storm, 2002).

Depression

Considered as a group, mental health problems show little difference in prevalence between males and females. However, when considered by specific disorder,
life cycle stage, or environmental and cultural causes, gender-related influences
become more apparent. For example, childhood mental health concerns tend to
be more prevalent in boys, whereas in later life, women are more likely than men
to experience poor mental health. Women in Western industrialized countries are
roughly twice as likely to experience depression as men, who in turn experience
rates of substance abuse at three times the rate of women (Patel, 2005).

Although the prevalence of depression is higher for females in most community-based studies conducted around the world, enough cross-cultural variability
exists to prevent researchers from attributing this difference to simple biological
or hormonal explanations (Patel, 2005). In her 1990 review of depression studies
conducted outside the United States, Nolen-Hoeksema found a mean 2-to-1
female-to-male ratio of depression in Western industrialized nations but found no
significant differences between the sexes in developing nations. Depression rates
vary not only between cultures but also within cultural subgroups; populations
with low social status and income levels generally experience higher depression
rates (Murakumi, 2002; Patel & Kleinmann, 2003). Patel (2005) suggests that some
of the reasons for higher rates of depression among women are that they are more
likely to be denied educational and occupational opportunities than men and so
have fewer options available when faced with economic and social challenges. In
addition, the social gradient in wealth is heavily gendered, and women bear the
burden of poverty disproportionately, possibly increasing their vulnerability to depression. Furthermore, this issue is not limited merely to the amount of money
coming into a household but extends to whether a woman can access that money
and exercise some control over how it is spent (Patel, 2005).

Similarly, Patel (2005) proposes that greater exposure to stressors, particularly
negative life events, explains part of the prevalence of depression among females.
As we noted earlier, women are more likely than men to become victims of intimate partner violence, and violence is often a precursor to mental health distress.
One in three female rape victims develops posttraumatic stress disorder and depression (Astbury, 2001). Not only do women experience more traumas in their
lives than men, but according to Nolen-Hoeksema (2000), they also tend to "ru-

minate," a psychological process that may further enhance their likelihood of developing depression. "Men and women experience different degrees and types of negative events in their lifetimes and are taught to react to these events in gender-specific ways" (Murakumi, 2002, p. 33).

Developing her reasoning further, Murakumi (2002) presents results from a study by Hammen and Peters (1978), who found that depressed female students who reached out to their roommates received concerned, nurturing reactions in response. In contrast, depressed male students who attempted to engage their roommates with similar behavior were met with social isolation and sometimes hostility. When this study was repeated fourteen years later (Joiner, Alfano, & Metalsky, 1992), researchers obtained similar results, leading Murakumi (2002) to conclude that "since men are taught that it is not acceptable to express their feelings of depression to others, they may seek comfort from other sources, such as alcohol. Indeed, one argument in support of the idea that the different rates of depression between men and women are illusionary is that alcoholism is twice as common in men as in women. If we think of alcoholism as the male version of depression, then we would not need to account for any differences in rates of depression between genders. There is, however, limited evidence in support of this theory" (p. 28).

Finally, men and women who do not comply with culturally endorsed, heterosexual, gendered behaviors may be at greater risk for depression and suicide. Approximately 30 percent of gay and lesbian youth attempt suicide (double or triple the rate for all youth), and young men with more feminine gender-role characteristics face the highest risk of self-destructive behavior (Remafedi, Farrow, & Deisher, 1991). A large percentage of suicides are considered to be the outcome of a variety of mental disorders, the most common of which is depression (Krug, Dahlberg, Mercy, Zwi, & Lozano, 2002).

Implications for Prevention. Although research evidence provides a reasonable understanding of how factors related to gender may shape differences in prevalence, much less is known about how sex and gender interact to influence help-seeking behaviors, treatment, and outcomes of depression (Patel, 2005). For instance, Culbertson (1997) points out that it is not known whether the depressive experience is similar in men and women. In addition, it is unclear whether the gender of a mental health professional affects the evaluation of depression and other patient problems. Effective primary prevention includes acknowledging that risk factors for depression may be gender-specific and that gender-based violence, discrimination, and stereotyping need to be addressed in legislation and policy development as well as in intervention programs (WHO, 2002c).

An example of a program that addresses depression from a primary prevention perspective is the Youth Leadership Academy on Mental Health Policy (YLA), a joint project of several agencies including the California Adolescent Health Collaborative. YLA trains young people throughout California in policy development and includes youth voices in recommendations on mental health issues. The project also brings youth and their ideas to state policymakers to advocate for change. The focus of the program is developing effective policies that not only increase treatment for youth but also address stigma and create environments that support adolescent mental health (California Adolescent Health Collaborative, 2005).

Another example is the Washington State Suicide Prevention Plan, which in 1999 created the Youth Suicide Prevention Program (YSPP) with funding from the state legislature. YSPP has three primary areas of focus: public awareness (suicide warning signs and reducing stigma associated with mental health issues), training for adults who work with youth on a regular basis, and community organizing aimed at helping communities identify assets and needs and development of necessary resources. The overarching theme of the program's efforts is the creation of environments and communities that support youth and positive youth development. Five years after the plan's implementation, the suicide rate in Washington had dropped by 33 percent (YSPP, 2004).

Strategies and Recommendations

A facilitator's guide to gender, health, and development created by the Pan American Health Organization (PAHO) discusses the differences between practical gender approaches (PGA) and strategic gender approaches (SGA) when creating health promotion programs (PAHO, 1997). A practical gender approach responds to the health needs of women and men within their socially accepted roles in society without attempting to modify gender inequities. A strategic gender approach is aimed at redistributing the roles, responsibilities, and power between the genders to reduce inequities that harm health and health-seeking behavior, in addition to responding to the concrete health needs of men and women.

Due to evidence that supports changing gender roles in order to bring long-term and sustainable benefits to women and families, the strategic gender approach is favored by the WHO's Interagency Gender Working Group (IGWG). In 2005, the IGWG reviewed twenty-five international health interventions that integrated gender in their delivery, had measurable health outcomes, and had previously been evaluated. Several programs sought to transform gender relations using the following methods (WHO, 2005):

- Encouraging critical awareness of gender roles and norms
- Promoting the position of women relative to men

- Challenging the imbalance of power, distribution of resources, and allocation of duties between women and men
- Addressing the unequal power relationships between women and health care providers

The IGWG also contends that to enhance equitable gender relations, programs must include both men and women in the development and implementation of health interventions. For example, a program designed to prevent unintended pregnancy in Peru engaged women and their husbands in sociodramas, storytelling, body mapping, and problem tree exercises about pregnancy prevention. At postintervention, contraceptive use among participants increased from 58.4 percent to 71.8 percent, with a reported increase in fourteen out of fifteen gender-equitable attitudes and practices. The IGWG evaluated programs that focused on reproductive health, but the strategies used to transform gender relations could be applied to other areas of prevention, education, and policy development that potentially could broaden the scope of prevention efforts.

Conclusion

Gender is implicated in behavior, social and institutional discrimination, and is interactive with other social determinants. As public health practitioners move beyond individually focused behavior change to consider gender as part and parcel of the human experience, we are moving toward a primary prevention model of public health practice that may bring long-term and sustainable benefits to both women and men. If we are to promote primary prevention as a way to bring about a more just and equitable society, members of the future public health workforce must consider the larger social context within which individuals are nested and of which gender is a key component.

References

Abbey, M., Owen, A., Suzakawa, M., Roach, P., & Nestel, P. J. (1999). Effects of menopause and hormone replacement therapy on plasma lipids, lipoproteins, and LDL-receptor activity. *Maturitas, 33,* 259–269.

Aboelata, M. J., Mikkelsen, L., Cohen, L., Fernández, S., Silver, M., & Fujie Parks, L. (2004). *The built environment and health: 11 profiles of neighborhood transformation.* (J. DuLong, Ed.). Oakland, CA: Prevention Institute.

Addis, M. E., & Mahalik, J. R. (2003). Men, masculinity, and the contexts of help seeking. *American Psychologist, 58,* 5–14.

Ajzen, I. (2001). Nature and operation of attitudes. *Annual Review of Psychology, 52,* 27–58.

American Heart Association. (2006). *Go Red for Women: About the movement.* Retrieved March 26, 2006, from http://www.goredforwomen.org/about_the_movement/index.html

Annandale, E., & Clark, J. (1996). What is gender? Feminist theory and the sociology of human reproduction. *Sociology of Health and Illness, 18,* 17–44.

Astbury, J. (2001). Gender disparities in mental health. In World Health Organization, *Mental health. A call for action by world health ministers* (pp. 73–92). Geneva: WHO.

Barrett-Connor, E. (1997). Sex differences in coronary heart disease: Why are women so superior? The 1995 Ancel Keys Lecture. *Circulation, 95,* 252–264.

Bell, D. M., & Nappi, J. (2000). Myocardial infarction in women: A critical appraisal of gender differences in outcomes. *Pharmacotherapy, 20,* 1034–1044.

Berkman, L. F., & Syme, S. L. (1979). Social networks, host resistance, and mortality: A nine-year follow-up study of Alameda County residents. *American Journal of Epidemiology, 109,* 186–204.

Berkowitz, A. D. (2003). Applications of social norms theory to other health and social justice issues. In H. W. Perkins (Ed.), *The social norms approach to preventing school- and college-age substance abuse* (pp. 259–279). San Francisco: Jossey-Bass.

Beyene, Y. (1989). *From menarche to menopause: Reproductive lives of peasant women in two cultures.* Albany: State University of New York Press.

Brunner, E., Shipley, M. J., Blane, D., Davey Smith, G., & Marmot, M. G. (1999). When does cardiovascular risk start? Past and present socioeconomic circumstances and risk factors in adulthood. *Journal of Epidemiology and Community Health, 53,* 757–764.

California Adolescent Health Collaborative. (2005, June). *Adolescent mental health policy news.* Retrieved July 28, 2006, from http://www.californiateenhealth.org/amhpn_overview_main.asp

California Friday Night Live. (2006). *About CFNLC.* Retrieved July 28, 2006, from http://www.fridaynightlive.org/About/About.htm

Campbell, J. C. (2002). Health consequences of intimate partner violence. *The Lancet, 359,* 1331–1336.

Centers for Disease Control and Prevention. (2000). Cigarette smoking among adults—United States, 1998. *Morbidity and Mortality Weekly Report, 49,* 881–884.

Centers for Disease Control and Prevention, Office of Public Health Research. (2004, March). *Community-based participatory prevention research grants: Men as Navigators for Health.* Retrieved June 26, 2006, from http://www.cdc.gov/od/ophr/awards/grants/grant53.htm

Centers for Disease Control and Prevention, Division of Heart Disease and Stroke Prevention. (2005). *Prevention works: Strategies for a heart–healthy and stroke–free America.* Retrieved May 16, 2006, from http://www.cdc.gov/dhdsp/library/prevention_works/index.htm#10

Cohen, L., Davis, R., & Graffunder, C. (2006). Before it occurs: Primary prevention of intimate partner violence and abuse. In P. R. Salber & E. Taliaferro (Eds.), *The physician's guide to intimate partner violence and abuse.* Volcano, CA: Volcano Press, 2006.

Courtenay, W. H. (2000a). Behavioral factors associated with disease, injury, and death among men: Evidence and implications for prevention. *Journal of Men's Studies, 9,* 81–142.

Courtenay, W. H. (2000b). Constructions of masculinity and their influence on men's well-being: A theory of gender and health. *Social Science and Medicine, 50,* 1385–1401.

Courtenay, W. H (2000c). Engendering health: A social constructionist examination of men's health beliefs and behaviors. *Psychology of Men and Masculinity, 1,* 4–15.

Courtenay, W. H. (2000d). Teaming up for the new men's health movement. *Journal of Men's Studies, 8,* 387–392.

Courtenay, W. H. (2003). Key determinants of the health and well-being of men and boys. *International Journal of Men's Health, 2*, 1–30.

Courtenay, W. H. (2004). Making health manly: Social marketing and men's health. *Journal of Men's Health & Gender, 1*(2–3), 275–276.

Cubbin, C., Sundquist, K., Ahlén, H., Johansson, S. E., Winkleby, M. A., & Sundquist, J. (2006). Neighborhood deprivation and cardiovascular disease risk factors: Protective and harmful effects. *Scandinavian Journal of Public Health, 34*, 228–237.

Culbertson, F. (1997). Depression and gender: An international review. *American Psychologist, 52*, 25–31.

Dalstra, J. A., Kunst, A. E., Borrell, C., Breeze, E., Cambois, E., Costa, G., et al. (2005). Socioeconomic differences in the prevalence of common chronic diseases: An overview of eight European countries. *International Journal of Epidemiology, 34*, 316–326.

Dejoy, D. M. (1992). An examination of gender differences in traffic accident risk perception. *Accident Analysis and Prevention, 24*, 237–246.

Doyal, L. (1995). *What makes women sick? Gender and the political economy of health.* New Brunswick, NJ: Rutgers University Press.

Eastwood, J., & Doering, L. V. (2005). Gender differences in coronary artery disease. *Journal of Cardiovascular Nursing, 20*, 340–351.

Elliot, D. (1987). Self-reported driving while under the influence of alcohol/drugs and the risk of alcohol/drug-related accidents. *Alcohol, Drugs and Driving, 3*(304), 31–43.

Ernst, A. A. (2006). Intimate partner violence: Steps for future generations. *Annals of Emergency Medicine, 47*, 200–202.

Frasure-Smith, N., Lesperance, F., Juneau, M., Talajic, M., & Bourassa, M. G. (1999). Gender, depression, and one-year prognosis after myocardial infarction. *Psychosomatic Medicine, 61*, 26–37.

Galdas, P. M., Cheater, F., & Marshall, P. (2005). Men and health help-seeking behavior: Literature review. *Journal of Advanced Nursing, 49*, 616–623.

Galobardes, B., Davey Smith, G., & Lynch, J. W. (2006). Systematic review of the influence of childhood socioeconomic circumstances on risk for cardiovascular diseases in adulthood. *Annals of Epidemiology, 16*, 91–104.

Gergen, K. (1985). The social constructionist movement in modern psychology. *American Psychologist, 40*, 266–275.

Gerlock, A. A. (1999). Health impact of domestic violence. *Issues in Mental Health Nursing, 20*, 373–385.

Golding, J. M. (1999). Intimate partner violence as a risk factor for mental disorders: A meta-analysis. *Journal of Family Violence, 14*, 99–132.

Hammen, C., & Peters, S. (1978). Interpersonal consequences of depression: Responses to men and women enacting a depressed role. *Journal of Abnormal Psychology, 87*, 322–332.

Hanna, C. (2000). Bad girls and good sports. *Hastings Constitutional Law Quarterly, 27*, 667–713.

Harre, N., Field, J., & Kirkwood, B. (1996). Gender differences and areas of common concern in the driving behaviors and attitudes of adolescents. *Journal of Safety Research, 27*, 163–173.

Hawkley, L. C., Masi, C. M., Berry, J. D., & Cacioppo, J. T. (2006). Loneliness is a unique predictor of age-related differences in systolic blood pressure. *Psychological Aging, 21*, 152–164.

Heise, L. L. (1998). Violence against women: An integrated ecological framework. *Violence Against Women, 4*, 262–290.

Heise, L. L., Ellsberg, M., & Gottmoeller, M. (2002). A global overview of gender-based violence. *International Journal of Gynecology and Obstetrics, 78*, S5–S14.

Hemard, J. B., Monroe, P. A., Atkinson, E. S., & Blalock, L. B. (1998). Rural women's satisfaction and stress as family health care gatekeepers. *Women and Health, 28,* 55–77.

Insurance Institute for Highway Safety. (2004). *Fatality facts 2004: Gender.* Arlington, VA: Author. Retrieved October 9, 2006, from http://www.iihs.org/research/fatality_facts/pdfs/gender.pdf

Joiner, T. E., Jr., Alfano, M. S., & Metalsky, G. I. (1992). When depression breeds contempt: Reassurance seeking, self-esteem, and rejection of depressed college students by their roommates. *Journal of Abnormal Psychology, 10,* 165–173.

Krieger, N. (2003). Genders, sexes, and health: What are the connections—and why does it matter? *International Journal of Epidemiology, 32,* 652–657.

Krug, E. G., Dahlberg, L. L., Mercy, L. A., Zwi, A. B., & Lozano, R. (2002). *World report on violence and health.* Geneva: World Health Organization.

Lane, S. D., & Cibula, D. A. (1999). Gender and health. In S. C. Scrimshaw & G. L. Albrecht (Eds.), *Handbook of social studies in health and medicine* (pp. 136–152). Thousand Oaks, CA: Sage.

Lock, M. (1993). *Encounters with aging: Mythologies of menopause in Japan and North America.* Berkeley: University of California Press.

Lorber, J. (1997). *Gender and the social construction of illness.* Thousand Oaks, CA: Sage.

Martin, E. (1992). *The woman in the body: A cultural analysis of reproduction.* Boston: Beacon Press.

Mayo Clinic. (2005). *Cardiovascular disease 101: Know your heart and blood vessels.* Retrieved May 30, 2006, from http://www.mayoclinic.com/health/cardiovascular-disease/HB00032

McDonough, P., & Walters, V. (2001). Gender and health: Reassessing patterns and explanations. *Social Science and Medicine, 52,* 547–559.

Men Can Stop Rape. (n.d.-a). *What's new: The Men of Strength (MOST) Club.* Retrieved July 28, 2006, from http://www.mencanstoprape.org

Men Can Stop Rape. (n.d.-b). *Who we are: Our mission, vision, and values.* Retrieved July 28, 2006, from http://www.mencanstoprape.org/info-url_nocat2701/info-url_nocat.htm

Morgen, S. (2006). Movement-grounded theory: Intersectional analysis of health inequalities in the United States. In A. J. Schulz & L. Mullings (Eds.), *Gender, race, class, and health: Intersectional approaches* (pp. 394–423). San Francisco: Jossey-Bass.

Mosca, L. (2002). Epidemiology and prevention of heart disease. In P. S. Douglas (Ed.), *Cardiovascular health and disease in women* (2nd ed., pp. 23–28). Philadelphia: Saunders.

Mosca, L., Jones, W., King, K., Ouyang, P., Redberg, R. F., & Hill, M. N. (2000). Awareness, perception, and knowledge of heart disease risk and prevention among women in the United States. *Archives of Family Medicine, 9,* 506–515.

Mosca, L., McGillen, C., & Rubenfire, M. (1998). Gender differences in barriers to lifestyle change for cardiovascular disease prevention. *Journal of Women's Health, 7,* 711–715.

Murakumi, J. (2002). Gender and depression: Explaining the different rates of depression between men and women. *Perspectives in Psychology, 5,* 27–34.

Murphy, A. (2006). The next stage. *Sports Illustrated, 104,* 60–69.

National Center for Health Statistics. (2005). *Health, United States, 2005: With chartbook on trends in the health of Americans.* Hyattsville, MD: Author.

National Women's Law Center. (n.d.). *Exercise my rights: Athletics.* Retrieved July 14, 2006, from http://www.titleix.info/content.jsp?content_KEY=185&t=athletics.dwt

Nolen-Hoeksema, S. (1990). *Sex differences in depression.* Stanford, CA: Stanford University Press.

Nolen-Hoeksema, S. (2000). The role of rumination in depressive disorders and mixed anxiety/depressive symptoms. *Journal of Abnormal Psychology, 109,* 504–511.

O'Brien, R., Hunt, K., & Hart, G. (2005). "It's caveman stuff, but that is to a certain extent how guys still operate": Men's accounts of masculinity and help seeking. *Social Science and Medicine, 61,* 503–516.

O'Keefe, M. (1997). Predictors of dating violence among high school students. *Journal of Interpersonal Violence, 12,* 546–568.

Östlin, P., George, A., & Sen, G. (2001). Gender, health and equity: The intersections. In T. Evans, M. Whitehead, F. Diderichsen, A. Bhuiya, & M. Wirth. (Eds.), *Challenging health inequities: From ethics to action* (pp. 175–189). New York: Oxford University Press.

Pan American Health Organization. (1997). *Workshop on gender health and development.* Washington, DC: Author.

Patel, V. (2005). *Gender in mental health research.* Geneva: World Health Organization.

Patel, V., & Kleinman, A. (2003). Poverty and common mental disorders in developing countries. *Bulletin of the World Health Organization, 81,* 609–615.

Petty, R. E., Wegener, D. T., & Fabrigar, L. R. (1997). Attitudes and attitude change. *Annual Review of Psychology, 48,* 609–647.

Phillips, G. B. (2005). Is atherosclerotic cardiovascular disease an endocrinological disorder? The estrogen-androgen paradox. *Journal of Clinical Endocrinology and Metabolism, 90,* 2708–2711.

Phillips, S. P. (2005). Defining and measuring gender: A social determinant of health whose time has come. *International Journal for Equity in Health, 4,* 1–4.

Remafedi, G., Farrow, J., & Deisher, R. (1991). Risk factors for attempted suicide in gay and bisexual youth. *Pediatrics, 87,* 869–876.

Rieker, P. P., & Bird, C. E. (2005). Rethinking gender differences in health: Why we need to integrate social and biological perspectives. *Journal of Gerontology, Series B, 60B* (Special Issue 2), 40–47.

Rosser, S. (1994). *Women's health: Missing from U.S. medicine.* Bloomington: University of Indiana Press.

Schiebinger, L. (2003). Women's health and clinical trials. *Journal of Clinical Investigation, 112,* 973–977.

Schmitz, J. (2003). Smoking cessation in women with cardiac risk. *American Journal of Medical Science, 326,* 192–196.

Schoenborn, C. A., Adams, P. F., Barnes, P. M., Vickerie, J. L., & Schiller, J. S. (2004). Health behaviors of adults, United States, 1999–2001. *Vital Health Statistics, 10*(219).

Siegrist, J. (2002). Commentary: Work stress and coronary heart disease—A gender (role) specific association? *International Journal of Epidemiology, 31,* 1154.

Staples, R. (1995). Health among African American males. In D. F. Sabo & D. F. Gordon (Eds.), *Men's health and illness: Gender, power, and the body* (pp. 121–138). Thousand Oaks, CA: Sage.

Storm H. (2002, June 22). Title IX offers fair play for all. *Chicago Sun-Times,* p. 12.

Tjaden, P., & Thoennes, N. (2000a). Prevalence and consequences of male-to-female and female-to-male intimate partner violence as measured by the national violence against women survey. *Violence Against Women, 6,* 142–161.

Tjaden, P., & Thoennes, N. (2000b). *Prevalence, incidence, and consequences of violence against women: Findings from the National Violence Against Women Survey.* Washington, DC: National Institute of Justice.

Turner, C., & McClure, R. (2003). Age and gender differences in risk-taking behaviour as an explanation for high incidence of motor vehicle crashes as a driver in young males. *Injury Control and Safety Promotion, 10,* 123–130.

United Nations. (1993). *Declaration on the elimination of violence against women.* New York: Author.

Vaccarino, V., Krumholz, H. M., Yarzebski, J., Gore, J. M., & Goldberg, R. J. (2001). Sex differences in two-year mortality after hospital discharge for myocardial infarction. *Annals of Internal Medicine, 134,* 173–181.

Waldron, I. (1995). Contributions of changing gender differences in behavior and social roles to changing gender differences in mortality. In D. F. Sabo & D. F. Gordon (Eds.), *Men's health and illness: Gender, power, and the body* (pp. 22–45). Thousand Oaks, CA: Sage.

Whitehead, T. L. (1997). Urban low-income African American men, HIV/AIDS, and gender identity. *Medical Anthropology Quarterly, 11,* 411–447.

Williams, J. E., Paton, C. C., Siegler, I. C., Eigenbrodt, M. L., Nieto, F. J., & Tyroler, H. A. (2000). Anger proneness predicts coronary heart disease risk: Prospective analysis from the Atherosclerosis Risk in Communities (ARIC) study. *Circulation, 101,* 2034–2039.

Wilson, R. (1966). *Feminine forever.* New York: Evans.

Wingood, G. M., & DiClemente, R. J. (2000). Application of the theory of gender and power to examine HIV-related exposures, risk factors, and effective interventions for women. *Health Education and Behavior, 27,* 539–565.

World Health Organization. (2002a.) *World report on violence and health.* Geneva: WHO.

World Health Organization. (2002b). *Gender and road traffic injuries.* Geneva: Department of Gender and Women's Health, WHO.

World Health Organization. (2002c). *Gender in mental health research.* Geneva: WHO.

World Health Organization. (2005). *Multi-Country Study on Women's Health and Domestic Violence Against Women.* Retrieved March 15, 2006, from http://www.who.int/gender/violence/who_multicountry_study/en

Yagil, D. (1998). Gender- and age-related differences in attitudes toward traffic laws and traffic violations. *Transportation Research, Part F, 1,* 123–135.

Youth Suicide Prevention Program. (2004). *Prevention works!* Retrieved October 9, 2006, from http://www.yspp.org/preventionWorks/preventionWorks.htm

CHAPTER FOUR

THE HOPE OF PREVENTION

Individual, Family, and Community Resilience

Bonnie Benard

A major breakthrough in both prevention research and practice occurred in the late 1980s and early 1990s, a discovery that offers the "hope of prevention" to all who care about improving the lives of individuals, families, and communities. This hope lies in the growing field of *resilience* research and practice. This field has evolved from the study of how individuals, families, and communities, facing multiple risks, challenges, and adversities, have not only successfully adapted but have even grown stronger through overcoming these obstacles. A classic definition of resilience is "a class of phenomena characterized by patterns of positive adaptation in the context of significant adversity or risk" (Masten & Reed, 2002, p. 75; see also Luthar, 2003). Resilience research and practice provides the prevention field with nothing less than a fundamentally different knowledge base, one offering the promise of transforming interventions. The identification of the attributes of individuals who have succeeded despite early stress and trauma; the characteristics of families, schools, and communities that facilitated this success; and the factors that lead communities as a whole to overcome challenging circumstances create a new paradigm for both research and practice, one that is based on entirely different assumptions and that asks entirely different questions. Resilience research provides a powerful rationale for moving our focus in the social and behavioral sciences from risk to resilience, from a concern with individual deficit and pathology to an examination of the strengths individuals, families, and communities have brought to bear in promoting healing and health.

Risk-Based Approaches

Initially, discussion and research examining the predictive impact of risks on individual lives was an important and exciting development. Risk-based approaches offer a way to identify social factors that are correlated with negative outcomes such as drug abuse, mental illness, and criminal behavior and get away from blaming individuals for their poor life outcomes. The implications were great for public policies addressing the most pervasive risks, such as poverty and educational opportunity. The promise existed that through exploratory research, all of the risks for a given pathology could be identified and remedied, and the pathology itself could be eliminated.

To a field desperate to have a research base, risk-focused prevention has been hailed as a breakthrough. According to the Institute of Medicine, "The concept of risk reduction is at the heart of prevention research" (Mrazek & Haggerty, 1994, p. 6). In fact, the institute's report, *Reducing Risks for Mental Disorders: Frontiers for Preventive Intervention Research,* is so named "because of the power of the risk reduction model" (p. 6). However, to prevention practitioners and researchers concerned with digging deeper into causality and not just correlation, this risk-focused research base is sometimes problematic and harmful at worst.

Historically, the social and behavioral sciences have followed a problem-focused approach to studying human and social phenomena. This "pathology" model of research traditionally examines problems, disease, illness, maladaptation, incompetence, deviance, and so on. The emphasis has been placed on identifying the "risk factors" for individual problems such as alcoholism and mental illness, family problems such as intimate partner violence and child abuse, and community problems such as poverty and violence. Most of the research has been retrospective in design involving a onetime historical assessment of individuals, families, and communities with these existing identified problems—a research design that perpetuates a problem perspective and implicates an inevitability of negative outcomes. For example, researchers have found that among adults who have abused their children, a higher percentage experienced abuse in their childhoods than is found in the general population. Similarly, a greater percentage of adults who abuse alcohol have been found to have grown up in an alcoholic family themselves. In general, risk-focused research has usually found that the risk factors are cumulative: as the number of risk factors increases, so does the likelihood of negative outcomes. Similarly, the predictive power of risks is also influenced by the chronicity, intensity, and duration of the stressors and risk conditions (Rutter, 1989).

For prevention practitioners, this research base raises several concerns. First, the study and identification of risk factors for a condition, such as violence or mental illness, does not answer the key questions that practitioners care about: "How does knowing that my student or client grew up with a mentally ill (or drug-using or criminal) mother or father help me help this person? What can I do Monday morning to improve the chances for this person?" In other words, risk-focused studies do not generally give us research-based *answers* or strategies for doing prevention. According to Norman Garmezy, the "grandfather" of resilience research, this pathology model of research has "provided us with a false sense of security in erecting prevention models that are founded more on values than facts" (quoted in Werner & Smith, 1982, p. xix).

A second concern is that while risk is a statistical concept applicable to the study of groups, it does not account for individual variation within the risk group. Risk research has been transferred to clinical and educational settings wherein individuals—even whole groups of people such as adolescents, their families, and their communities—are identified and subsequently labeled according to their perceived deficit, be it hyperactive, emotionally unstable, dysfunctional, disadvantaged, at-risk, high-risk, or a plethora of others. Regardless of the original benevolent intention, such as getting help to individuals, families, or communities who are hurting, the application of risk-factor-focused research usually leads to the labeling and stigmatizing of youth, their families, and their communities as "at-risk" and "high-risk," as well as to the implementation of drastic public policy practices like zero tolerance in schools and incarceration in our communities.

Perhaps most deleterious of all, as you'll see later in the light of resilience practice, this deficit approach has encouraged prevention practitioners and other helping professionals to view, identify, and name children, families, and communities exclusively through a deficit lens. This "glass-is-half-empty" perspective blocks helpers' ability to see and engage the capacities and strengths of individuals, families, and communities; to see the whole person or environment; and to hear the whole story, thus creating stereotypes or myths about who people, families, and communities really are and promulgating the self-fulfilling prophecy of finding exactly what you're looking for. Ultimately, according to longtime prevention researcher Richard Jessor, our "univocal preoccupation with risk tends to homogenize and caricature those who are poor" (1993, p. 121).

In terms of risk-focused research, two problems predominate. First of all, the examination of the correlates of problems such as violence tend to focus on individual and family risk factors—because they are easier to measure—and ignore the larger societal or environmental risk factors such as poverty and racism. Policymakers, politicians, the media, and often researchers have personalized "at-riskness," locating it in youth and their families, thereby avoiding difficult discussions about the impact of environmental conditions. In fact, more than forty years of social science research has clearly identified poverty—the direct result of public abdication of responsibility for human welfare—as the factor most likely to put a person "at risk" for social ills such as drug abuse, teen pregnancy, child abuse, violence, and school failure, not to mention being imprisoned, having no health care, attending poor schools, being unemployed, lacking recreational facilities, and having no housing (Currie, 1994; Males, 1996; Swadener & Lubeck, 1995).

A second concern is that even researchers doing retrospective or correlational studies of risk factors for the development of problem behaviors were stymied by the issue of whether risk factors in people already diagnosed as schizophrenic, criminal, violent, or alcoholic were the *causes* or the *consequences* of their condition. In other words, which came first, and which is the true risk? Is mental illness a risk factor for poverty, or vice versa? It is this research question that ultimately paved the way for what is now called resilience research.

The Gift of Resilience Research

With the exception of a few earlier studies, beginning in the 1950s and on into the 1960s and 1970s, a handful of researchers decided to circumvent the causality-correlation dilemma by studying individuals postulated to be at high risk for developing certain disorders—children growing up under conditions of great adversity such as neonatal stress, poverty, neglect, abuse, physical handicaps, war, and parental schizophrenia, depression, alcoholism, and criminality. This second wave of risk research therefore used a *prospective* research design, which is developmental and longitudinal, assessing children at various times during the course of their lives in order to better understand the nature of the risk factors that result in the development of a disorder. Although much of the research on both risk and resilience focuses on children (based on their ability to change, the perceived moral injustice of youth suffering, and the relative ease of studying youth over time and in settings such as schools), the frameworks and lessons learned can, in general, be applied to all individuals.

As the children studied in various longitudinal projects grew into adolescence and adulthood, a consistent—and amazing—finding emerged: although a certain percentage of these high-risk children developed various problems (a higher percentage than in the normal population), a greater percentage of the children became "competent, confident, and caring" youths and adults (Werner & Smith, 1982, 1992, 2001). For example, one early study found that only 9 percent of children of schizophrenic parents became schizophrenic, while 75 percent developed into healthy adults (Watt, Anthony, Wynne, & Rolf, 1984). Similarly, whereas one out of four children of alcoholic parents develops alcohol problems—compared to one out of ten in the general population—three out of four of these children do not. In fact, in most studies, the figure seems to hover around 70 to 75 percent resilience when exposed to a significant risk factor. This includes children who were placed in foster care (Fanshel, 1975; Festinger, 1984), were members of gangs (Vigil, 1990), were born to teen mothers (Furstenberg, 1999), were sexually abused (Higgins, 1994; Wilkes, 2002; Zigler & Hall, 1989), had substance-abusing or mentally ill families (Beardslee & Podoresfky, 1988; Chess, 1989; Watt et al., 1984; Werner, 1986; Werner & Smith, 2001), and grew up in poverty (Clausen, 1993; Schweinhart, Barnes, & Wiekart, 1993; Vaillant, 2002). In absolute worst-case scenarios, when children experience multiple and persistent risks, still half of them overcome adversity and achieve good developmental outcomes (Rutter, 1989, 2000).

Researchers Emmy Werner and Ruth Smith, in their seminal community-wide epidemiological study of risk and individual resilience (1982, 1992, 2001), followed nearly seven hundred children growing up with risk factors (one-third of whom had multiple risk factors) from birth to adulthood. As the cohort of children aged, they grew increasingly more like their peers without risk factors. Werner and Smith report, "One of the most striking findings of our two follow-ups in adulthood, at ages thirty-two and forty, was that most of the high-risk youths who did develop serious coping problems in adolescence had staged a recovery by the time they reached midlife. . . . They were in stable marriages and jobs, were satisfied with their relationships with their spouses and teenage children, and were responsible citizens in their community" (2001, p. 167). In fact, only one out of six of the adult subjects at either age thirty-two or forty was doing poorly, "struggling with chronic financial problems, domestic conflict, violence, substance abuse, serious mental health problems, and/or low self-esteem" (p. 37).

These findings challenge a core belief of many risk-focused social scientists—that risk factors for the most part predict negative outcomes. Instead, individual resilience research suggests that risk factors are predictive of outcomes for only about 20 to 49 percent of a given high-risk population. In contrast, *protective factors*, the supports and opportunities that buffer the effect of adversity and enable development to proceed, appear to predict positive outcomes in anywhere from 50 to 80 percent of a high-risk population. According to Werner and Smith, "Our findings and those by other American and European investigators with a life-span perspective suggest that these buffers [that is, protective factors] make a more profound impact on the life course of children who grow up under adverse conditions than do specific risk factors or stressful life events. They [also] appear to transcend ethnic, social class, geographical, and historical boundaries. Most of all, they offer us a more optimistic outlook than the perspective that can be gleaned from the literature on the negative consequences of perinatal trauma, care-giving deficits, and chronic poverty" (1992, p. 202). In other words, the protective factors that foster resilience do indeed offer the "hope of prevention."

The gift of resilience research to the prevention—and intervention—community is essentially that in contrast to risk-focused prevention, it actually does provide a knowledge base for practice since it does answer the question, "What works to promote health and healing, even in the face of challenge and risk?" The *protective factors or processes* within individuals, families, and communities that support the resilience of individuals can be incorporated into the repertoire of not only prevention practitioners but also parents, teachers, neighbors, child protective workers, youth workers, counselors, therapists, and anyone else at their work, at home, and in the community. These protective factors encompass the critical developmental supports and opportunities of caring relationships, high-expectation messages, and opportunities for meaningful participation and contribution that are found in healthy families, effective schools, and competent and caring communities (Benard, 1991, 2004) (see Table 4.1).

TABLE 4.1. PROTECTIVE FACTORS AND PROCESSES IN FAMILIES, SCHOOLS, AND COMMUNITIES.

Caring Relationships	High Expectations	Opportunities for Participation or Contribution
Being there	Belief in people's resilience	People focus
Paying attention	People focus	Engaging, challenging, interesting experiences
Showing interest	Challenge using support messages	Active learning
Respect	Guidance without coercion	Cooperative and inclusive small group activities
Loving support	Freedom with structure and safety	Reflection and dialogue
Compassion	Rituals and rites of passage	Creative expression
Nonjudgmental listening	Focus on strengths	Decision making and planning
Patience	Reframing	Responsibilities
Getting to know interests, strengths, dreams	Demonstrating innate resilience	Leadership
Trust		Service, giving back

Positive development and successful outcomes in any human system depend on the quality of the relationships, beliefs, and opportunities for participation. Keep in mind that these three protective "factors" are not separate entities; rather they are three aspects or components of a dynamic protective "process" in which they work synergistically. For example, caring relationships without high expectations or opportunities for meaningful participation foster dependence and codependence, not positive human system development. High expectations without caring relationships and support to help people meet them are a cruel "shape up or ship out" approach associated with negative outcomes. And caring relationships with high-expectation messages but no opportunities for active participation and contribution create a frustrating situation that blocks the natural process of human development in any system.

Similarly, the resilience *strengths* that are demonstrated by individuals in the face of challenges have also been clearly identified (Benard, 1991, 2004) (see Table 4.2). Identification of these strengths provides us with a language for both research and practice that motivates positive change by drawing the focus away from deficits, dysfunction, and problems and toward strengths, assets, and competencies present in all individuals, even those facing multiple challenges. For example, having a language of strengths helps practitioners and caregivers working with youth begin to look for and find strengths in the young people they serve and then to name and reflect the strengths they have witnessed. This positive language helps practitioners and caregivers *reframe* how they see their clients, to begin to shift from seeing only risk to seeing resilience, especially among those facing a range of challenges

TABLE 4.2. RESILIENCE STRENGTHS: HOW TO RECOGNIZE RESILIENCE IN INDIVIDUALS, FAMILIES, AND COMMUNITIES.

"Much of the task of prevention in this new century," predicts Martin Seligman (2002, p. 5), "will be to create a science of human strengths whose mission will be to understand and learn how to foster these virtues in young people"—and in their families, schools, and communities as well.

Resilience strengths are the characteristics, also called internal assets or competencies, associated with healthy individual, family, and community development. They are not the causes of resilience but rather are the positive developmental *outcomes* demonstrating that human systems are engaging their innate resilience. These strengths are what resilience looks like!

Four categories of often overlapping strengths can be consistently found in resilience and other related literature as follows (Benard, 1991, 2004).

Social Competence	Problem Solving	Autonomy	Sense of Purpose
Responsiveness	Planning	Positive identity	Goal direction
Communication	Flexibility	Internal locus of control	Achievement motivation
Empathy	Resourcefulness	Initiative	Educational aspirations
Caring	Critical thinking	Self-efficacy	Special interests
Compassion	Insight	Mastery	Creativity
Altruism		Adaptive distancing	Imagination
Forgiveness		Resistance	Optimism
		Self-awareness	Hope
		Mindfulness	Faith
		Humor	Spirituality
			Sense of meaning

and adversity. In terms of the research community, having a nomenclature helps legitimate the study of strengths, to empirically measure developmental outcomes from prevention and education interventions, and to better understand what works and what does not. The positive psychology movement, with leadership from Christopher Peterson and Martin Seligman, has compiled the *Character Strengths and Virtues: A Handbook and Classification* (2004), which is intended to be psychology's positive response to psychiatry's *Diagnostic and Statistical Manual* of human "dysfunctions."

A point to clarify in terms of resilience strengths is that they are not fixed personality traits that result in resilience. Research instead suggests that human beings are biologically driven to develop these strengths and to use them for survival. In fact, an elegantly simple definition of resilience is that of Robert J. Lifton (1993), who refers to resilience as the capacity of human systems to transform and change. What appears to be driving this process of adaptation is an internal force, an amazing developmental wisdom often referred to as *intrinsic motivation.* Human beings are intrinsically motivated to meet basic developmental needs, including needs for belonging and affiliation, competence, autonomy, safety, and meaning (Baumeister & Leary, 1995; Deci, 1995; Maslow, 1954). *How* these needs are expressed and met varies, of course, not only within a person and over time but from person to person and from culture to culture. The bottom line for resilience theory and practice is that these psychological needs are givens. These needs are increasingly referred to by developmentalists as "fundamental protective human adaptational systems" (Masten & Reed, 2002, p. 82). All human beings are compelled to meet these needs throughout their lives. For young people, whether these needs are allowed expression in positive, prosocial ways depends to a great extent on the people, places, and experiences they encounter in their families, schools, and communities.

A key point for prevention practitioners and researchers is that because these strengths are intrinsic, dynamic, contextual, and culturally expressed, they are not learned, for the most part or in a lasting way, through a social skills program or a life skills curriculum that attempts to teach them directly. A long history of prevention program evaluation (Kohn, 1997; Kreft & Brown, 1998) testifies to the short-lived effects of eight-week life skills programs. That this approach still predominates in both education and prevention speaks to the strong hold that behaviorism—in terms of focusing on individual behavior change—and "kid-fixing" have over our culture and institutions.

Although researchers and writers often use differing names for these strengths, the categories have continued to hold up under the scrutiny of a decade and a half of research. In fact, as Masten states, "Recent studies continue to corroborate the importance of a relatively small set of global factors associated with resilience" (2001, p. 234) that are both personal and environmental. These competencies and strengths appear to transcend ethnicity, culture, gender, geography, and time and apply at the deeply human level as essential thriving skills. According to an Institute of Medicine report on youth development, "The little available evidence suggests that most of these characteristics are important in all cultural groups" (Eccles & Gootman, 2002, p. 81).

As depicted in Table 4.3, resilience research provides a powerful rationale for moving our focus in the prevention field from a risk approach to a resilience approach. This requires a different paradigm, looking with new eyes, that ultimately changes what we believe, what we do, and how we do it. The good news is that the resilience paradigm gives all who work with despairing individuals, families, and communities the ultimate gift of dwelling in possibility, of working for change with hope in their hearts.

Resilience, Youth Development, and Community Development

Resilience research has played a pivotal role in providing a research base for many of the strengths-based movements currently gaining momentum such as youth development, asset building, positive psychology, strengths-based social work practice, personalized learning environments (in high school reform), and social capital (the amount and strength of associations and networks within communities that produce social cohesion, trust, and a willingness to engage in community

TABLE 4.3. PARADIGMS FOR PREVENTION.

	Risk	**Resilience**
Focus and language:	Deficits	Assets and strengths
Goal:	Problem prevention	Healthy development
Attitude toward people:	People as problems	People as resources
Attitude toward diversity:	Eurocentric	Multicultural
Attitude toward learning:	Mechanistic	Constructivist
Strategic emphasis:	Program and content	People and places
Locus of control:	External	Internal
Philosophy:	Control	Connectedness
Needs being met:	Bureaucracies'	People's
Feelings:	Despair	Hope and motivation

activities), to name a few. It also validates the long-standing approach in public health known as health promotion and the interdisciplinary field of community development.

What all of these approaches share is their focus on a language of assets and strengths; healthy development of human systems as the goal; the viewing of people as resources and not problems; an embracing of diversity as a strength; the understanding that people are constructors of their own knowledge and "stories"; strategies that move beyond programs and curricula to the deep restructuring of the relationships, beliefs, and participation within a system; the development of internal "locus of control" or empowerment; and a philosophy not of control but of connectedness. It is ultimately this underlying philosophy—that acknowledges the interconnectedness of human systems (and other living systems for that matter) and their innate resilience, their potential and capacity to transform and change and the developmental wisdom that is motivating their behavior—that drives this *developmental* paradigm and unites the approaches that go by the names of resilience, youth development, and community development. Without this philosophy, approaches like youth development and community development result in new wine being poured into old bottles; that is, they evolve into the same old deficit-based stuff.

Recognizing Resilience in Communities

Longitudinal studies conducted during the past two decades indicate that while the absence of a strong community is devastating for young people, the reverse is also true: positive community contexts can be transformational (Carnegie Task Force, 1992; McLaughlin, 2000; McLaughlin, Irby, & Langman, 1994; Werner & Smith, 1992). As with the other two major settings in which children are socialized, the family and school, the community that supports the positive development of young people promotes the building of the strengths and competencies associated with healthy development and resilience—social competence, problem solving, autonomy, and a sense of purpose and future. Social scientists refer to the capacity of a community to build resilience in its members as community competence or capacity.

Perhaps the most obvious manifestation of the protective factors at the community level is the availability of resources necessary for healthy human development: health care, child care, housing, education, job training, employment, and recreation. Resilient communities exert not only a *direct* influence on the lives of young people but also, perhaps even more important, a profound influence on the lives of the families, schools, and youth-serving neighborhood-based organizations

Reasons to Adopt a Community Resilience Approach

- For individuals to be healthy, they need healthy communities.

  Communities have strengths and assets that can provide an environment that promotes health and well-being.

- Health disparities, by definition, affect groups or whole populations of people, not individuals.

  A community resilience approach allows for community-level action that will benefit the population within the community.

- The absence of risk does not equal health; a community resilience approach goes beyond risk.

  Addressing risk factors results in the absence of factors that threaten health and safety; however, it does not necessarily achieve conditions that support health.

- A community approach minimizes "blaming the victim."

  Behavior is typically constructed in individualist terms, leaving many to conclude that poor health is the result of poor or ill-informed choices. However, researchers are increasingly recognizing the relationship between behavior and environment in determining health outcomes, acknowledging the limits of efforts that focus solely on individual behavior change.

- A community approach means ensuring that fewer people get sick, not just that more people get well.

  Addressing the ways in which root factors play out at the community level creates opportunities to ensure that people do not get sick in the first place, thereby reducing disparities.

- A resilience approach is based on the unique culture of the community.

  Different ethnic and racial groups have unique values, perspectives, assets, and living styles. A resilience approach builds on what is already working within cultures and is tailored to the community's strengths.

- A community resilience approach is responsive to the range of developmental needs.

  Every community must address a range of developmental needs, from the very young to the elderly. A community resilience approach enables communities to develop solutions that benefit all.

- A community resilience approach meets community needs for well-being by strengthening the overall environment within a community.

  Such an approach identifies the needs within a community that support overall well-being. The approach acknowledges the direct impact of the environment on health as well as its impact on behavior, which in turn affects health outcomes.

(Continued)

- A community resilience approach changes conditions shaped by oppression, poverty, and economic disparity.

  The root factors of health disparities, such as oppression, discrimination, and poverty, play out at the community level, which results in the populations of some communities being at higher risk for a range of poor health and safety outcomes. By strengthening key community factors, communities can build their own capacity to effect change where they see need. By empowering communities to take action, the impact of these root factors will be minimized.

- Multiple health and safety concerns are addressed simultaneously and before the onset of symptoms.

  By going "upstream" from injury and illness, a community resilience approach enables communities to design effective strategies that prevent multiple health and safety problems. Such an approach creates community norms that are focused on being healthy, not on protection from illness, and can therefore address the causes of multiple health issues. A focus before the onset of symptoms translates into more cost-effective interventions.

Source: Prevention Institute.

within their domain and thus also *indirectly*—but powerfully—affect the outcome for children and youth. According to most researchers, the greatest protection we could give children is ensuring that they and their families have access to these basic necessities (Coleman, 1987; Garmezy, 1991; Long & Vaillant, 1989; Sameroff, Barocas, & Seifer, 1984; Wilson, 1987). Conversely, the greatest risk factor for the development of nearly all problem behaviors is poverty, a condition characterized by the lack of these basic resources.

The fact that the rate of child poverty has remained hovering around 25 percent for the past two decades clearly testifies to the lack of national political will to provide the opportunities for all children to succeed. In light of this national neglect of children and families, the imperative falls to local communities to fill the gap. And the only way communities can succeed and have succeeded in this endeavor is through the building of social networks—both formal and informal—that reweave the social fabric, that is, that link not only families and schools but agencies and organizations throughout the community with the common purpose of collaborating to address the needs of children and families (Coleman, 1987; Putnam, 2000; Putnam & Feldstein, 2003; Schorr, 1988, 1997). In a resilient community, community members and organizations support and work in partnership with families, youth, and schools. Families support youth, volunteer in their community, and work in partnership with schools. Schools not only support and work in partnership with their students but also support and work in partnership with families and with community groups, especially with their community-based organization partners.

A major finding of almost every successful youth-serving entity is that its success was enhanced by creating partnerships. For example, mentoring by a community organization is more successful when the family is also a partner and when schools are cooperative. After-school programs run by community organizations but located in schools benefit from the commitment of the school and from involved parents. By contrast, the absence of partnerships and collaboration has the opposite effect. According to the Institute of Medicine report, "Both quantitative and qualitative implementation data also tell us a great deal about why programs fail. These studies make it clear how the programs are nested into larger social systems that need to be taken into account. When adequate supports are not available in these larger systems, it is unlikely that specific programs will be able to be implemented well and sustained over time" (Eccles & Gootman, 2002, p. 221).

Formal community-building or change efforts are now recognizing the truth of White and Wehlage's argument: supporting a community's informal social networks and relationships is key to successful prevention efforts (1995). The Rockefeller Foundation's report on successful community initiatives concluded that "while community building is more an art than a science, research shows that relationships are key to turning lives around. . . . Building on this insight to develop networks of social support in low-income neighborhoods cannot help but yield positive change" (Walsh, 1997, p. vi).

The Project on Human Development in Chicago Neighborhoods, led by Robert Sampson and his colleagues, even found that the informal networks in poor neighborhoods served as protective factors against youth crime and violence (Sampson, Raudenbush, & Earls, 1997). They use the term *collective efficacy* to describe communities where residents consistently interact in ways that are positive and cooperative. As Sampson explains, "It's a sense of shared expectations among neighbors. It's the social networks people have, the values that they share and whether or not they trust each other" (quoted in Owens, 2002, p. 5). When these characteristics exist, regardless of a community's poverty level, neighbors look out for the young people in the community, hold them to "orderly" behavior, and take collective action—for example, to get rid of a local drug hangout. The Chicago Neighborhoods researchers reported that rates of violence differed dramatically in poor communities with similar demographics, depending on the level of collective efficacy. "At the neighborhood level, the willingness of local residents to intervene for the common good depends in large part on conditions of mutual trust and solidarity among neighbors" (Sampson et al., 1997, p. 919).

Mapping Community Assets

In other words, the heart of community can be found at the relational level. Any attempt to rebuild a sense of community connection for young and old must begin with caring relationships that communicate high expectations through positive beliefs in the capacities of young people and their families, focusing on strengths and assets. In every model of successful community change, the initiatives start not with an inventory of risks and problems but with a mapping of the community's assets and strengths. A couple of examples illustrate this high-expectations approach.

Roger Mills's Community Health Realization initiatives (1993) start with helping community members directly recognize their innate wisdom and resilience and develop a sense of self-efficacy, which in turn results in their feeling powerful and hopeful enough to take action with others to improve their community themselves. The approach of asset-based community development is to begin with a "community assets map." According to John McKnight (1992), "The starting point for any serious development effort is the opposite of an accounting of deficiencies. Instead there must be an opportunity for individuals to use their own abilities to produce. Identifying the variety and richness of skills, talents, knowledge, and experience of people in low-income neighborhoods provides a base upon which to build new approaches and enterprises" (p. 10). Creating a community assets map thus begins the process of neighborhood regeneration, which "locates all of the available local assets, begins connecting them with one another in ways that multiply their power and effectiveness, and begins harnessing those local institutions [and individuals] that are not yet available for local development" (Kretzmann & McKnight, 1993, p. 6).

The natural outcome of having high expectations for people, especially for viewing youth as resources and not as problems, is the creation of opportunities for them to be contributing members of their community. Just as healthy human development involves the process of bonding to the family and school through the provision of opportunities to be involved in meaningful and valued ways in family and school life, developing a sense of belonging and attachment to one's community also requires opportunities to participate in the life of the community. Once again, resilience research has found that young people who have opportunities in their communities to be part of clubs, teams, work apprenticeships, mentoring programs, neighborhood-based youth development organizations, and community service-learning programs are able to overcome other challenges in their lives and become healthy and successful adults (McLaughlin et al., 1994; Werner & Smith, 1992). A sine qua non in creating effective communitywide initiatives for all people, young and old, is engaging their active involvement. Youth, just like adults, need to have ownership and active roles in the life of their community if the community is to serve as a protective factor.

A Focus on Community Resilience

In addition to the power that communities have to support individual resilience, communities themselves demonstrate resilience. Although it is vital to foster resilience in individuals, the opportunity for a broader impact is being missed. The range of health, safety, and social ills that afflict families, schools, and communities are too broad to be simply addressed one individual at a time. Rather, what is needed to complement individual work is a multifaceted approach that strengthens the overall environment. Communities have an enormous capacity to contribute to the resolution of their own problems, building on strengths that may previously have been obstructed. In addition, in the same way that focusing on risk can lead to blaming the victim, focusing on community support for individual resilience can lead to blaming the community for not providing adequate opportunity for assets and strengths to emerge. By focusing on community resilience, the responsibility is placed even more broadly on all of us to create the conditions and policies that support the emergence of community assets and strengths.

According to the National Charrette Institute (2002), resilient communities that promote health and safety often work toward improving the social, economic, and physical well-being of their people, places, and natural environments. These communities work to enhance existing resilience factors such as daily physical activity, social cohesion and trust, safe streets (including walking paths and trails for residents), and transportation options that reduce automobile congestion and encourage economic, social, environmental, and cultural sustainability.

A resilient community, like a resilient individual, can be described as having social competence, problem-solving capacity, a sense of identity, and hope for the future. A resilient community provides the same triad of protective factors as resilient families and schools: caring relationships, high expectations, and opportunities for participation. Sociologists have recently begun describing community protective factors in terms of the concept of *social capital*, "social networks, norms of reciprocity, mutual assistance, and trustworthiness" (Putnam & Feldstein, 2003, p. 2).

A resilient community is characterized by mutually caring relationships, high expectations in the form of shared positive beliefs and respect for all citizens—especially those on the margin, such as young people—and active participation and contribution on the part of everyone. It is a community in which young people, families, schools, and other community members and organizations work *as partners* to ensure not only that individuals receive the critical supports and opportunities necessary for healthy development but also that community strengths are supported and developed. Fostering the kind of community that supports individuals requires paying attention to a broad range of factors. Prevention Institute did an extensive examination of the literature and research and developed the Toolkit for Health and Resilience in Vulnerable Environments (THRIVE) for the U.S. Department of Health and Human Services' Office of Minority Health. THRIVE outlines four clusters of community factors that directly affect resilience: *built environment* factors such as housing, environmental quality, and transportation; *social capital* factors such as collective efficacy, social cohesion, and social norms; *structural* factors such as economic capital, racial relations, and media and marketing; and *service and institution* factors such as education, cultural opportunities, and public safety (http://www.charretteinstitute.org/healthy.html).

Evaluators of the New Futures venture, an ambitious communitywide initiative to benefit young people in five large communities, warn that we neglect the qualities of the immediate caregiving environment at our peril. On-site evaluators of the five-year initiative, which was funded by the Annie E. Casey Foundation, attribute the failure of these early communitywide collaborations to the finding that systems and organizations talked only to each other; they did not, for example, bring in the families or youth they served, nor did they invite teachers to the table. According to these evaluators, Julie White and Gary Wehlage (1995), "It is the strengthening of neighborhoods from the inside that is vital, something that traditional social services have not succeeded in doing" (p. 35). The authors go on to state that if the goal becomes one of "building social capital, the criteria for a successful collaborative would shift from delivering services more efficiently to success in fostering community. Social capital contributes to community by fostering networks of interdependency within and among families, neighborhoods, and the larger community." Furthermore, they argue, "the shift from delivering services to individual clients to investing in the social capital of whole groups of people appears to be essential if collaboratives are to ultimately improve the life chances of generations of at-risk children" (p. 35).

A Framework for Resilience and Community and Youth Development

Getting youth involved as partners in change efforts to improve their conditions and opportunities is an important and powerful strategy. Community youth development (CYD), an emerging movement, places the emphasis on young people themselves becoming community change agents, fully capable of improving their communities not only for the young but also for families and other community members. For example, the California Wellness Foundation funds community-based initiatives in which, according to foundation president Gary Yates, "young people work in leadership roles alongside of adults to determine what changes are needed in their physical, social and chemical environments to promote health and wellness in their communities" (California Wellness Foundation, 1999).

In contrast to other community development approaches, CYD holds that healthy communities cannot be built without a youth development approach, one that actively enlists young people in the change effort. The ultimate goal of this approach is the creation of "safe, just, prosperous communities, countries, and world where young people are partners and contributors working with adults to positively influence the conditions affecting the security and quality of their lives" (Curnan & Hughes, 2002, p. 33). This approach is exemplified in the Ford Foundation's Community Youth Development Initiative (Cutler & Edwards, 2002), Stanford University's Gardner Center for Youth and Community (McLaughlin, 2000), the Annie E. Casey Foundation (Hyman, 1999), the Innovation Center for Community and Youth Development at the University of Wisconsin (2002), and the National 4-H Council (2002), to name just a few.

As illustrated in Figure 4.1, the CYD approach recognizes that youth participation and contribution (in the context of caring relationships and high-expectation messages) not only benefit young people themselves by promoting positive developmental outcomes but also that youth participation and contribution are critical and necessary if we are to actually improve communities not just for young

FIGURE 4.1. THE COMMUNITY YOUTH DEVELOPMENT PROCESS: RESILIENCE IN ACTION.

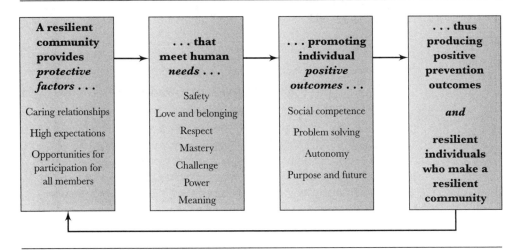

people but for everyone. CYD recognizes the web of interconnectedness that defines a resilient community, reminding prevention practitioners and supporters that besides taking "a whole village to raise a child," it also takes "a child to raise a whole village" (Kretzmann & Schmitz, 1999).

Youth Development, Resilience, and Primary Prevention

The framework in Figure 4.1 not only illustrates the interconnectedness of the fields of resilience, community development, and youth development but also presents a theory of change that postulates that prevention outcomes are best achieved by the community youth development process. This process starts by enhancing community support for resilience by helping communities provide the protective factors of caring relationships, high expectations, and opportunities for participation at the community level that meet youth needs both directly and indirectly through supporting families and schools. Protective factors promote young people's positive social, emotional, cognitive, and moral and spiritual development (individual resilience strengths), resulting in positive prevention outcomes (reductions in problem behaviors across the board). These healthy and successful young people feed right back into their communities, in turn strengthening the resilience of the community.

When communities fail to provide the critical protective factors that meet developmental needs, young people can be drawn to seek support elsewhere, often from groups that prey on youthful needs for affiliation and belonging, such as gangs. It is past time for the prevention field to move from its dominant risk-based paradigm, especially from the current focus on narrow "evidence-based programs" designed to fix "high-risk youth," to embrace a community youth development approach that embraces the resilience and other innate gifts that every young person possesses.

The Healthy-Immigrant Paradox

First-generation immigrants tend to be healthier than U.S.-born populations of the same race and ethnicity (National Institutes of Health [NIH], 2003). This holds true even when the immigrant populations have characteristics that are associated with poorer health outcomes, such as low socioeconomic status. This phenomenon, known as the *healthy-immigrant paradox,* can be seen in U.S. immigrant and migrants. Significantly, the protective influence of immigration tends to dissipate with acculturation to mainstream U.S. culture—second-generation immigrant populations are less healthy than their elders.

Theories postulated to explain the healthy-immigrant paradox include the notions that immigrants are a self-selected group and that healthier people tend to immigrate. A study of infant health among Puerto Rican migrants provides some evidence for these theories. Puerto Ricans are not immigrants; they are native-born U.S. citizens, but they share many characteristics with immigrants. Despite their relatively low socioeconomic status, Puerto Rican migrants to the U.S. mainland have relatively low levels of infant mortality. In fact, infant mortality is lower for new migrants to the mainland than among families who remain in Puerto Rico, suggesting that selective migration is an important explanatory factor. But among migrants to the mainland, infant mortality rates rise as time on the mainland increases; the positive association between infant mortality and length of stay on the mainland increases when other behavioral, demographic, and socioeconomic factors are controlled (NIH, 2003).

Another theory posited for healthy immigrants is that they bring with them cultural practices from their home countries that are protective for some adverse health outcomes (Guendelman et al., 1999). Birth outcomes among Mexican-born women might provide evidence for this theory. Immigrant Mexican women tend to face significant challenges to their health during pregnancy, but their babies tend to be healthier on average than other demographics in the United States. Immigrant Mexican women have high rates of fertility, low incomes, and delayed access to prenatal care—all significant contributors to infant mortality (Guendelman et al., 1999). However, rates of infant mortality are lower for babies born to Mexican-born women than for population groups that face fewer correlated risks (Guendelman, Thornton, Gould, & Hosang, 2005), and birth outcomes for second-generation Mexican American women are worse than for their mothers.

The explanation for these differences may lie in cultural practices. Although first-generation Mexican American women hold lower socioeconomic status than second-generation or non-Hispanic white women, they average a higher average intake of protein, vitamins A and C, folic acid, and calcium than the other two groups. In fact, intake of these nutrients was highest for first-generation Mexican women and lowest in their second-generation counterparts. While low incomes correlate with less healthy diets for non-Hispanics, low incomes are associated with healthier diets for first-generation Mexicans (Guendelman & Abrams, 1995).

In addition, an NIH study shows that mothers of Mexican origin born in the United States are more than twice as likely to smoke during pregnancy than Mexican-born mothers, and a review of related research shows that a higher level of U.S. cultural assimilation is associated with worse birth and prenatal outcomes (prematurity, low birthweight, teen pregnancy, and neonatal mortality), as well as with undesirable prenatal and postnatal behaviors (smoking and drug

(Continued)

use during pregnancy and decreased number of breastfeeding mothers) (Marie-lena, Gamboa, Kahramanian, Morales, & Bautista, 2005). Hence babies born to Mexican-born women are less likely to have adverse birth outcomes associated with cigarette smoking. Less quantifiable factors in the relative health of Latino babies may also include positive cultural attitudes toward pregnant women, strong family ties, kinship networks, religious faith, and cultures that promote the consumption of whole foods.

Public health practitioners can use this kind of information to build on the cultural strengths of Mexican-born women to prevent the development of health problems that may put their children at risk. Furthermore, by identifying populationwide characteristics that offset high risks, practitioners may be in a better position to direct their public health efforts in a way that would have the greatest impact. By shifting the focus of our public health approach from one that is centered around individuals to an approach that focuses on larger communities, it is possible to effectively promote the health and well-being of entire at-risk populations that face health disparities in the United States.

Source: Prevention Institute.

Creating a Resilience Perspective

Much progress has been made bringing a strengths perspective to the table. Unfortunately, many human service professions—education, criminal justice, social services, and even public health—often still reflect a deficit perspective. How do we influence caregivers (service providers) and, even more important, transform human service systems so that they take a positive, community youth development or resilience approach to prevention?

This question is similar to the question that has been at the heart of the resilience movement: How do we transform risk into resilience? One important answer and starting point is to help caregivers recognize their *own* resilient nature. This allows them to reframe their experience and see themselves and their lives in new ways. Over a decade of research has shown that this reframing is facilitated by the protective factors of caring relationships, high expectations, and opportunities for participation and contribution. Providing organizational supports and opportunities to the caregivers of youth and others thus becomes the ultimate starting point for resilience-based efforts. A supportive and nurturing climate for youth and community development is exponentially enhanced when governments, communities, and schools support the "health of the helpers." Healthy helpers model in their own lives and work the resilience strengths of social competence, problem solving, autonomy, and sense of purpose.

Other strategies include directly disseminating and teaching what we know about resilience both to adult caregivers and to our children and youth. A resilience study group is a powerful strategy for helping people learn about their resilience, the power they have to see themselves and their lives in new ways. In these groups, service providers, youth, and community members learn about resilience research and about other people's successes and share their own histories. All of these stories of resilience create hope. As Werner and Smith (1992) write, "The life stories of the resilient youngsters now grown into adulthood teach us that competence, confidence, and caring can flourish, even under adverse circumstances, if children encounter persons who provide them with the secure basis for the development of trust, autonomy, and initiative. From odds successfully overcome springs hope—a gift each of us can share with a child—at home, in the classroom, on the playground, or in the neighborhood" (p. 209).

Directly teaching both caregivers and youth about their personal resilience is also a major strategy for engendering a belief in resilience. For example, the Health Realization and Community Resilience work of Roger Mills (see Mills & Spittle, 2001) is being used in schools, communities, workplaces, and organizations nationally and internationally to help parents, teachers, managers, youth workers, and law enforcement officers recognize their own resilience so that they can in turn see the resilience of the populations they serve. Resilience classes (Vasquez, 2001) and insight meditation (Lozoff, 2000) are becoming more commonplace in juvenile halls and prisons for *both* caregivers and inmates—with transformational results (Donnenfield, 2000; Menahemi & Ariel, 1997). The National Resilience Resource Center at the University of Minnesota is using this health-of-the-helper model of change in schools and communities around the country (Marshall, 1998). Meditation and mindfulness programs are also often critical components of programs focused on reducing the stress of caregivers and even young people themselves so that they can see the health in themselves and others (Kabat-Zinn, 1995).

Caregivers who learn about and model their own resilience are also able to directly teach young people about their own resilient nature. According to Barrera and Prelow (2000), "An important direction for future research would be to investigate how support provision affects the well-being of the support provider (e.g., mentor). . . . The well-known helper-therapy principle would suggest that the benefits for the support providers are at least as great as the benefits for the support recipients" (p. 333). Instead of burning out or developing a strong case of compassion fatigue, this research may just find that having a resilient attitude— a belief in one's own innate capacity as well as in the capacities of one's children, students, or clients—is a protective factor supporting caregiver self-efficacy, optimism, and hope—and, in turn, young people's resilience strengths.

The Challenges for Public Health Professionals

The challenge to the research community is to focus more time and resources on the study of resilience in communities and individuals. "Our choices about what to research and how to go about it are conditioned by where we hope to go in the broadest sense. Our ideas about values, aesthetics, politics, and normal behavior and preferences are integral to educational [and public health] research, its interpretation, and its utilization. Science and research cannot determine or validate these values, visions, and ideas. Science and research can only be used to help us develop effective methods for working toward our values, visions, and ideas" (Shannon, 1995, p. 127).

The challenge to practitioners and caregivers is to get in touch with their own innate resilience, to understand it so that they can model it and recognize it in the communities and people they serve. The "power of one" is clearly a major finding of four decades of resilience research, validating the influence each of us has in every interaction with people both young and old, to nurture or block—their innate resilience.

Yet as important as our individual relationships with people are, they are not enough, especially in the face of the barriers to change within the bureaucracies of the human services and public health. So a third challenge is to our human-serving systems and bureaucracies. In *Common Purpose* (1997), Lisbeth Schorr analyzes why half of the successful programs for children and families that she had reported on in her previous book, *Within Our Reach* (1988), were defunct five years later and none had been expanded or replicated. She concluded that "when effective programs aiming to reach large numbers encounter the pressures exercised by prevailing attitudes and systems, the resulting collision is almost always lethal to the effective programs. Their demise can be prevented only by changing systems and public perceptions to make them more hospitable to effective efforts to change lives and communities" (1997, p. 20).

What Schorr is ultimately advocating is the importance of trusting local knowledge and capacity and building resilient communities. The final challenge requires the attention of everyone, not only public health professionals. Farsighted economists and political scientists view the rebuilding of our communities as the key to our future survival as a nation, world, and even species. In his seminal book, *The End of Work* (1995), Jeremy Rifkin writes that as we entered the twenty-first century, the world was in the throes of the third Industrial Revolution, a revolution transforming our industrial age into a "postmarket economy," a "new phase in world history," and "one in which fewer and fewer workers will be needed to produce the goods and services for the global population." Rifkin concludes that "only by building strong, self-sustaining local communities will people in every country be able to withstand the forces of technological displacement and market globalization that are threatening livelihoods and survival of much of the human family" (p. xvi).

Similarly, John Gardner writes prophetically in his classic essay *Building Community* (1991) that "without the continuity of the shared values that community provides, freedom cannot survive. . . . [Only] strong and resilient communities can stand between the individual and any government that tries to impose dictatorial solutions from the right or left. Undifferentiated masses never have and never will preserve freedom against usurping power" (p. 5).

Just as the resilience paradigm focuses on the "glass half full" versus the risk paradigm of the "glass half empty," Gardner states that it is the generative rather than the disintegrative functions "that deserve our closest attention": "The regenerative powers of human society have not weakened. The capacity of humankind to create and re-create social coherence is always there—enduring and irrepressible" (1991, p. 9). As noted many times in this chapter, one of the major assumptions of resilience theory is that human systems are innately resilient. At the individual level, this means we are genetically wired with the capacities for social competence and caring, problem solving and change, autonomy and identity, and hope and meaning. At the community level, this translates into communities also having this inherent transformative capacity to adapt and change.

"Passive allegiance isn't enough today. The forces of disintegration have gained steadily and will prevail unless individuals see themselves as having a positive duty to nurture their community and continuously reweave the social fabric" (Gardner, 1991, p. 11). What has become apparent is that just as the degenerative forces at work today have grown, so has the importance of the intentional work done by public health practitioners in building or emerging community. What is at stake is not only the support provided to those in need but the ability of all of us and our communities to grow and thrive.

References

Barrera, M., & Prelow, H. (2000). Interventions to promote social support in children and adolescents. In D. Cicchetti, J. Rappaport, I. Sandler, & R. P. Weissberg (Eds.), *The promotion of wellness in children and adolescents* (pp. 309–339). Washington, DC: Child Welfare League of America Press.

Baumeister, R., & Leary, M. (1995). The need to belong: Desire for interpersonal attach-
  ments as a fundamental human motivation. *Psychological Bulletin, 117,* 497–529.
Beardslee, W., & Podoresfky, D. (1988). Resilient adolescents whose parents have serious
  affective and other psychiatric disorders: The importance of self-understanding and relationships. *American Journal of Psychiatry, 145,* 63–69.
Benard, B. (1991). *Fostering resiliency in kids: Protective factors in the family, school, and community.*
  Portland, OR: Northwest Regional Educational Laboratory.
Benard, B. (2004). *Resiliency: What we have learned.* San Francisco: WestEd.
California Wellness Foundation. (1999, Summer). Youth lead the way to healthier communi-
  ties. *TCWF Newsletter,* p. 1. This is available in hard copy by calling The California Well-
  ness Foundation at (818) 702-1900.
Carnegie Task Force on Youth Development and Community Programs. (1992). *A matter of
  time: Risk and opportunity in the nonschool hours.* New York: Carnegie Corp.
Chess, S. (1989). Defying the voice of doom. In T. F. Dugan & R. Coles (Eds.), *The child in our
  time: Studies in the development of resiliency* (pp. 179–199). New York: Bruner/Mazel.
Clausen, J. A. (1993). *American lives: Looking back at the children of the Great Depression.* New York:
  Free Press.
Coleman, J. (1987). Families and schools. *Educational Researcher, 16*(6), 32–38.
Curnan, S., & Hughes, D. (2002). Towards shared prosperity: Change-making in the CYD
  movement. *CYD Journal, 3,* 25–33.
Currie, E. (1993). *Reckoning: Drugs, the cities, and the American future.* New York: Hill & Wang.
Cutler, I., & Edwards, S. (2002). Linking youth and community development: Ideas from the
  Community Youth Development Initiative. *CYD Journal, 3,* 17–23.
Deci, E. L. (with R. Flaste). (1995). *Why we do what we do: Understanding self-motivation.* New
  York: Putnam.
Donnenfield, D. (2000). *Changing from the inside* [Video]. San Francisco: David Donnenfield
  Productions.
Eccles, J. S., & Gootman, J. A. (Eds.). (2002). *Community programs to promote youth development.*
  Washington, DC: National Academy Press.
Fanshel, D. (1975). Status changes of children in foster care: Final results of the Columbia
  University Longitudinal Study. *Child Welfare, 555,* 143–177.
Festinger, T. (1984). *No one ever asked us: A postscript to the foster care system.* New York: Columbia
  University Press.
Furstenberg, F. F., Jr., Cook, T. D., Eccles, J., Elder, G. H., Jr., & Sameroff, A. (1999). *Manag-
  ing to make it: Urban families and adolescent success.* Chicago: University of Chicago Press.
Gardner, J. (1991, September). *Building community.* Paper prepared for the Leadership Studies
  Program. Washington, DC: INDEPENDENT SECTOR.
Garmezy, N. (1991). Resiliency and vulnerability to adverse developmental outcomes associ-
  ated with poverty. *American Behavioral Scientist, 34,* 416–430.
Guendelman, S., & Abrams, B. (1995). Dietary intake among Mexican-American women:
  Generational differences and a comparison with white non-Hispanic women. *American
  Journal of Public Health, 85,* 20–25.
Guendelman, S., Buekens, P., Blondel, B., Kaminski, M., Notzon, F. C., & Masuy-Stroobant,
  G. (1999). Birth outcomes of immigrant women in the United States, France, and Bel-
  gium. *Maternal and Child Health Journal, 3,* 177–187.
Guendelman, S., Thornton, D., Gould, J., & Hosang, N. (2005). Social disparities in mater-
  nal morbidity during labor and delivery between Mexican-born and U.S.-born white
  Californians, 1996–1998. *American Journal of Public Health, 95,* 2218–2224.

Higgins, G. O. (1994). *Resilient adults: Overcoming a cruel past.* San Francisco: Jossey-Bass.

Hyman, J. (1999). *Spheres of influence: A strategic synthesis and framework for community youth development.* Baltimore: Annie E. Casey Foundation.

Innovation Center for Community and Youth Development. (2002). *Mission and goals.* Madison: University of Wisconsin.

Jessor, R. (1993). Successful adolescent development among youth in high-risk settings. *American Psychologist, 48,* 117–126.

Kabat-Zinn, J. (1995). *Wherever you go, there you are: Mindfulness meditation in everyday life.* New York: Hyperion.

Kohn, A. (1997, Summer). The limits of teaching skills. *Reaching Today's Youth,* pp. 14–16.

Kreft, I., & Brown, J. (Eds.). (1998). The zero effects of drug prevention programs: Issues and solutions. *Evaluation Review, 22*(Special issue).

Kretzmann, J. P., & McKnight, J. L. (1993). *Building communities from the inside out: A path toward finding and mobilizing a community's assets.* Evanston, IL: Northwestern University, Center for Urban Affairs and Policy Research.

Kretzmann, J. P., & Schmitz, P. H. (1999). It takes a child to raise a whole village. *Resiliency in Action, 4*(2), 1–4.

Lifton, R. J. (1993). *The protean self: Human resilience in an age of fragmentation.* New York: Basic Books.

Long, J. V., & Vaillant, G. E. (1989). Escape from the underclass. In T. F. Dugan & R. Coles (Eds.), *The child in our time: Studies in the development of resiliency* (pp. 200–213). New York: Brunner/Mazel.

Lozoff, B. (2000). *It's a Meaningful Life—It Just Takes Practice.* New York: Viking.

Luthar, S. S. (Ed.). (2003). *Resilience and vulnerability: Adaptation in the context of childhood adversities.* New York: Cambridge University Press.

Males, M. (1996). *The scapegoat generation: America's war on adolescence.* Monroe, ME: Common Courage Press.

Marielena, L., Gamboa, C., Kahramanian, M. I., Morales, L. S., & Bautista, D. E. (2005). Acculturation and Latino health in the United States: A review of the literature and its sociopolitical context. *Annual Review of Public Health, 26,* 367–397. Retrieved July 25, 2006, from http://www.rand.org/pubs/reprints/RP1177

Marshall, K. (1998). Reculturing systems with resilience/health realization. *Promoting positive and healthy behaviors in children: Fourteenth annual Rosalynn Carter Symposium on Mental Health Policy* (pp. 48–58). Atlanta: The Carter Center.

Maslow, A. (1954). *Motivation and personality.* New York: HarperCollins.

Masten, A. (2001). Ordinary magic: Resilience processes in development. *American Psychologist, 56,* 227–238.

Masten, A., & Reed, M. (2002). Resilience in development. In C. R. Snyder and S. J. Lopez (Eds.), *Handbook of positive psychology* (pp. 74–88). New York: Oxford University Press.

McKnight, J. L. (1992, Winter). Mapping community capacity. *New Designs for Youth Development,* pp. 9–15.

McLaughlin, M. W. (2000). *Community counts.* New York: Public Education Network.

McLaughlin, M. W., Irby, M. A., & Langman, J. (1994). *Urban sanctuaries: Neighborhood organizations in the lives and futures of inner-city youth.* San Francisco: Jossey-Bass.

Menahemi, A., & Ariel, E. (Dirs.). (1997). *Doing time, doing Vipassana* [Video]. Tel Aviv, Israel: Karuna Films.

Mills, R. (1993). *The Health Realization model: A community empowerment primer.* Alhambra: California School of Professional Psychology.

Mills, R., & Spittle, E. (2001). *Wisdom within.* Auburn, WA: Lone Pine Publishing.

Mrazek, P., & Haggerty, R. (Eds.). (1994). *Reducing risks for mental disorders: Frontiers for preventive intervention research.* Washington, DC: National Academy Press.

National 4-H Council. (2002). *The national conversation on youth development in the 21st century: Final report.* Chevy Chase, MD: National 4-H Council.

National Charrette Institute. (2002). *Healthy communities.* Retrieved October 4, 2002, from http://www.charretteinstitute.org/healthy.html

National Institutes of Health, National Institute of Child Health and Human Development. (2003). Demographic and Behavioral Sciences Branch, NICHD: Report to the NACHHD Council, 2003. Retrieved October 10, 2006, from http://www.nichd.nih.gov/publications/pubs/ upload/council_dbsb_2003.pdf

Owens, J. (2002, February 20). Breaking new ground: Two neighborhood studies on crime, children aim to change policy, improve lives. *Chicago Tribune,* p. 5.

Peterson, C., & Seligman, M.E.P. (2004). *Character strengths and virtues: A handbook and classification.* New York: Oxford University Press.

Putnam, R. D. (2000). *Bowling alone: The collapse and revival of American community.* New York: Simon & Schuster.

Putnam, R. D., & Feldstein, L. M. (2003). *Better together: Restoring the American community.* New York: Simon & Schuster.

Rifkin, J. (1995). *The end of work: The decline of the global labor force and the dawn of the post-market era.* New York: Tarcher.

Rutter, M. (1989). Pathways from childhood to adult life. *Journal Child Psychology and Psychiatry, 30,* 23–51.

Rutter, M. (2000). Resilience reconsidered: Conceptual considerations, empirical findings, and policy implications. In J. P. Shonkoff & S. J. Meisels (Eds.), *Handbook of early childhood intervention* (pp. 651–682). New York: Cambridge University Press.

Sameroff, A., Barocas, R., & Seifer, R. (1984). The early development of children born to mentally ill women. In N. F. Watt, E. J. Anthony, L. C. Wynne, & J. E. Rolf (Eds.), *Children at risk for schizophrenia: A longitudinal perspective* (pp. 482–514). New York: Cambridge University Press.

Sampson, R. J., Raudenbush, S. W., & Earls, F. (1997). Neighborhoods and violent crime: A multilevel study of collective efficacy. *Science, 277,* 918–924.

Schorr, L. B. (with D. Schorr). (1988). *Within our reach: Breaking the cycle of disadvantage.* New York: Doubleday.

Schorr, L. B. (1997). *Common purpose: Strengthening families and neighborhoods to rebuild America.* New York: Anchor Books.

Schweinhart, L. J., Barnes, H. V., & Wiekart, D. P. (1993). *Significant benefits: The High/Scope Perry Preschool Study through age 27.* Ypsilanti, MI: High/Scope Press.

Seligman, M.E.P. (2002). Positive psychology, positive prevention, and positive therapy. In C. R. Snyder & S. J. Lopez (Eds.), *Handbook of positive psychology* (pp. 3–9). New York: Oxford University Press.

Shannon, P. (1995). *Text, lies, and videotape: Stories about life, liberty, and learning.* Portsmouth, NH: Heinemann.

Swadener, B. B., & Lubeck, S. (Eds.). (1995). *Children and families "at promise": Deconstructing the discourse of risk.* Albany: State University of New York Press.

Vaillant, G. E. (2002). *Aging well: Surprising guideposts to a happier life from the landmark Harvard Study of Adult Development.* Boston: Little, Brown.

Vasquez, G. (2000). Resiliency: Juvenile offenders recognize their strengths to change their lives. *Corrections Today, 62,* 106–110, 125.

Vigil, J. D. (1990). Cholos and gangs: Culture change and street youth in Los Angeles. In R. Huff (Ed.), *Gangs in America: Diffusion, diversity, and public policy* (pp. 146–162). Thousand Oaks, CA: Sage.

Walsh, J. (1997). *Stories of renewal: Community building and the future of urban America.* New York: Rockefeller Foundation.

Watt, N. F., Anthony, E. J., Wynne, L. C., & Rolf, J. E. (Eds.). (1984). *Children at risk for schizophrenia: A longitudinal perspective.* New York: Cambridge University Press.

Werner, E. E. (1986). Resilient offspring of alcoholics: A longitudinal study from birth to age 18. *Journal of Studies on Alcohol, 14,* 34–40.

Werner, E. E., & Smith, R. S. (1982). *Vulnerable but invincible: A longitudinal study of resilient children and youth.* New York: Adams, Bannister, & Cox.

Werner, E. E., & Smith, R. S. (1992). *Overcoming the odds: High-risk children from birth to adulthood.* Ithaca, NY: Cornell University Press.

Werner, E. E., & Smith, R. S. (2001). *Journeys from childhood to the midlife: Risk, resilience, and recovery.* Ithaca, NY: Cornell University Press.

White, J. A., & Wehlage, G. G. (1995). Community collaboration: If it is such a good idea, why is it so hard to do? *Educational Evaluation and Policy Analysis, 17,* 23–28.

Wilkes, G. (2002). Abused child to nonabusive parent: Resilience and conceptual change. *Journal of Clinical Psychology, 58,* 261–278.

Wilson, W. J. (1987). *The truly disadvantaged: The inner city, the underclass, and public policy.* Chicago: University of Chicago Press.

Zigler, E., & Hall, N. W. (1989). Physical child abuse in America: Past, present, and future. In D. Cicchetti & V. Carlson (Eds.), *Child maltreatment: Theory and research on the causes and consequences of child abuse and neglect* (pp. 38–75). New York: Cambridge University Press.

PART TWO

KEY ELEMENTS OF EFFECTIVE PREVENTION EFFORTS

Part Two provides in-depth descriptions of strategies and methods for current and future practitioners of primary prevention. Each of its six chapters covers a skill set that, when effectively put to use, helps primary prevention efforts succeed.

People coming together and insisting on their community well-being is as important a factor in achieving it as any scientific or technical capacity. Health is no different; there is a rich history of community organizing for primary prevention, of people gathering to develop effective strategies that prevent a range of health and social issues, such as widespread youth violence, epidemic acute and chronic illnesses, and the ever-expanding gap between the powerful and the powerless that underlies so much illness and injury. In Chapter Five, "Community Organizing for Health and Social Justice," authors Vivian Chávez, Meredith Minkler, Nina Wallerstein, and Michael Spencer examine community organizing in local settings and its effect in building people's capacity and relationships and creating action for community change. They offer a historical context and a perspective on women's organizing and youth activism, and they emphasize the notion of "cultural humility," which advocates nonpaternalistic partnerships with self-reflection. The "wheel of community organizing"—a set of principles to create, put into practice, and evaluate prevention initiatives—and a list of essential qualities for organizing are provided as practical frameworks.

The term *framing* relates to how an approach is communicated in order to elicit the most supportive response. A key component of primary prevention is reaching decision makers and the public with a message that resonates with their own values. Lori Dorfman, Lawrence Wallack, and Katie Woodruff, the authors of Chapter Six, "More Than a Message: Framing Public Health Advocacy to Change Corporate Practices," describe how prevention advocates must use their messaging to articulate values and a social justice framework that resonates with decision makers as it motivates activists and consumers. They discuss the ways in which primary prevention supporters can challenge a culture of individual responsibility and market justice. Although the focus is on advocacy efforts aimed at changing harmful corporate practices, the insights apply to any primary prevention effort.

There are numerous examples of collaborations achieving significant primary prevention outcomes that would not have been possible by one group alone. In fact, the formation of a coalition often marks the beginning of significant prevention efforts. At the same time, not everyone knows how to collaborate effectively; collaboration is a skill that should not be taken for granted.

Chapter Seven, "Working Collaboratively to Advance Prevention," by Larry Cohen and Ashby Wolfe, focuses on coalitions, which are one particular form of collaboration. The authors detail the steps necessary to ensure that coalitions are diverse and effective and that they add to, rather than risk detracting from, quality prevention efforts. A sidebar describes how to address common coalition turf struggles, noting that turf issues are a natural element of many partnerships and should be dealt with up front rather than ignored or feared. The information presented is applicable to both leaders and participants in all types of coalitions, whether newly initiated or already existing.

Public policy development is an important tool for primary prevention because policy shapes the environment in which we live, work, and play. Makani Themba-Nixon, the author of Chapter Eight, "Making Change: The Power of Local Communities to Foster Policy," describes basic elements for developing policy initiatives and offers specific advice to overcome common challenges. The chapter focuses in particular on local policy development for historically disfranchised communities. Local policy development is ideal for primary prevention efforts because so many community efforts are organized locally, and it provides realistic and achievable means to address large-scale community health issues. In addition, decisions made at the local level are easier to monitor and evaluate and often act as a catalyst for statewide and national change.

Media are more than educational or public relations tools. Media advocacy provides the voice prevention advocates need to reach key decision makers and alter public opinion. Without effective approaches to media, primary prevention efforts will continually fall short of their potential. In Chapter Nine, "Using Media

Advocacy to Influence Policy," Lori Dorfman describes the basic elements of developing a strategic plan for media advocacy, noting that it is much more than a method for information dissemination. It is also a process of developing media literacy, effective messaging, and political and cultural savvy. From efforts seeking to eliminate tobacco advertising to those restricting the sale of handguns, media advocacy is a natural complement to community-organizing and coalition-building efforts aimed at primary prevention.

A common yet unfounded criticism of primary prevention efforts is that they cannot be evaluated. The argument is based on a belief that primary prevention efforts are too diffuse and aren't applied to sufficiently discrete populations. Dan Perales, author of Chapter Ten, "Primary Prevention and Program Evaluation," dispels this notion, providing examples of primary prevention evaluation. Yet evaluation of primary prevention does have unique challenges. Prevention efforts are aimed at large populations, involve collaborations, and are by definition long-term processes, so having a clear strategy and the ability to see if it is being effectively followed is very important. Evaluators of primary prevention must have the tools as well as the theoretical understanding of how preventive evaluations differ from traditional models. The author describes some of the most useful tools and principles, including community-based participatory research, as part of his emphasis that a respectful evaluation process is as important as achieving results.

CHAPTER FIVE

COMMUNITY ORGANIZING FOR HEALTH AND SOCIAL JUSTICE

Vivian Chávez, Meredith Minkler,
Nina Wallerstein, Michael S. Spencer

C ommunity organizing—these two words, woven together, evoke vivid images and provoke an emotional response. The concept of community organizing is neither neutral nor easy to define. The term carries a deep history intricately tied to oppression, struggle, and resistance. The words *community* and *organizing* are contextualized with stories from people, places, and events that make up the diverse face of the United States. Community organizing includes persons of color demanding civil rights and claiming their equality through nonviolent marches, boycotts, and sit-ins. Community organizing is workers creating unions and making agreements about their humanity and their labor. It is women speaking painful truths about their private lives so that violence is made into a public issue. Community organizing is about gay, lesbian, bisexual, and transgender people lifting the veil of secrecy and stigma around sexual identity and sexual health. It's young people marching and participating in protests, mobilizing to get tobacco ads targeting youth of color removed from their communities and in other ways being civically engaged in efforts to promote change in spite of not being old enough to vote.

The label "community organizing" has been attached to a variety of activities drawing on disparate traditions and historical periods. Community organizing is

Portions of this chapter are adapted from M. Minkler and N. Wallerstein, "Improving Health Through Community Organization and Community Building: A Health Education Perspective," in M. Minkler (Ed.), *Community Organizing and Community Building for Health*, © 2004 by M. Minkler.

about primary prevention—people coming together to effectively ward off a range of health and social problems, including youth violence, chronic illness, skyrocketing medical costs, and the ever-expanding gap between rich and poor. Of course, community organizing can also be used to promote agendas that are not conducive to good health, as in the case of anti-immigrant organizing or denial of civil rights on the basis of sexual orientation or efforts to limit women's reproductive rights.

However, this chapter intentionally focuses on the positive, examining community organizing that occurs in local settings, to empower individuals, build relationships, and create action for community change (Beckwith, 1997; Bobo, Kendall, & Max, 1991; Kahn, 1991; Minkler, 2004; Stall & Stoecker, 1998).

We limit our analysis primarily to the United States while recognizing that community organizing methods are used internationally to address health disparities, hunger, and poverty. We describe community organizing as a major primary prevention strategy linked to personal and community well-being. As the Canadian health promotion leader Ronald Labonte (1994) reminds us, we are careful not to "romanticize" community.

After providing background on definitions and terminology, the chapter offers a brief historical summary, a perspective on women's organizing and youth activism, and an overview of the notion of "cultural humility." The "wheel of community organizing" is then explored as a conceptual framework and practical guide to the application of prevention methodologies. The chapter concludes with a list of essential qualities for organizing and a critique of empowerment as a key concept for future directions in the field.

Definitions and Terminology

"Definitions," observes bell hooks (2000), "are vital starting points for the imagination. A good definition marks our starting point and lets us know where we want to end up. As we move toward our desired destination we chart the journey, creating a map" (p. 14).

Community

Often we think of community in terms of homogeneous groups—people like ourselves, of similar background, from the same class, religion, race, ethnicity, and language. We define community, beyond exclusivity, as a group of people who have identified common interests and act together to achieve them. A community's ability to act together may have existed for centuries or may be triggered in a very short time by an urgent problem. The World Health Organization defines community as a group of people, often living in a defined geographical area, who share a common culture, values, and norms (1998, p. 5). While typically thought of in geographical terms, communities may also be identified with no particular locality and based instead on shared interests or characteristics, such as race or ethnicity, language, sexual orientation, age, or occupation (Fellin, 2001). Members of a community gain their personal and social identity by sharing common beliefs. They exhibit awareness of their identity as a group and share common needs and a commitment to meeting them. Communities sustain life and ensure human survival. Although each person is a unique individual, people need others not merely for sustenance or company but also to add meaning to their lives (Peck, 1987). A community is "a group that has learned to transcend its individual differences" (p. 62). Contrary to the myth of rugged individualism, community recognizes and strives for interdependence. As Bellah and his associates (1985) noted, the tension between individualism and community is central to understanding social tensions in the United States. People need to be recognized as individuals as much as they need to unite with others for collective well-being.

Community Organizing

Community organizing is defined here as a dynamic process that encompasses a wide range of community engagement strategies. In its best practice, it is a long-term approach that includes people defining their community, identifying common problems or goals they wish to address, defining the solutions they wish to pursue and the methods they will use to mobilize resources, and implementing strategies for reaching the goals they have collectively set (Minkler & Wallerstein, 2004). Community organizing is a craft that requires building an enduring network of people, who identify with common ideals and who can engage in social action (Stall & Stoecker, 1998). A critical dimension of community organizing is a power analysis of social change rooted in political economy and concerned with dynamics of oppression and privilege. Such an analysis carefully considers the role of factors such as race, class, gender, and sexual orientation that help determine how health and social problems are defined, treated or ignored (Minkler & Wallerstein, 2004).

Community organizing involves advocacy and organized activism in direct favor of or opposition to an issue. The term includes the notions of community building and asset-based approaches (Kretzmann & McKnight, 1993; McKnight, 1995) that focus on solutions and resilience as opposed to a strict negative focus on problems. Community building is concerned as much with interpersonal relationships as it is with the identification, nurturing, and celebration of community strengths (Walters, 2004) and the integration of personal experience (hooks, 1984).

Although the terms *organizer, activist,* and *advocate* are often used loosely and interchangeably, some experts in the field differentiate in the following ways: *Advocates* tend to be professionals working on behalf of or for a community that may not be able to represent themselves (Stoecker, 2001). *Activist,* a term people are either proud of or shy away from, tends to imply militancy, protest, and social movement (Prokosch & Raymond, 2002). *Community organizer* tends to describe a range of experiences, from someone working behind the scenes to support the community voice to a campaign or program manager, coordinator, or prevention planner.

Civic Engagement

Ehrlich (2000) defines civic engagement as working to make a difference in the civic life of the community and developing the combination of knowledge, skills, values, and motivation to make that difference, that is, promoting the quality of life in a community through both political and nonpolitical processes. With examples from college campuses, churches, and neighborhood associations, Ehrlich (2000) notes that a "civically responsible individual recognizes himself or herself as a member of a larger social fabric and therefore considers social problems to be at least partly his or her own; such an individual is willing to see the moral and civic dimensions of issues, to make and justify informed moral and civic judgments, and to take action when appropriate" (p. xxvi). Civic engagement encompasses a large range of activities such as working in a soup kitchen, writing a letter to an elected official, and voting (Putnam, 1996). However, a criticism of the language of civic engagement is that it is increasingly being used to promote individual volunteerism as a means of helping shore up the safety net sagging under the weight of government cutbacks in health and human services (Martinson & Minkler, 2006). Therefore, from a primary prevention context, we prefer the term *community organizing,* as it includes fighting the politics of retrenchment that makes people dependent on charity in the first place (Martinson & Minkler, 2006). We argue that a civically responsible individual must recognize himself or herself as a member of a larger social fabric and therefore consider social problems to be at least partly his or her own. Such an individual is willing to see the moral and civic dimensions of issues, to make and justify informed moral and civic judgments, and to take action when appropriate.

Historical Context

The expression *community organizing* was first used by American social workers in the late 1800s to describe their efforts to coordinate health and social services for European immigrants and the poor through the settlement house movement

(Minkler & Wallerstein, 2004). Garvin and Cox (2001) point out, though, that while community organizing is often described as having begun with the settlement house movement, several important milestones outside of social work must be included. For example, the post-Reconstruction period organizing by African Americans fighting white supremacy and Jim Crow segregation laws in the last two decades of the nineteenth century; the Populist movement that started in the late nineteenth century among farmers and became a multisectoral coalition and a national political force; and direct social action organizing from the labor movement that taught the importance of forming coalitions around issues and the use of conflict as a means of bringing about change.

Direct social action organizing was pioneered in Chicago's old stockyards neighborhood by Saul Alinsky in the late 1930s. A criminologist by training, Alinsky is often credited with leading strikes that led to better health and work conditions for all factory workers. Direct social action organizing emphasizes redressing power imbalances, building communitywide identification, and helping members devise winnable goals and nonviolent conflict strategies as means to bring about change. Although the Alinsky tradition was historically dominated by white male organizers, many of whom eschewed critical analyses of race and gender, the community organizing model was adapted throughout the 1960s and 1970s in communities of color (Pintado-Vertner, 2004).

Fisher and Romanofsky (1981) divide community organizing into four historical periods (see Table 5.1): organizing European immigrants through settlement houses, national-level organizing, direct social action, and local organizing. The sociologist Aldon Morris (1984) notes that the tactics of direct social action organizing were refined by the civil rights movement in the South through the

TABLE 5.1. FOUR HISTORICAL PERIODS IN COMMUNITY ORGANIZING.

Period	Activities
1890–1920	Organizing European immigrant neighborhoods. Building community through settlement houses, service delivery, and social work.
1920–1940	Organizing on a national scale, especially during the Great Depression, because the nation's economic problems did not seem solvable at the community level.
1940–1960	Direct social action organizing. Federal involvement in reshaping communities through post–World War II urban renewal programs and the War on Poverty.
1960–1980	Local organizing. Thoughtful responses among activists and theorists in the early 1970s informing broader social change objectives through the civil rights, women's health, gay rights, antiwar, student, and disability rights movements.

Source: Adapted from Fisher and Romanofsky (1981).

mobilization of networks of local black churches, NAACP chapters, and black colleges. The legacy of social action traveled to California, where César Chávez and Dolores Huerta combined Saul Alinsky's and Mahatma Gandhi's strategies with their profound commitment to agricultural workers to develop a network of organizations and founded the United Farm Workers union (Ferris & Sandoval, 1997). Communities of color found community organizing to be an especially powerful strategy for challenging racial oppression (Sen, 2003). As noted by Gary Delgado (1987), cofounder of Center for Third World Organizing, organizers in communities of color brought a new level of analytical sophistication, emphasizing issues of race, class, and gender and developing indigenous leadership.

In the health field, a historical example of community organizing was the work of the Medical Committee for Human Rights in the Mississippi Delta in the 1960s when Jack Geiger and others linked health to the consequences of racism and poverty.

Dr. Jack Geiger

℞: *So Much Milk, So Much Meat, So Many Vegetables, So Many Eggs*
—H. JACK GEIGER, "THE UNSTEADY MARCH," p. 9

"We always need colleagues in other disciplines. Doctors aren't very good as community organizers. We are trained in hierarchical systems, and it's hard for us to get over that. We don't have the same skills that are necessary for activism, so we need to find ways to work with community organizers, health educators, nurses, clinical psychologists, social workers, labor leaders and others who have the skills to supplement the skills that we have—with lawyers, with other forms of human rights activists" (Geiger, 2005, p. 8).

In 1965, H. Jack Geiger, physician and civil rights activist, opened one of the first two community health centers in the United States in Mound Bayou, Mississippi (Geiger Gibson Program, n.d.). The invention of the double-row cotton-picking machine had recently replaced the need for an entire population of sharecroppers, causing massive unemployment and exacerbating poverty (Caplan & Rodberg, 1994). Geiger's community health work has left a distinct imprint on the world of public health, changing acceptable methodologies for achieving health and eliminating health disparities by addressing poverty and racism directly.

To assess the needs of the community, the Mississippi health center began by holding a series of meetings in homes, churches, and schools. As a result of these meetings, residents created ten community health associations, each with its own perspective and priorities. Some communities needed clean drinking water without having to walk 3 miles; others needed child care or elder care. Community participation played a central role in broadening traditional conceptions of health. In the beginning, the health center saw an enormous amount of malnutrition, stunted growth, and infection among infants and young children. Geiger and his colleagues linked hunger, a health issue, to acute poverty and linked poverty to the massive unemployment that had turned an entire population into squatters.

Instead of just treating individual cases, Geiger and his colleagues addressed the problem of malnutrition, first by writing prescriptions for food. Health center workers recruited local black-owned grocery stores to fill the prescriptions and reimbursed the stores out of the health center's pharmacy budget. "Once we had the health center going, we started stocking food in the center pharmacy and distributing food—like drugs—to the people. A variety of officials got very nervous and said, 'You can't do that.' We said, 'Why not?' They said, 'It's a health center pharmacy, and it's supposed to carry drugs for the treatment of disease.' And we said, 'The last time we looked in the book, the specific therapy for malnutrition was food'" (Geiger, 2005, p. 7).

The health center then sought to prevent hunger and began urging people to start vegetable gardens. The health center used a grant from a foundation to lease 600 acres of land to start the North Bolivar County Cooperative Farm. By pooling their labor to grow vegetables instead of cotton, members of a thousand families owned a share in the crops. In the first two years, scores of tons of vegetables were grown. Health center workers also repaired housing, dug protected wells and sanitary privies (Geiger, 2005, pp. 7–8), and later even started a bookstore focused on black history and culture.

By addressing the roots of illness drawn from community concerns, these health centers pioneered an effective methodology for approaching health care in underserved communities. They explored environmental conditions such as housing, food, income, education, employment, and exposure to environmental dangers and linked them to health outcomes. Then, in an effort to prevent poor health outcomes, they moved upstream to change the conditions that led to those outcomes.

"You can do more than bail out these medical disasters after they have occurred, and go upstream from medical care to forge instruments of social change that will prevent such disasters from occurring in the first place. One of those disasters is the combination of racism and poverty," said Geiger (2005, p. 4) some forty years later, speaking to a graduating class of medical students.

Today there are almost a thousand community health centers in the United States, making health care accessible for more than 11.5 million patients each year (Fairchild, 2005).

Source: Prevention Institute.

Another health-related illustration of community organizing efforts was the World Health Organization's adoption of a new approach to health promotion that stressed increasing people's control over the determinants of their health (WHO, 1986). The WHO-initiated Healthy Cities/Healthy Communities movement grew to involve thousands of localities worldwide. It aims to create sustainable environments and processes in which the governmental and nongovernmental sectors work in partnership to create healthy public policies, achieve high-level participation in community-driven projects, and ultimately reduce health disparities (Norris & Pittman, 2000). More recently, as Makani Themba-Nixon notes in Chapter Eight, prevention specialists and health advocates have organized against the alcohol and tobacco industries' irresponsible advertising and marketing to young people and communities of color.

In the past twenty years, the Internet has enhanced communication for community organizing efforts around the world (Hick & McNutt, 2002; Van de Donk, Loader, Nixon, & Rucht, 2004). Groups across the political spectrum go online to build community and to identify and organize supporters on a mass scale (Herbert, 2005). Prevention specialists, community organizers, and other advocates today must actively rely on their computers and other forms of media to research, learn skills, plan, solve problems, and connect with others (Fawcett, Schultz, Carson, Renault, & Francisco, 2003). Although community organizing continues to be based heavily on direct interaction among physically present people, direct interaction is complemented by media (billboards, newsletters, newspapers, television, and radio) and other communications technologies (computers, cell phones). (For specific information on community organizing through the media, see Chapter Nine.)

Women's Health and Organizing

The women's health movement of the 1960s and 1970s in the United States was a grassroots movement that challenged medical authority in many aspects of women's health, health access, and health care delivery. Community organizing methods were used to transform women's health knowledge, health politics, and the health care service systems. Women's health organizing was based on interactive reflection linking health status, personal experience, and political processes (Evans, 1980). This type of organizing came out of the consciousness-raising education genre with the explicit political agenda of reducing women's isolation, building community empowerment, and shifting the site of knowledge creation (Naples, 2002). Through community building, organizing, and education, the women's health movement has addressed many issues, including abortion, battering, rape, and contraception. Movement participants developed self-help manuals such as *Our Bodies, Ourselves* (Boston Women's Health Book Collective, 1973, 2005) and founded birth centers run by midwives.

Women of color and working-class women have created and sustained numerous protest efforts and organizations to alter living conditions or policies that threaten their families and communities (Gutierrez & Lewis, 1992; Naples, 2002; Stall & Stoecker, 1998). Stall and Stoecker (1998) examine two strains of community organizing, distinguished by philosophy and often by gender and influenced by the historical division of American society into public and private spheres. They compare the well-known Alinsky model, which focuses on communities organizing for power, with what they call the women-centered model, which focuses on organizing relationships to build community. The women-centered model cannot be attributed to a single person or movement. Although it has a long history, it has received attention from feminist researchers and organizers only in the past two decades (Barnett, 1993; Gutierrez & Lewis, 1992, Stall & Stoeker, 1998). The model can be traced back to African American women's efforts to sustain home and community under slavery (Davis, 1981) and to the women's health movement (Evans, 1980). In women-centered organizing, power is gained by bringing people together to resolve disputes and build relationships within their own community. The goal of women-centered organizing is empowerment through changes in women's health, reproductive rights, body awareness, sexual and domestic violence prevention, legislation, and knowledge of their own bodies as well as change of norms in relationships, sexuality, work, and family (Evans, 1980).

Youth Organizing

"Since time immemorial, young people have often been on the front lines of social movements, bravely questioning what others merely accepted, and energetically demanding—if not always winning—justice, equality and freedom" (Mohamed & Wheeler, 2001, p. 11).

Youth organizing is an innovative developmental and social justice strategy that trains young people in community organizing and assists them in employing these skills to alter power relations and create meaningful institutional change in their communities (Pintado-Vertner, 2004). Young people are and have long been innovative members of society who can create community change (Checkoway et al., 2003). Despite generally being politically disempowered and denied access to the decision-making process, youth are nevertheless protesting unfair laws, getting school clinics built, defeating curfew laws, changing school curricula to make them more reflective of diversity, and working on environmental justice campaigns (Maira & Soep, 2004). Engaging in social change helps to develop transferable skills such as writing, public speaking, critical thinking, and improved group skills (Mohamed & Wheeler, 2001). The efforts of this burgeoning youth movement are slowly and systematically being knitted together with inclusive principles and strategies that view youth as producers, contributors, creators, and leaders.

The field of youth organizing is the outgrowth of three important elements: the legacy of traditional organizing models informed by Saul Alinsky, the progressive social movements of the 1960s and 1970s, and the rise of positive youth development (Pintado-Vertner, 2004). Youth organizing pays attention to culture and identity as it studies political systems and structures and values sustained relationships with caring adults and expanded opportunities for youth leadership. Community organizing strategies have particular promise for youth who are negatively affected by racism, sexism, classism, or discrimination based on immigrant status or sexual orientation. Youth from poor and working-class communities of color are particularly likely to conclude that they are society's lowest priority just by looking around critically at the neighborhoods in which they live, the buses they ride, the parks they play in, and the schools they attend.

Youth can be among our greatest teachers in terms of primary prevention. The process through which youth critically analyze their circumstances and then develop both a personal and a collective response can be deeply empowering (Mohamed & Wheeler, 2001). For example, in Oakland, California, the Environmental Prevention in Communities (EPIC) program effectively involved youth in the process of educating businesses and community organizations to reduce crime and alcohol and tobacco use in Oakland's economically depressed communities. Youth from these affected communities identified an overconcentration of alcohol outlets and advertising in their neighborhoods as a major roadblock to their personal and academic success. EPIC youth organized with community residents, retailers, and city officials to make changes in their community to resolve and prevent alcohol problems (Environmental Prevention in Communities, 2006). Like other youth activists all over the country (Checkoway et al., 2003), they conducted surveys and facilitated workshops in the community. The skills and knowledge learned through activism prepared them to create a youth-initiated prevention campaign. Similarly, the Youth Leadership Institute program YO! Mateo is organizing to ban the on-campus sale of products from subsidiaries of tobacco companies. These youth organizers want their school district to recognize that the same multinational corporations that sell tobacco products also make huge profits from subsidiaries that sell nontobacco products, including many food items available in high school cafeterias and vending machines (Youth Leadership Institute, 2006). Such efforts are important not only for their tangible results in schools and communities but also for empowering youth participants, for whom community organizing for social change may become an important lifelong commitment.

Culture

Culture includes beliefs, values, attitudes, and behaviors shared by members of a social group or organization. It shapes and is shaped by language, relationships, religion, and material goods. Our perceptions are informed by the cultures we are born into, grow up around, and are socialized by.

Culture affects health, disease, and health care by encouraging certain health behaviors and discouraging others, by providing definitions for personal experience and prescribing idioms of distress, and by providing a social context. Cultural variations across communities are numerous and complex even within the same ethnic group. To avoid misleading reductionism or stereotypes, it is important to recognize that it is not possible to predict the beliefs and behaviors of individuals based on their race, ethnicity, or national origin. In fact, one can never become truly "competent" or "proficient" in another's culture.

Beyond Cultural Competence and Cultural Proficiency

The United States is a nation of many cultures; it is a country of immigrants, forced migration, and extermination. It has had policies—responses to immediate needs or political pressures—that are often contradictory and inadequate to cope with the size and diversity of its racial and ethnic populations (Crawford, 2004). In the United States, there are "two languages of race" (Blauner, 2001), one in which members of communities of color see the centrality of race in history and everyday experience and another in which whites see race as a peripheral reality and do not perceive themselves as racist. "Whites tend to locate racism in color consciousness and find its absence in color-blindness. In so doing, they see the affirmation of difference and racial identity among racially defined minority students as racist. Black students, by contrast, see racism as a system of power and correspondingly argue that they cannot be racist because they lack power" (Omi, 2000, p. 257).

In this increasingly multicultural society, issues of culture, race, ethnicity, racism, and privilege are vital to recognize and address when organizing for primary prevention in the community. The concept of cultural competence emphasizes the ability to function effectively with members of different groups through cultural awareness and sensitivity when delivering services to culturally diverse populations. *Competence* implies having the capacity to function effectively as an individual and an organization within the context of the cultural beliefs, behaviors, and needs presented by the community as well as the ability to foster respectful and effective interactions with people of many cultures (Cross, 1989; Lynch & Hanson, 1998). Within the context of health care, cultural competence is the ability "to recognize and respond to health-related beliefs and cultural values, disease incidence and prevalence, and treatment efficacy" (U.S. Department of Health and Human Services, Office of Minority Health, 2001). Nonetheless, despite widespread popularity, cultural competence remains a vaguely defined goal with no explicit criteria established for its accomplishment or assessment (Hunt, 2001). Lindsey, Robbins, and Terrell (2003) argue that educators and advocates must learn as much as possible about culture and go beyond cultural competence to become culturally proficient in order to meet the needs of our diverse population. They define cultural proficiency as "the policies and practices of an organization or the values and behaviors of an individual that enable the agency or person to interact effectively in a culturally diverse environment." (p. 21). They offer a "cultural proficiency continuum" to illustrate the major concepts (see Figure 5.1). This model has been infused with the notion of cultural humility.

Cultural Humility

Whereas cultural proficiency is used to gain awareness of and sensitivity toward others, cultural humility emphasizes the need to gain a greater awareness of and sensitivity to one's own worldview and the cultural implications of one's own identity group membership. Cultural humility connotes a deference of one's own cultural beliefs and assumptions, which can be clouded by hegemony and racism. Cultural humility has been described by Tervalon and Murray-Garcia (1998) as a lifelong commitment to self-evaluation and self-critique, redressing power imbalances, and developing and maintaining mutually respectful dynamic partnerships based on mutual trust. In this model, the most serious barrier to culturally appropriate care is not a lack of knowledge of the details of any given cultural orientation but the failure to develop self-awareness and a respectful attitude toward diverse points of view and ways of living. Following the principle of cultural humility, community organizers are open and flexible enough to be able to identify the presence and importance of differences between their own orientation and that of each community member and to explore compromises and possibilities acceptable to both.

Central to cultural humility is the need to develop individual critical reflection skills, involving awareness of self and others. Several important elements of critical reflection are necessary when working with diverse communities. The first

FIGURE 5.1. THE CULTURAL PROFICIENCY CONTINUUM: FROM CULTURAL DESTRUCTIVENESS TO CULTURAL HUMILITY.

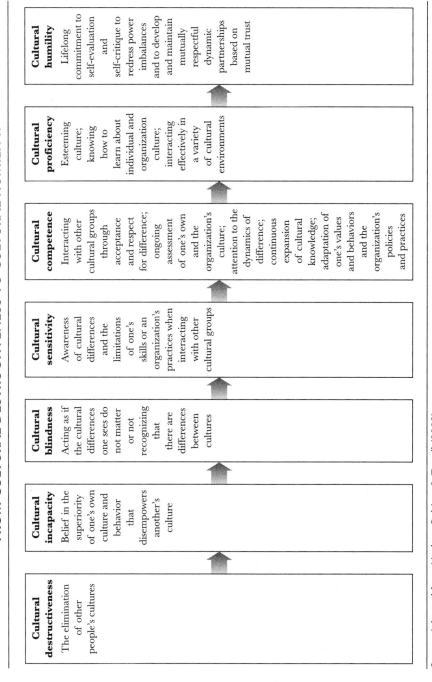

Cultural destructiveness	Cultural incapacity	Cultural blindness	Cultural sensitivity	Cultural competence	Cultural proficiency	Cultural humility
The elimination of other people's cultures	Belief in the superiority of one's own culture and behavior that disempowers another's culture	Acting as if the cultural differences one sees do not matter or not recognizing that there are differences between cultures	Awareness of cultural differences and the limitations of one's skills or an organization's practices when interacting with other cultural groups	Interacting with other cultural groups through acceptance and respect for difference; ongoing assessment of one's own and the organization's culture; attention to the dynamics of difference; continuous expansion of cultural knowledge; adaptation of one's values and behaviors and the organization's policies and practices	Esteeming culture; knowing how to learn about individual and organization culture; interacting effectively in a variety of cultural environments	Lifelong commitment to self-evaluation and self-critique to redress power imbalances and to develop and maintain mutually respectful dynamic partnerships based on mutual trust

Source: Adapted from Lindsey, Robins, & Terrell (2003).

is an awareness and value of people's strengths and their daily contributions. Rather than viewing people as problems or challenges to tolerate we must take into account their contributions. These contributions may come in the form of caring for younger siblings, interpretation and translation skills for parents who are not literate or not proficient in English, housework, mediating with public institutions, or working outside the home (Orellana, 2001).

A second aspect of critical self-reflection is an understanding of our own diversity. Lum (2003) uses a framework of diversity developed by Schriver (2001) to explore our own understanding of diversity. He asks that organizers be able to articulate their own diversity perspective and worldview (values and beliefs, culture, family, gender, sexual orientation, socioeconomic class, spirituality, ability status, and so on), the intersection between these perspectives (the implications of our membership in multiple groups), and the interrelatedness and interconnectedness to other people (our similarities and differences). Through the examination and exploration of our own multiple identities, we are able to situate ourselves within our world in relation to others and become better aware of our own biases and assumptions.

Finally, in the context of community organizing for social justice, cultural humility entails social transformation. It requires that we move beyond cultural competence toward social justice. Organizing racially and culturally diverse communities is certain to be a difficult task until we act within a framework of social justice. This requires a moral and ethical attitude toward equality and possibility and a belief in the capacity of people as agents who can transform their world. The Brazilian educator Paulo Freire (1970) notes that we must begin by examining the contradictions between our espoused social principles and our lived experience. If we are unable to perceive and resolve social, political, and economic contradictions in our own lives, we will have great difficulty organizing communities to take action toward social justice. In summary, cultural humility in community organizing for prevention and social justice promotes social transformation first through our work to transform ourselves and then by extending this process through our work in both the education and the empowerment of others.

The Wheel of Community Organizing

The process of community organizing does not happen in predictable steps; nevertheless, the "wheel of community organizing" offers a set of cyclical principles that an organizer can use to support the crafting, implementation, and evaluation of comprehensive prevention initiatives. It was developed from the Marin Institute publication *Community Organizing for the Prevention of Problems Related to Alcohol*

FIGURE 5.2. THE WHEEL OF COMMUNITY ORGANIZING.

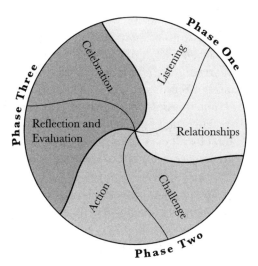

and Other Drugs (Wechsler & Schnepp, 1993) and applied to teach community organizing and public health at San Francisco State University (Chávez & Turalba, 2006; Chávez, Turalba, & Malik, 2006). The model is based on seven organizing principles: listening, relationships, challenge, action, reflection, evaluation, and celebration, structured in beginning, middle, and ending phases (see Figure 5.2). These principles are cyclical in that they are repeated, each time building on assessments of earlier successes, errors, and lessons learned. The wheel provides a map to build an organized community where members are mutually invested in learning from one another. Its framework is not bottom-up, community-based, or grassroots in origin but aims at bottom-up, community-based, or grassroots strengthening as its goal; it promotes community participation in controlling the decision making for all actions affecting the community as a whole. The main steps are logically linked with each other and to the cycle as a whole. They are all needed; absence of any one will seriously weaken its impact.

Phase One: Listening and Building Relationships

We are trained in a culture that values personal expression and speech over listening (Rosenberg, 2003). Communities are made up of individuals who are often discouraged by a mainstream culture of individualism and mistrust. The strategy of community organizing requires listening not simply with one's ears but with one's heart. Listening with one's heart entails the use of empathy, genuineness, and sincerity. Listening is starting where the people are; it enables the organizer to become familiar with the community, its history, its demographics, its geography, and its political leadership. Entering a community requires listening and learning from norms of the community as well as developing personal relationships. An organizer meets first with people individually, rather than trying to meet everyone in a group to assess community goals. Conversations and information gathering are an important part of this phase of community organizing, as they lay the foundation for all the work that comes after. The organizer must learn to hear what community concerns are and find out what community members identify as problems, not tell the community what the problems are. This phase is basic to building trust and promoting community involvement. Outreach includes asking questions, participating in formal community events, and engaging in many casual activities to demonstrate respect and cultural humility. A word of caution: even if organizers attempt to genuinely "start where the people are" (Nyswander, 1956), they may lack access to the "hidden discourse" in a community and misinterpret situations or conversations because of their own lack of cultural competence, lack of access to cultural translators, or lack of self-reflection on the problematic nature of power dynamics between themselves and community members (Chávez, Duran, Baker, Avila, & Wallerstein, 2003; Scott, 1990). Hidden discourse may also be important to recognize as an inevitable reality between outsiders and insiders, even with the closest of relationships, and reminds us of our humility in doing this work.

Phase Two: Challenge and Action

What are the challenges faced by the community? What are the root causes of these problems? This phase requires every organizer not just to answer these questions but to move beyond with action steps and realistic tasks that build on community strengths. Once the group has identified its goals, the organizer's responsibility is to keep the momentum of the group moving forward. One of the most important steps in community organizing practice involves the effective differentiation between problems, or things that are troubling, and issues the community feels strongly about (Miller, 1985). The difference between identifying a problem and selecting an issue is the movement from challenge to action. As Mike Miller (1985) suggests, a good issue must meet several important criteria. It must be winnable to ensure that working on the campaign doesn't simply reinforce fatalistic attitudes and beliefs. It must be simple and specific so that any member of the group can explain it clearly in a sentence or two. It must unite members of the group and involve them in a meaningful way in achieving resolution. It affects many people and is part of a larger plan or strategy that builds community capacity (Minkler & Wallerstein, 2004). An approach to issue selection that has proved especially helpful is the use of Freire's educational strategies to identify the core themes, which in turn generate social and emotional commitment for starting organizing efforts (Carroll & Minkler, 2000; Giroux, 1992; Hope & Timmel, 1984; Shor, 1995; Wallerstein & Auerbach, 2004). Key to this approach is being in touch with community "stakeholders" and operating in partnership with them. Stakeholders include any person or organization with an interest in the action, such as parents, children, customers, owners, employees, associates, and others who can affect or who are affected by achievement of a group's objectives.

Phase Three: Reflection, Evaluation, and Celebration

As the action is designed and implemented, it is important to carefully review progress, ensure that it is on track, and evaluate the community organizing efforts, limitations, and contributions. The goal is to understand what went right or wrong and to learn lessons for the future. Reflective questions include

What was accomplished?

What still needs to be done?

What was done well?

What could have been done better?

Finally, every community organizing process ideally concludes with celebration. Celebration helps create a sustainable community. Phil Bartle (2005), in a series of training modules designed for community empowerment, suggests that celebration is more than a public party—it is a ceremony of completion that confirms the legitimacy and appropriateness of community participation and empowerment for social justice. Completion of a community project is an important element of community organizing and community building where the community is publicly recognized for successfully engaging in local action. It is also an opportunity to start another mobilization cycle. Si Kahn, in *How People Get Power* (1970), notes that as the organizing cycle is completed, the organizer must be sure folks in the community are ready and trained to sustain future efforts. Sustainability needs to be addressed at the start of the organizing effort, continue through capacity-building efforts, and be part of the reflective process.

Essential Qualities

The cyclical principles at the heart of community organizing are enacted by individuals who possess essential qualities of inclusion, trustworthiness, leadership development, and self-reflection. Community organizers are required to clearly communicate their values, interests, and motivations. They "must constantly examine life, including [their] own, to get some idea of what it is all about, and [they] must challenge and test [their] own findings. Irreverence, essential to questioning, is a requisite. Curiosity becomes compulsive. The most frequent word is 'why?'" (Alinsky, 1971, p. 11). The Marin Institute (2006) notes that not all of us are well suited to be organizers: "community organizers think strategically about their work while always keeping the final goal in mind and continually making contributions to the goal." The institute suggests that the following qualities go hand in hand with the practice of community organizing:

Imagination

Sense of humor

Organized personality

A free and open mind

A strong sense of self

Blurred vision of a better world

The ability to create something new out of the old

Furthermore, leadership development is a cornerstone of community organizing. As Beckwith (1997) notes, community organization "provides people with a lot of opportunities to practice, to try it out, to learn by doing. A broad team of folks who can lead is built by constantly bringing new people into leadership roles and supporting them in learning from this experience" (p. 8). The W. K. Kellogg Foundation (1995), after years of studying how to develop and sustain community organizations, found that a new kind of leadership is required. The "old structure that exalted control, order, and predictability has given way to a non-hierarchical order in which all individuals' contributions are solicited and acknowledged, and in which creativity is valued over blind loyalty." The foundation's report identifies the qualities of collaborative leaders, noting that they are global thinkers, multi-culturally literate, creative and innovative, participative and inclusive, good communicators and networkers, encouraging and supportive, energetic, and adept at using conflict resolution skills.

Empowerment

As the great Chinese philosopher Lao-tzu noted some 2,600 years ago, ". . . With the best leaders, when the work is done, the task is accomplished, the people will say, 'We have done it ourselves.'"

More than an essential quality of community organizing, empowerment is a core value and developmental process that includes building skills through repetitive cycles of action and reflection that evoke new skills and understandings, which in turn provoke new and more effective actions (Kieffer, 1984). It is a process by which people, organizations, and communities gain mastery over the issues that are important to them (Rappaport, 1987). Empowerment includes the development of self-confidence, a critical worldview, and the cultivation of individual and collective skills and resources for social and political action. Empowerment is a multilevel construct involving "participation, control, and critical awareness" at the individual, organizational, and community levels (Zimmerman, 2000). From a social justice perspective, empowerment has also been defined as having the capacity to identify problems and solutions (Cotrell, 1976), and participatory self-competence in political life (Wandersman & Florin, 2000) and embodies both social change processes and outcomes of transformed conditions (Wallerstein, 2006).

Regrettably, empowerment is also a concept that has become common political rhetoric with a flexibility of meaning so broad that it is in danger of losing its inherent activist roots. At the core of the concept of empowerment is the idea of power, resistance to domination and social change. Power exists within the context of relationships between people and institutions. Because power is created in relationships, power and power relationships can change. Empowerment is thus a process of change. This is important to recognize when generalizing what empowerment means cross-culturally. How *empowerment* translates into other languages raises the question of whether this concept is relevant, meaningful, and portable across cultures (Erzinger, 1994). A broad definition of empowerment highlights the ability to create change on the personal, interpersonal, and political levels. "Power from within" and "power with others" are moral, spiritual, and skill-based sources of power that can constantly expand as people empower themselves. While empowerment includes the dimension of transferring power to others, the organizer cannot directly empower the community; empowerment is something people do for themselves. Further, organizers must let go of their power and their need to control in order to make power more available to others.

Empowerment is strengthened by building critical consciousness, or "conscientization," a concept that comes from Freire (1970). Darder, Baltodano, and Torres (2003) explain conscientization as a process that questions oppression and social privilege, builds empowerment, and works toward social change. They note that Freire developed conscientization to teach illiterate peasants to read by teaching them to "read" their political and social reality. Freire's theory and method of combining community organizing with popular education and community research is basic to the goal of empowerment. His methodology of listening, dialogue, and action strengthens the community organizing cycles of reflection and action (Wallerstein & Auerbach, 2004). Freire's work has been a catalyst worldwide for programs in adult education, health, and community development (Carroll & Minkler, 2000; Hope & Timmel, 1984; Tran et al., 2004; Wallerstein & Bernstein, 1994; Wallerstein & Weinger, 1992). Freire's theories are relevant to community organizers and prevention specialists in the United States as we experience heath inequities among communities of color and a growing gap between the rich and poor.

Conclusion

The current system of power relations in the United States is unjust and challenging for most people in their quest to lead healthy and fulfilling lives. The problem is systemic, institutional, and also deeply personal. This chapter outlined broad themes of community organizing practice as well as the fundamental purpose of community organizing—to help discover and enable people's shared goals, as informed by values, knowledge, culture, and experience. Examples from women's health and youth organizing perspectives introduced community organizing as a strategy to change the balance of power and create new power bases at local, statewide, or national levels. Effective organizing leads to the levels of community engagement and empowerment that are vital for successful primary prevention efforts targeting environmental determinants of health. Community organizing is about resistance to domination, developing self-awareness and cultural humility and about meeting people where they are. It is activism bringing people together who want to work out common solutions that include the community every step of the way.

References

Alinsky, S. (1971). *Rules for radicals.* New York: Vintage Books.

Barnett, B. (1993). Invisible southern black women leaders in the civil rights movement: The triple constraints of gender, race, and class. *Gender and Society, 7,* 162–182.

Bartle, P. (2005). *Community empowerment training modules.* Retrieved September 20, 2005, from http://www.scn.org/cmp

Beckwith, D. (with Lopez, C.). (1997). *Community organizing: People power from the grassroots.* Retrieved October 11, 2006, from http://comm-org.wisc.edu/papers97/beckwith.htm

Bellah, R. N., Madsen, R., Sullivan, W. M., Swidler, A., & Tipton, S. M. (1985). *Habits of the heart: Individualism and commitment in American life.* Berkeley: University of California Press.

Blauner, B. (2001). *Still the big news: Racial oppression in America.* Philadelphia: Temple University Press.

Bobo, K., Kendall, J., & Max, S. (1991). *Organizing for social change: A manual for activists in the 1990s.* Santa Ana, CA: Seven Locks Press.

Boston Women's Health Book Collective. (1973) *Our bodies, ourselves: A book by and for women.* New York: Simon & Schuster.

Boston Women's Health Book Collective. (2005) *Our bodies, ourselves: A new edition for a new era.* New York: Simon & Schuster.

Caplan, R., & Rodberg, L. (1994, Fall). Rx: Federal support for community health: An innovative community-based approach to preventive health. *In Context,* p. 58. Retrieved July 25, 2006, from http://www.context.org/ICLIB/IC39/Caplan.htm

Carroll, J., & Minkler, M. (2000). Freire's message for social workers: Looking back, looking ahead. *Journal of Community Practice, 8,* 21–36.

Chávez, V., Duran, B., Baker, Q. E., Avila, M. M., & Wallerstein, N. (2003). The dance of race and privilege in community-based participatory research. In M. Minkler & N. Wallerstein (Eds.), *Community-based participatory research for health* (pp. 81–97). San Francisco: Jossey-Bass.

Chávez, V., & Turalba, R.-A. N. (2006). Pedagogy of collegiality. In J. L. Perry & S. G. Jones (Eds.), *Quick hits for educating citizens* (pp. 26–27). Bloomington: Indiana University Press.

Chávez, V., Turalba R.-A. N., & Malik, S. (2006). Teaching public health through a pedagogy of collegiality. *American Journal of Public Health, 96,* 1175–1180.

Checkoway, B., Richards-Schuster, K., Abdulla, S., Aragon, M., Facio, E., Figueroa, L., et al. (2003). Young people as competent citizens. *Community Development Journal, 38,* 298–309.

Cotrell, L. S. (1976). The competent community. In B. H. Kaplan, R. N. Wilson, & A. Leighton (Eds.), *Further explorations in community psychiatry.* New York: Basic Books.

Crawford, J. (2004). *Educating English learners: Language diversity in the classroom* (5th ed.). Los Angeles: Bilingual Educational Services.

Cross, T. L. (1989). Towards a culturally competent system of care. *A monograph of effective services for children who are severely emotionally disturbed* (Vol. I). Washington, DC: Georgetown University Child Development Center.

Darder, A., Baltodano, M., & Torres, R. (2003). *The critical pedagogy reader.* New York: Routledge Falmer.

Davis, A. (1981). *Women, race, and class.* New York: Random House.

Delgado, G. (1987). *Organizing the movement: The roots and growth of ACORN.* Philadelphia: Temple University Press.

Ehrlich, T. (2000). *Civic engagement, civic responsibility, and higher education.* Westport, CT: Oryx Press.

Environmental Prevention in Communities. (2006). Retrieved November 1, 2006, from http://www.marininstitute.org/take_action/epic.htm

Erzinger, S. (1994). Empowerment in Spanish: Words can get in the way. *Health Education Quarterly, 21*(3), 417–419.

Evans, S. (1980). *Personal politics: The roots of women's liberation in the civil rights movement and the New Left*. New York: Vintage Press.

Fairchild, P. (2005). *Community health centers in the United States: Expanding the power of community health centers in rural Indiana*. Retrieved July 25, 2006, from http://www.jsi.com/JSIInternet/DITL/US/Community_Health_Centers_in_the_United_States.cfm

Fawcett, S. B., Schultz, J. A., Carson, V. L., Renault, V. A., & Francisco, V. T. (2003). Using Internet-based tools to build capacity for community-based participatory research and other efforts to promote community health and development. In M. Minkler & N. Wallerstein (Eds.), *Community-based participatory research for health* (pp. 155–178). San Francisco: Jossey-Bass.

Fellin, P. (2001). Understanding American communities. In J. Rothman, J. L. Erlich, & J. E. Tropman (Eds.), *Strategies of community intervention* (6th ed., pp. 118–133). Belmont, CA: Wadsworth.

Ferris, S., & Sandoval, R. (1997). *The fight in the fields: Cesar Chavez and the farmworkers movement*. Orlando, FL: Harcourt.

Fisher, R., & Romanofsky, P. (1981). Introduction. In R. Fisher & P. Romanofsky (Eds.), *Community organization for social change* (pp. xi–xviii). Westport, CT: Greenwood Press.

Freire, P. (1970). *Pedagogy of the oppressed*. New York: Seabury Press.

Garvin, C. D., & Cox, F. M. (2001). A history of community organizing since the Civil War with special reference to oppressed communities. In J. Rothman, J. L. Erlich, & J. E. Tropman (Eds.), *Strategies of community intervention* (6th ed., pp. 65–100). Belmont, CA: Wadsworth.

Geiger, H. J. (2005). The unsteady march. *Perspectives in Biology and Medicine, 48*, 1–9. Retrieved July 25, 2006, from www.phrusa.org/racial_disparities/pdf/geiger_unsteadymarch.pdf

Geiger Gibson Program in Community Health Policy. (n.d.). *Dr. H. Jack Geiger*. Washington, DC: George Washington University, School of Public Health and Health Services, Department of Health Policy. Retrieved October 11, 2006, from http://www.gwumc.edu/sphhs/healthpolicy/ggprogram/geiger.html

Giroux, H. *Border crossings*. New York: Routledge, 1992.

Gutierrez, L. M., & Lewis, E. (1992). A feminist perspective on organizing with women of color. In F. G. Rivera & J. L. Erlich (Eds.), *Community organizing in a diverse society*. Boston: Allyn & Bacon.

Herbert, S. (2005). Harnessing the power of the Internet for advocacy and organizing. In M. Minkler (Ed.), *Community organizing and community building for health* (2nd ed.). New Brunswick, NJ: Rutgers University Press.

Hick, S., & McNutt, J. G. (2002). *Advocacy, activism, and the Internet: Community organization and social policy*. Chicago: Lyceum Books.

hooks, b. (1984). *Feminist theory from margin to center*. Boston: South End Press.

hooks, b. (2000). *All about love: New visions*. New York: Perennial.

Hope, A., & Timmel, S. (1984). *Training for transformation: A handbook for community workers*. Gweru, Zimbabwe: Mambo.

Hunt, L. M. (2001, November-December). Beyond cultural competence: Applying humility to clinical settings. *Park Ridge Center Bulletin, 24*, 3–4.

Kahn, S. (1970). *How people get power: Organizing oppressed communities for action*. New York: McGraw-Hill.

Kahn, S. (1991). *Organizing: A guide for grassroots leaders*. Silver Springs, MD: NASW Press.

Kieffer, C. H. (1984). Citizen empowerment: A development perspective. *Prevention in Human Services, 3*, 9–36.

Kretzmann, J. P., & McKnight, J. L. (1993). *Building communities from the inside out.* Evanston, IL: Northwestern University, Center for Urban Affairs and Policy Research.

Labonte, R. (1994). Health promotion and empowerment: Reflections on professional practice. *Health Education Quarterly, 21*, 253–268.

Lindsey, R., Robbins, K., & Terrell, R. (2003). *Cultural proficiency: A manual for school leaders* (2nd Ed.). Thousand Oaks, CA: Sage Publications.

Lum, D. (2003). *Social work practice and people of color: A process-stage approach* (4th ed.). Belmont, CA: Wadsworth.

Lynch, E., & Hanson, M. (1998). *Developing cross-cultural competence: A guide for working with children and their families.* Baltimore: Brooks.

Maira, S., & Soep, E. (2004). *Youthscapes: The Popular, the national, the global.* Philadelphia: University of Pennsylvania Press.

Marin Institute. (2006). *Take action: Community organizing action packs.* Retrieved October 11, 2006, from http://www.marininstitute.org/action_packs/community_org.htm

Martinson, M., & Minkler, M. (2006). Civic engagement and older adults: A critique. *The Gerontologist, 46*, 318–324.

McKnight, J. L. (1995). Regenerating community. In J. L. McKnight, *The careless society: Community and its counterfeits* (pp. 161–172). New York: Basic Books.

Miller, M. (1985). *Turning problems into actionable issues.* San Francisco: Organize Training Center.

Minkler, M. (Ed.). (2004). *Community organizing and community building for health* (2nd ed.). New Brunswick, NJ: Rutgers University Press.

Minkler, M., & Wallerstein, N. (2004). Improving health through community organization and community building: A health education perspective. In M. Minkler (Ed.), *Community organizing and community building for health* (2nd ed., pp. 30–52). New Brunswick, NJ: Rutgers University Press.

Mohamed, I., & Wheeler, W. (2001). *Broadening the bounds of youth development: Youth as engaged citizens.* New York: Ford Foundation & Innovation Center for Community and Youth Development.

Morris, A. D. (1984). *Origins of the civil rights movement: Black communities organizing for change.* New York: Free Press.

Naples, N. A. (2002). The dynamics of critical pedagogy, experiential learning, and feminist praxis. In N. A. Naples & K. Bojar (Eds.), *Teaching feminist activism: Strategies from the field* (pp. 9–21). New York: Routledge.

Norris, T., & Pittman, M. (2000). The healthy communities movement and the Coalition for Healthier Cities and Communities. *Public Health Reports, 113*, 118–124.

Nyswander, D. B. (1956). Education for health: Some principles and their application. *Health Education Monographs*, 13, 65–70.

Omi, M. A. (2000). The changing meaning of race. In N. J. Smelser, W. J. Wilson, & F. Mitchell (Eds.), *America becoming: Racial trends and their consequences* (Vol. 1, pp. 243–263). Washington, DC: National Academy Press.

Orellana, M. F. (2001). The work kids do: Mexican and Central American immigrant children's contributions to households and schools in California. *Harvard Educational Review, 71*(3), 366–389. Peck, M. S. (1987). *The different drum: Community making and peace.* New York: Simon & Schuster.

Pintado-Vertner, R. (2004). *The West Coast story: The emergence of youth organizing in California.* New York: Funders Collaborative on Youth Organizing.

Prokosch, M., & Raymond, L. (2002). *The global activist's manual: Local ways to change the world.* New York: Thunder's Mouth Press/Nation Books.

Putnam, R. D. (1996). The strange disappearance of civic America. *The American Prospect, 24,* 34–48.

Rappaport, J. (1987). Terms of empowerment/exemplars of prevention: Toward a theory for community psychology. *American Journal of Community Psychology, 15,* 121–148.

Sen, R. (2003). *Stir it up.* San Francisco: Jossey-Bass.

Rosenberg, M. B. (2003). *Nonviolent communication: A language of life* (2nd ed.). Encinitas, CA: PuddleDancer Press.

Schriver, J. M. (2001). *Human behavior and the social environment: Shifting paradigms in essential knowledge for social work practice.* Boston: Allyn & Bacon.

Scott, J. C. (1990). *Domination and the arts of resistance: Hidden transcripts.* New Haven, CT: Yale University Press, 1990.

Shor, I. (1993). Education is politics: Paulo Freire's critical pedagogy. In P. McLaren & P. Leonard (Eds.), *Paolo Freire: A critical encounter* (pp. 25–35). New York: Routledge.

Stall, S., & Stoecker, R. (1998). Community organizing or organizing community? Gender and the crafts of empowerment. *Gender and Society, 12,* 729–756.

Tervalon, M., & Murray-Garcia, J. (1998). Cultural humility versus cultural competence: A critical distinction in defining physician training outcomes in multicultural education. *Journal of Health Care for the Poor and Underserved, 9,* 17–25.

Tran, A. N., Haidet, P., Street, R. L., O'Malley, K. J., Martin, F., & Ashton, C. M. (2004). Empowering communication: A community-based intervention for patients. *Patient Education and Counseling, 52,* 113–121.

U.S. Department of Health and Human Services, Office of Minority Health. (2001). *National standards for culturally and linguistically appropriate services in health care.* Washington, DC: Author.

Van de Donk, W., Loader, B. D., Nixon, P. G., & Rucht, D. (Eds.). (2004). *Cyberprotest: New media, citizens, and social movements.* New York: Routledge.

Wallerstein, N. (2006). The effectiveness of empowerment strategies to improve health. Copenhagen: World Health Organization. Available from http://www.euro.who.int/HEN/Syntheses/empowerment/20060119_10

Wallerstein, N., & Auerbach, E. (2004). *Problem posing at work: Popular educators' guide.* Edmonton: Grassroots Press.

Wallerstein, N., & Bernstein, E. (Eds.). (1994). Community empowerment, participatory education, and health. *Health Education Quarterly, 21,* 141–148.

Wallerstein, N., & Weinger, M. (Eds.). (1992). Special issue: Empowerment approaches to worker health and safety education. *American Journal of Industrial Medicine, 22*(5).

Walters, C. L. (2004) Community building practice: A conceptual framework. In M. Minkler (Ed.), *Community organizing and community building for health* (2nd ed., pp. 66–81). New Brunswick, NJ: Rutgers University Press.

Wandersman, A. H., & Florin, P. (2000). Citizen participation and community organizing. In J. Rappaport & E. Seidman (Eds.), *Handbook of community psychology* (pp. 247–272). New York: Plenum.

Wechsler, R., & Schnepp, T. (1993). *Community organizing for the prevention of problems related to alcohol and other drugs.* San Rafael, CA: Marin Institute.

W. K. Kellogg Foundation. (1995). *Sustaining community-based initiatives: Developing community capacity.* In partnership with The Healthcare Forum. Retrieved November 1, 2006, from www.wkkf.org/pubs/Health/Pub657.pdf

World Health Organization. (1986). *Ottawa charter for health promotion.* Retrieved November 1, 2006, from http://www.euro.who.int/aboutwho/policy/20010827_2

World Health Organization. (1998). *Health promotion glossary.* Geneva: WHO.

Youth Leadership Institute. (2006). *Prevention.* Retrieved July 28, 2006, from http://www.yli.org/prevention

Zimmerman, M. (2000). Empowerment theory: Psychological, organizational, and community levels of analysis. In J. Rappaport & E. Seidman (Eds.), *Handbook of community psychology* (pp. 43–63). New York: Plenum.

CHAPTER SIX

MORE THAN A MESSAGE

Framing Public Health Advocacy to Change Corporate Practices

Lori Dorfman, Lawrence Wallack, Katie Woodruff

If they can get you asking the wrong questions, they don't have to worry about the answers.

—THOMAS PYNCHON, *GRAVITY'S RAINBOW* (1973), p. 251.

Public health educators are often confronted by challenging arguments from companies that produce harmful products. Tobacco companies say they sell a legal product. Alcohol companies insist that most people drink responsibly and that the companies should not be blamed if some people abuse their products. Junk food purveyors say that it is the parents' responsibility to control what children eat. Car companies say that the key to greater safety on the road is changes in drivers' behavior.

Public health educators often struggle to respond to such arguments. They are put on the defensive, and the language does not come easily. It is no wonder, after all, that each industry argument is truthful, if incomplete. One reason public health advocates have difficulty responding may be that they do not understand that public health language needs to be rooted in a framework of values. The good news is that in fact, public health has a clear, consistent set of values that can guide health educators' messages. Just as the corporate arguments are organized along

The authors thank Makani Themba-Nixon of the Praxis Project and George Lakoff and Pamela Morgan of the Rockridge Institute for their insights and innovative thinking about how to frame public policy battles. Dr. Wallack's work on this article was supported in part by an innovator's grant from the Robert Wood Johnson Foundation.

This chapter is reprinted from *Health Education and Behavior*, Vol. 32, No. 3, pp. 320–336. Copyright © 2005 by the Society for Public Health Education.

a consistent set of values, public health advocates can reframe issues with the same level of confidence and consistency to reflect broader public health goals.

Public Health and Social Justice

For more than a generation, public health practitioners have been guided by the work of Beauchamp (1976), who argues that the ethic of public health is social justice. "Public health should be a way of doing justice," Beauchamp wrote, "a way of asserting the value and priority of all human life" (p. 521). Beauchamp called for newly constructed collective definitions of public health problems that clearly communicate "that the origins of [death and disability] lie beyond merely individual factors" (p. 522), despite the fact that individual factors must, of course, be acknowledged.

The biggest barrier to achieving social justice is the competing ethic of market justice. Market justice is rooted in the basic notion of Adam Smith's (1776/2000) invisible hand, the idea that the market will naturally respond to the desires of the people and so the unfettered marketplace is the best way to serve those desires. Market justice ideals have long dominated political and cultural life in the United States. Much of the debate on policy issues concerns whether or how to restrain the marketplace with regulation. Regulation is always seen as a constraint on the free market, to be tolerated only in limited circumstances.

It is no surprise then that market justice dominates current thinking and practice in public health. Politicians' focus on tax cuts as a means of unleashing market power and solving societal problems is a good example of how public health suffers when market justice predominates. Services for helping people and policies for protecting people are left unfunded as tax cuts are embraced and available funds disappear. Without a shift to social justice, says Beauchamp (1976), progress in public health will be thwarted. A shift to stronger social justice values would bring greater public health gains for communities and individuals because policies to ensure equitable public health outcomes would be put in place to counter the ill effects of the market (see Table 6.1).

The fight against tobacco can be seen as one clearly successful example of the shift that Beauchamp (1976) advocated. Tobacco has been fundamentally redefined from an individual problem called smoking to a public issue called tobacco, from a focus on blaming the smoker to a focus on the role of industry and the government. Consequently, strategies are now directed toward creating rules that hold the tobacco industry disproportionately, but fairly, accountable for the death and disability it has caused. A new definition of the problem exposed the limits of the norm of individual responsibility, challenged the market justice ethic driving pub-

TABLE 6.1. MARKET JUSTICE VALUES COMPARED TO SOCIAL JUSTICE VALUES.

Market Justice	Social Justice
Self-determination and self-discipline	Shared responsibility
Rugged individualism and self-interest	Interconnection and cooperation
Benefits based solely on personal effort	Basic benefits should be assured
Limited obligation to collective good	Strong obligation to the collective good
Limited government intervention	Government involvement is necessary
Voluntary and moral nature of behavior	Community well-being supersedes individual well-being

Source: Beauchamp (1976).

lic policy, and made room for a shift toward collective solutions emphasizing social justice. Public health is, arguably, a long way from completing its task, but surely, the tide has turned and we are headed toward a world with less tobacco, not more.

Practitioners working in other public health arenas are now eyeing tobacco control enviously, wondering if similar tactics will work to advance fairer policy approaches to obesity and other public health problems. Certainly, this is possible and there is much to learn from successes, and failures, in tobacco control. Fundamentally, however, the shift must be tied to a core set of values, and for public health, those values should reflect social justice. As Beauchamp (1976) explains:

> The central problems remain the injustice of a market ethic that unfairly protects majorities and powerful interests from their fair share of the burdens of prevention, and of convincing the public that the task of protecting the public's health lies categorically beyond the norms of market justice. This means that the function of each different redefinition of a specific problem must be to raise the common and recurrent issue of justice by exposing the aggressive and powerful structures implicated in all instances of preventable death and disability, and further to point to the necessity for collective measures to confront and resist these structures. [p. 523]

The aggressive and powerful structures implicated in market justice forces can often be traced to corporate actors. This understanding does not negate the value of individual liberty in our society, but it does suggest that those values must be balanced with other values that emphasize the common good, including health.

Public health advocates often argue that individual freedom is taken to the extreme when companies are permitted to profit regardless of the consequences for health and safety, whereas industries insist that they have the right to promote products that are legal. How public advocates make the case for their position will influence which ethic comes to dominate public health policy, because how they argue for change, including the language they use, can either reinforce social justice values or undermine them.

The Language of Public Health

The dominant language, what sociologists Bellah, Madsen, Sullivan, Swidler, and Tipton (1985) called the first language, of America is individualism and personal responsibility. The central idea is that rugged individualism, self-discipline, and self-determination are the key variables for success in American society. Indeed, a recent Pew Research Center poll (2002) conducted in forty-four countries found that people in the United States were much more likely to believe that they are in control of their lives than to see their lives as subject to the effect of external forces. Thus, self-determination, personal discipline, and hard work are seen as dominant factors, reinforcing individualism. A shift to social justice demands a rebalancing of these values with others that Americans also hold (Wallack & Lawrence, 2005).

It is in this redefinition that language comes into play. Recent explorations by political scientists (Harrington, 1999; Reich, 1990; Tronto, 1994), sociologists (Gamson, 1992), and cognitive linguists (Lakoff, 1996) offer new tools to public health educators who want to communicate stronger social justice values.

Language is important to public health practitioners because how an issue is described, or framed, can determine the extent to which it has popular or political support. Language communicates thoughts and ideas, and certain words and phrases shape the way people think about issues. Framing battles in public health illustrates the tension in our society between individual freedom and collective responsibility, which Beauchamp (1976) articulated in terms of market justice and social justice. Recent analyses of language from various fields explain how frames influence public dialogue on social issues, with important consequences for public health. Using these new rubrics, we compare and contrast arguments used to oppose or support public health goals. We then identify the common public health frames across these issues to illustrate how clear, concise language, anchored in social justice values, can effectively reframe issues, concluding with lessons for health educators who need to frame public health issues effectively. Our focus is on debates involving corporate practices that harm health, but the principles apply in other contentious and controversial policy contexts.

A Caveat: Language Is Never First or Foremost

Although language is a crucial expression of public health values, it should never be an advocate's first and foremost consideration. Before determining what to say, public health advocates must determine what they want to change in concrete terms, the more specific, the better (Chapman, 2001; Themba, 1999). And advocates need to know how to create the change (Chapman & Lupton, 1994; Wallack, Dorfman, Jernigan, & Themba, 1993; Wallack, Woodruff, Dorfman, & Diaz, 1999). Only then should they turn to considerations of language. The language public health educators use needs to grow out of policy that needs first to be rooted in social justice values.

Still, close attention to language is necessary and important because it is how public health advocates make their case for the change they want and a key mechanism with which they communicate their values. Once the steps to a solution for a given public health problem have been identified and the mechanisms for instituting them have been determined, then language should be developed to communicate the solution and why it matters. That language, the specifics of the message, will then emerge from how the issue is being framed.

Framing: What It Is, Why It Matters

Framing means many different things to people. Some think of framing as finding the right word, whereas others believe that frames tap complex moral structures that trigger how people react to a whole constellation of social and public policy issues in our society. We describe two types of frames—conceptual frames and news frames—that we believe have the most bearing on how to create messages that emphasize public health as social justice.

Conceptual Frames

Lakoff (1996), a cognitive linguist, argues that frames are the conceptual bedrock for understanding anything. People are only able to interpret words, images, actions, or text of any kind because their brains fit those texts into an existing conceptual system that gives them order and meaning. Just a few cues, a word or an image, trigger whole frames that inspire certain interpretations in audiences. Frames are often expressed in metaphors that people routinely use to understand abstract issues: "Horse race metaphors are common in political campaigns; war metaphors are common in discussion of health threats; and sports and business metaphors are common in other areas" (Lakoff & Morgan, 2001, p. 18). For example, the California Chamber of Commerce regularly issues a list of job-killer legislation it tries to defeat. The term is simple and evocative. *Killer* implies that someone is coming after you and that the situation is threatening, even dire. Killers must be stopped. They must be punished. Their targets need immediate protection and defensive maneuvers. The frame evokes these ideas before we have even an inkling of what the specific legislation might be about. In fact, if the chamber is successful with its job-killer frame, it will not ever have to debate the merits of the bill. The frame will preempt any discussion about the benefits of the legislation.

Political scientist Gilliam (2003) explains that frames are the "labels the mind uses to find what it knows." Frames are a composition of elements—visuals, values, stereotypes, messengers—which together trigger an existing idea. They tell us what this communication is about. They signal what to pay attention to (and what not to), they allow us to fill in or infer missing information, and they set up a pattern of reasoning that influences decision outcomes. Framing, therefore, is a translation process between incoming information and the pictures in our heads (Gilliam, 2003).

It takes very few words to trigger a frame. Consider this example from a poll *The New York Times* conducted in 2000. By changing just a few words, pollsters registered a marked difference in audience response. When asked whether leaders in Washington should allocate an expected budget surplus to tax cuts or government programs, 60 percent chose tax cuts. But when asked the same question in a slightly different way, "should the money be used for a tax cut, or should it be spent on programs for education, the environment, health care, crime-fighting, and military defense?" (i.e., government programs), 69 percent chose the more tangible list. Small differences in the poll question elicited significantly different responses, illustrating the power of language. But more than just the word, it is the conceptual framework that the word *government* evokes that is critical here. Government, in this instance, triggers interpretations such as waste, inefficiency, or giving people something for nothing, all of which undermine the role of public health.

Framing Levels Move from Values to Strategy

Lakoff describes three conceptual levels for framing messages in the context of public health and other social or political issues (personal communication, June 2004). Level 1 is the expression of overarching values, such as fairness, responsibility, equality, equity, and so forth, the core values that motivate us to change the world or not change it. Level 2 is the general issue being addressed, such as housing, the environment, schools, or health. Level 3 is about the nitty gritty of those issues, including the policy detail or strategy and tactics for achieving change.

Messages can be generated from any level, but Level 1 is most important because it is at Level 1 that people connect in the deepest way. According to Lakoff (1996), people's support or rejection of an issue will be largely determined by whether they can identify and connect with the Level 1 value. Values are motivators and messages for social change should reinforce and activate values. Messages, therefore, should articulate Level 1 values and not get mired in Level 3 minutiae. Public health advocates must know the Level 3 details (e.g., what needs changing and how the change will occur), but those details need not be prominent in the message. In fact, if Level 3 details crowd out Level 1 values, Lakoff contends that the message will be less effective.

The difference between how Level 1 and Level 3 are expressed in messages is nicely illustrated in an example from how health care was discussed in the 2004 presidential campaign. Quotes from President George W. Bush and his Democratic challenger, Senator John Kerry, are easily recognizable as Level 1 and Level 3 messages. In a radio story early in the campaign, National Public Radio reporter Julie Rovner compares the health plans being touted by Bush and Kerry, noting the details and differences between them, including the fact that Kerry's plan will cover a far greater percentage of the uninsured than Bush's plan would. At different points in the story, she includes a statement, passionately delivered, from each man:

> *President Bush:* The debate is about whether or not the marketplace ought to have a function in determining the cost of health care or whether or not the federal government should make all decisions. I've made my stand. I believe that the best health care policy is one that trusts and empowers consumers, and one that understands the market.
>
> *Senator Kerry:* Have your co-pays gone up? Have your deductibles gone up? Then you need to tell this administration that we're fed up, and their time is up. . . . [My plan] will reduce the average premium by $1,000 a year and it will crack down on the skyrocketing drug prices we face today. [Rovner, 2004]

Rovner notes that President Bush's concern is less about the differences between the plans and more about values. Indeed, President Bush's statement about health care clearly reflects his Level 1 market justice values, whereas Senator Kerry's statement focuses on the details of the plan, a Level 3 frame. If the market justice perspective around reforming health care dominates debate at Level 1, reinforcing the idea that the market will solve the problem with minimal government action, it does not matter how forcefully advocates can argue the details of the policy at Level 3. This is because, as Lakoff (1996) says, frames trump facts, and the frame is set at Level 1. To compete with Bush's statement and reframe the debate, Kerry would have to make a similarly strong statement communicating his Level 1 values, perhaps based on what he believes is fair and right for Americans rather than the details of how the plan will operate.

Of course, simply because the Level 1 frame is asserted does not mean it will carry the day; there are many factors at play that influence the outcomes of elections and policy debate, and framing is only one, however important. It is also worth noting that unfortunately, advocates' tendency is to argue the fallacy of their opponent's Level 1 frame, in this case, the basic idea that an unfettered marketplace will solve the health care crisis. Cognitive linguists and other communication scholars suggest that advocates should resist this impulse because such arguments will only reinforce the existing frame. Thus, public health advocates will have the strategic advantage when they set the Level 1 frame themselves, not when they respond to an opponent's frame that has already been set.

The theoretical and empirical work on Level 1 values and how they affect messages is nascent but likely to be important and valuable to public health educators because, in general, many are more adept at describing Level 3 details than they are at integrating Level 1 values. Insofar as Level 1 values set the frame, the advantage will be with those groups who most easily and frequently trigger their values in key audiences.

Different Level 2 issues can share the same Level 1 values. Below are sample messages from three different issues—tobacco, alcohol, and affordable housing—that share the same Level 1 value, in this case, fairness and equity. The policies used here are examples, and at any given time, the specifics of the policy may change. When they do, the values statement may remain consistent, or it too may change.

For alcohol, with a Level 3 policy goal of limiting the number of places alcohol is sold, the message might be the following:

> Too many liquor stores detract from the quality of life. It is not fair that certain families are subjected to such degraded conditions. Every family should have the opportunity to raise its children in a healthy environment. The city should make a rule to limit the number of liquor stores allowed within a certain radius.

For tobacco, with a Level 3 policy goal of enacting clean indoor air laws across all sectors of the city, the message might be the following:

> While we have achieved great progress in reducing smoking, there are still large populations, primarily in low-income communities of color, that are regularly exposed to toxic secondhand smoke. It is not fair that some of our cities' workers are protected and others are not. We should enact uniform clean indoor ordinances to protect workers in all workplaces, including restaurants and bars.

For affordable housing, with a Level 3 policy goal of providing rent subsidies to low-income families, the message might be the following:

People who need housing can't get it even though they work two jobs. Without a place to live, basic family life is shattered. It is not fair that hardworking people cannot find an affordable home. The city council should pass the rent subsidy resolution immediately.

News Frames

Conceptual frames operate inside our heads to organize and interpret the cues we get from the world. But where do the cues come from? In greater numbers than ever before, people in our society get their information, especially what they know about any person or situation they don't personally experience, from the media, especially the news.

Although the entertainment media transmit ideas and mores through popular culture, the news is the site for our public conversation, the place where policy issues are debated and framed. As early as 1922, commentator Walter Lippmann warned that news was functioning to provide the pictures in our heads that were determining policy decisions. The news, then, is an important source of frames as well as the terrain on which public health policy is debated and so warrants a closer look. What we find is that the routines of producing news have shaped typical news frames in ways that make public health stories that communicate social justice values harder to tell.

In the context of news, frames organize the meaning in stories, delineating what is and is not important. Communications researcher Robert Entman (1993) suggests four functions of news frames:

Frames . . . *define problems*—determine what a causal agenda is doing with what costs and benefits, usually measured in terms of common cultural values; *diagnose causes*—identify the forces creating the problem; *make moral judgments*— evaluate causal agendas and their effects; and *suggest remedies*—offer and justify treatments for the problems and predict their likely effects. [p. 52]

Similar to a frame around a painting, the news frame draws attention to a specific picture and separates told from untold pieces of the story. Elements in the story are said to be in the frame; elements left out of the story are outside the frame and are thought to be unimportant or less legitimate.

News frames can also refer to the structure of a story. Sociologist Todd Gitlin (1980) notes that frames are "persistent patterns" by which the news media organize and present the news so that it concerns "the event, not the underlying condition; the person, not the group; conflict, not consensus; the fact that 'advances the story,' not the one that explains it" (p. 28). The structural pattern is evident in newspaper stories but is even more pronounced in local and network television news.

Political scientist and communications scholar Shanto Iyengar (1991) demonstrates that (1) most television news is framed in terms of individuals and events, what we call portraits and what he called "episodic," and (2) audiences interpret episodic stories in ways that tend to blame the victim.

According to Iyengar (1991), when people watch news stories that lack context, they focus on the individuals. Without any other information to go on, viewers tend to attribute responsibility to the people portrayed in the story for the problem and its solution. In other words, they blame the victim. Without a sense of the forces that brought the people in the story to this point, viewers are likely to distance themselves from the victims portrayed, assume that those portrayed in the story brought it on themselves, look to them to work harder to solve their own problem or accept the consequences of their behavior, and gain no insight into the larger social and political circumstances that contribute to the individual problem.

It is not surprising that the most prevalent news frames would inspire interpretations of personal responsibility in audiences. As an integral part of American culture, the media reflect the dominant values of that culture. So the first language of America, individualism, is also dominant in news portrayals.

To counter this dominant news frame, advocates must help reporters do a better job describing the landscape surrounding individuals and events so the context of public health problems becomes visible. Iyengar (1991) called these stories thematic.

Thematic stories may engage viewers with a personal story, but they also give them more: background, consequences, and other information that provides context. Iyengar (1991) found that viewers who see thematic stories understand that responsibility is shared between individuals and their institutions and found that viewers are more likely to recognize that the government or other institutions have a role in solving the problem.

Typical News Frames Are More Often Portraits Than Landscapes

A simple way to distinguish story types is to think of the difference between a portrait and a landscape (see Chapter Nine). In a news story framed as a portrait, audiences may learn a great deal about an individual or an event, with great drama and emotion. But it is hard to see what surrounds that individual or what brought him or her to that moment in time. A landscape story pulls back the lens to take a broader view. It may include people and events, but it connects them to the larger social and economic forces. News stories framed in such a manner are more likely to evoke solutions that do not focus exclusively on individuals but rather also focus on the policies, institutions, and conditions that surround and affect them.

The key value that is affected by portrait and landscape frames is responsibility. News stories focused on people or events evoke feelings of personal responsibility in audiences. Landscape stories evoke shared responsibility between individuals and institutions. Advocates should strive to make stories about the landscape as vivid and interesting as the portrait. This is not easy to do but is crucial. The framing challenge for public health educators is to create landscape stories that are as compelling as portraits and include Level 1 values statements.

There are economic imperatives in the media business that compel reporters to pursue portraits rather than landscapes. Corporate concentration has forced news outlets to abandon public interest goals to pursue profit in the form of larger audiences (Bagdikian, 2004). Stories framed as portraits serve that purpose better than landscapes because they are easier stories to tell and presumably attract a larger audience.

Framing Public Health

Public health issues, such as tobacco, alcohol, guns, and traffic safety, have all experienced a transition from a focus on behavior to attention to policy that affects the environments in which the behavior takes place. The issue of drinking and driving provides one example. In the 1950s, the issue was barely visible as a public health problem. Drivers had "one for the road" before they left the bar. Alcohol problems were personal problems, and the remedy was to drive defensively. The development of a national focus on alcohol problems coalesced in the 1970s with the formation of the National Institute on Alcohol Abuse and Alcoholism, which began concentrated government support for research and intervention. The issue gained greater visibility and began to mature in 1980 when Mothers Against Drunk Driving (MADD) was founded to support families of victims and advocate for cultural change regarding how society tolerated drunk drivers. Combining forces with public health advocates who investigated and promoted a variety of prevention strategies, MADD expanded its purpose and scope to focus on state policies across the country. The alcohol issue has matured during the past 50 years. Most states now have a 0.08 blood alcohol limit, and as a nation, we have a 21-year-old drinking age. Although many programs still focus on personal drinking behavior, others include such policy goals as reducing alcohol outlet concentration in the inner city, removing alcohol advertising that reaches kids, and raising excise taxes (Dorfman, Ervice, & Woodruff, 2002).

In fact, many health and social problems are related to conditions outside the individual's immediate control. A focus limited to personal behavior change ultimately fails us as a society because it narrows the possible solutions inappropriately. For example, individual children and their parents need to make healthy personal choices so they will grow up with strong bodies and sound minds. If they do that, we should have a healthier society. But the choices are difficult and sometimes impossible. How can children get adequate exercise—important for establishing good habits and preventing childhood obesity and adult cancer—if there are no safe places to play? Or if physical education is no longer an available part of the school curriculum? Or if there are insufficient resources for after-school sports? Personal choices are always made in the context of a larger environment. Prevention can address both ends of the spectrum.

The language problem that ensues for public health educators derives from the challenges inherent in advocating for prevention that requires social or environmental change. Inevitably, environmental changes are more controversial than changes in personal behavior because they generally require a shift in resources or responsibility. The changes tap into Level 1 values, such as fairness and responsibility, and how those values are interpreted. For example, is fairness about being able to choose any vehicle one wants, no matter how unsafe or gas-guzzling? Or is fairness about the government providing standards for products that protect health and safety? How should responsibility for auto safety be shared? These arguments will be contested in highly visible public settings, such as legislative hearings. (Personal behavior changes may also be contested but usually by individuals in private settings.) Typically, the debates surrounding the social changes, be they policies to restrict tobacco use, limit access to alcohol, change the way motor vehicles are manufactured, or ban certain firearms, will be carried out in the news.

Public Health Issues in the News

Research across various public issues has upheld Iyengar's (1991) findings that typical news stories are episodic, focused on individuals or events. Studies of childhood lead poisoning (Bellows, 1998), childhood nutrition policy (Woodruff, Dorfman, Berends, & Agron, 2003), immunizations and other children's health issues (Lawrence, 2002), injury and violence (Chávez & Dorfman, 1996; Dorfman & Schiraldi, 2001; Dorfman, Woodruff, Chávez, & Wallack, 1997; Jernigan & Dorfman, 1996; McManus & Dorfman, 2005), including the policy discussions surrounding guns (Woodruff & Villamin, 1997) and alcohol (Dorfman & Wallack, 1998), have found an emphasis on episodic stories, paralleling what Iyengar found on a variety of other issues in the news. Public health perspectives, in particular, are rare in news coverage. In one of the largest studies of local television news, more than 200 hours of local news broadcast across California in English and Spanish, only one story among 8,021 aired during a 12-day period, or about 2 minutes of news, was devoted to violence as a public health issue (see Chapter Nine).

Studies of children's issues in the news have found an abundance of news that mentions children's health but, similar to the violence coverage, a dearth of in-depth reporting on the consequences of ill health or poor conditions for children, their families, or society at large. One study of childhood nutrition policy, for example, designed to maximize the number of policy-related stories, found that advice to parents was the single largest subject in the sample. The study found advocates describing the problem of childhood obesity using environmental, upstream concepts (e.g., "supersizing," too much TV and sedentary activity, and fast food in schools), but when it came to describing solutions, they reverted to the individual and described personal behavior, generating individually oriented "news-you-can-use pieces," which reporters love but which may undermine a public health approach to childhood obesity (Dorfman et al., 2002). A follow-up study added childhood immunization, childhood injury, and children's health insurance to the mix and confirmed the earlier findings, going further to establish that although children's health policy is present in news stories, the values underlying the policies are rarely expressed (Lawrence, 2002).

Overall, the findings from the various studies suggest that public health issues are rarely portrayed in the news in ways that encourage audiences to comprehend and ponder the underlying causes of problems or their potential policy solutions. Health stories, similar to other news, reinforce values of individualism and personal responsibility that feed the market justice perspective. This perspective comes out clearly in the comments from industry spokespeople in news stories and constitutes one of the more difficult challenges that public health educators must address, or reframe, in their own messages.

Anticipating the Opposition Frames

Because corporations' goal, and fiduciary responsibility, is to sell more of their products, their statements reflect a market justice value system. As former U.S. Surgeon General Antonia Novello (1992) noted, "One of the fundamental paradoxes of market-oriented societies is that some entrepreneurs—even acting completely within the prescribed rules of business practice—will come into conflict with public health goals." Corporate actors use all the resources at their command, including vast advertising and public relations budgets, to actively promote their market justice values.

The statements corporate spokespeople make in the face of public health challenges are remarkably similar. Statements from various industry spokespeople opposing public health measures generally reflect Level 1 market justice values: first, what's needed is more personal responsibility, not government regulation; second, as a precursor to taking personal initiative, education can solve the problem; and third, if the issue involves children or youth, this is really the parent's responsibility (see Table 6.2).

TABLE 6.2. STATEMENTS FROM CORPORATE
SPOKESPEOPLE ON VARIOUS PUBLIC HEALTH ISSUES.

Industry	Statement	Level 1 Value
Toy industry (product safety)	"Legal products can enter the market, and the public rejection or acceptance determines what goes from there" (Douglas Thompson, personal communication, November 5, 1987).[a]	Market justice
Alcohol	"All our efforts are based on our belief that education and awareness are the best ways to build personal responsibility. Every individual chooses if and how he or she will use our products. In a free society, we can only encourage wise choices, legislating them has never worked" (from a full-page ad from Anheuser-Busch that appeared in *The New York Times*).[b]	Free will, personal responsibility
Advertising	"Only through education programs in schools at all levels, in the workplace, and through public awareness campaigns such as those sponsored by the Advertising Council and alcohol beverage manufacturers can our society make real progress against alcohol-related problems" (DeWitt F. Helm Jr., personal communication, December 10, 1990).[c]	Education will set you free
Fast food	"I wouldn't say we're part of the [obesity] problem. There are not good or bad foods. There are good and bad diets. This does come down to personal responsibility" (Steven Anderson, quoted in Barboza, 2003).[d]	Free will, personal responsibility
Guns	"Safety and education are the main components for addressing problems of this nature. You cannot legislate against accidents happening" (Dave Marshall, quoted in Wintemute, Teret, Kraus, Wright, & Bradfield, 1987).[e]	Education will set you free
Soda	"As with most public health challenges, more and better consumer education is the answer" (McBride, 2003).[f]	Education will set you free

[a]Douglas Thompson, president of the Toy Manufacturers Association of America, in a letter to Dr. Garen Wintemute regarding his request that they not support making toy guns that look identical to real guns.

[b]Anheuser-Busch ran a full-page ad claiming that it does not use television to increase consumption of its product but only "to build brand loyalty and to promote responsibility."

[c]DeWitt F. Helm Jr. is president of the Association of National Advertisers and wrote this in a letter to President George Bush protesting Surgeon General Novello's (1992) call for restrictions on alcohol advertising targeting youth.

[d]Steven Anderson is president of the National Restaurant Association, which represents big outlets, such as McDonald's and Burger King, as well as thousands of other restaurants.

[e]Dave Marshall is speaking for the National Rifle Association on KTXL Channel 40 in Sacramento, California, in response to Dr. Garen Wintemute's study on childhood injury from gunshots.

[f]Sean McBride is a spokesperson for the National Soft Drinks Association.

Public health advocates can use the insights from the framing literature to anticipate and counter these frames by constructing messages that incorporate their own Level 1 values into concise descriptions of the problem and what should be done to address it.

The Components of a Message

Advocates can influence interpretations in any context by triggering frames that connect to their values. They can influence interpretation of news stories by creating news that makes the context visible. Effective messages meld specific policy demands with value statements that are delivered by strategically chosen messengers to specific targets. They are framed to emphasize Level 1 values and illustrate the landscape. Advocates can structure their messages this way by clearly and simply specifying the components of a message using three questions: What's wrong? Why does it matter? What should be done about it?

The first question forces advocates to make a clear statement of concern. It flows directly from the overall strategy, which advocates should determine before they construct their message. Too often, advocates try to tell journalists everything they know about the issue, because they feel this may be their only opportunity to convey the enormity and importance of the problem. They should resist that urge. It is impossible to be comprehensive and strategic at the same time. Instead, public health advocates should focus narrowly on just one aspect of the problem and be able to describe it succinctly. Once that portion of the problem is being addressed, they will be able to shift their policy goal and message to focus on another aspect of the problem.

The second question represents the value dimension. This is the place for advocates to shout their Level 1 value, to say what is at stake. Several studies show that advocates do not do this enough. In news coverage, the value component is often absent (Chávez & Dorfman, 1996; Dorfman & Schiraldi, 2001; Dorfman & Wallack, 1998; Dorfman et al., 1997; Jernigan & Dorfman, 1996; Lawrence, 2002; McManus & Dorfman, 2005; Woodruff et al., 2003; Woodruff & Villamin, 1997). Values should be specific and clear and should describe why the target audience (often a single policymaker) should care. Advocates can use this part of the message to call on their target's sense of fairness, duty, or fiscal responsibility.

The third question articulates the policy objective. A common pitfall is that advocates expend so much energy communicating about the problem that when the inevitable question about the solution is asked, they are ill prepared to answer it. They give vague responses such as "Well, it is a very complex problem with many facets, so the solution is complicated" or "The community needs to all come together." Certainly these responses are truthful, but they are not strategic; they do not advance the issue toward a specific solution. More effective by far is to answer with a specific, feasible solution, even if it is an incremental step toward the larger goal. This is not to say that there is only one solution to complex and difficult public health problems but rather that solutions generally evolve from small steps throughout time.

As an example, consider this core message used to publicize a study of fast food sold in California high school cafeterias, the *California High School Fast Food Survey*, released by the Public Health Institute in 2000. The study highlighted the surprisingly high percentage of high schools with branded fast-food outlets on campus and called for institutional solutions at both the local school district and state government levels. The core message, used in discussing the results with journalists and policymakers, was developed by staff at California Project LEAN (Leaders Encouraging Activity and Nutrition), a project of the California Department of Health Services, and was as follows:

1. What's wrong? Fast food is widespread on high school campuses.
2. Why does it matter? Fast food on campus contributes to youth obesity and endangers the health of the next generation.
3. What should be done? Two solutions are key: (a) Schools must promote appealing, affordable healthy food options for students, and (b) the government must provide adequate funds for food service so that local school districts do not have to supplement their food service budgets by contracting with fast-food vendors.

Project LEAN's message reflects a strategic approach to communicating about obesity prevention. The problem statement does not attempt to describe every facet of life that may contribute to youth obesity; it focuses on the specific problem of fast food sold on high school campuses. The values statement, although it could be more explicit, calls for responsible action to protect the health of the next generation. The solution statement articulates two concrete policy actions that, although not intended to solve the entire problem of obesity, will certainly make a difference in the environment within which schools and students are making their nutrition-related decisions.

The benefit of developing and adhering to such a focused and strategic message statement was apparent in the news coverage that followed the release of the *2000 California High School Fast Food Survey*. The event resulted in substantive news articles and opinion pieces in many California newspapers, many of which reflected the frame of shared institutional responsibility for addressing the problem of youth obesity. By contrast, many of the other news pieces on nutrition issues appearing during the same period were more likely to be superficial food features that resorted to traditional, individual-oriented advice about diet and exercise habits (Woodruff et al., 2003).

A news story that features an important public health issue can do more harm than good if it reinforces a blaming-the-victim frame for the cause and treatment of the problem and excludes the role for government and other institutions in solving the problem. This means that public health advocates must (1) be aware of the limited reach of most news frames and (2) work harder to help reporters focus more broadly, including on the social conditions and historical context beyond the individual or event, if they want key audiences to understand that responsibility for solutions to health problems must be shared across individuals and institutions, including the government. Left to their own devices, reporters will opt for the simple but interesting story about individual triumph or tribulation. But as Iyengar (1991) reminds us, "By simplifying complex issues to the level of anecdotal evidence, television news leads viewers to issue-specific attributions of responsibility, and these attributions tend to shield society and government from responsibility" (pp. 136–137).

Lessons for Public Health Educators

Framing involves more than a message; knowing what change will advance public health interests comes first, followed by a clear analysis of what it will take to make the change happen. Once those fundamentals have been established, the next step will be developing a message strategy to make the case for the change because, if the change is significant, it will be contested. How the message is framed can either establish or bolster support for the change or reinforce the opposition. Public health educators can draw on three key lessons gleaned from the literature on framing and the news to increase their chances of making a winning case for social change:

1. Understand and be able to articulate the core values and beliefs motivating the desired change
2. Articulate the components of messages so they integrate those values with a concise description of a key aspect of the problem and its corresponding, immediate solution
3. Develop media skills to be able to deliver the message and compete effectively with adversaries, including the ability to make the landscape, or context, of the problem and solution visible to reporters

The concepts underlying these lessons are being put to the test in defense of public health policies across issues and communities. Tobacco control advocates have perhaps the most collective experience and willingness to confront a market justice perspective. By now, their arguments are familiar and comfortable as they have spent decades challenging the idea that tobacco is simply a matter of personal choice. Although the tobacco industry remains a formidable opponent to public health interests and the fight is not over for the leading cause of preventable death, in that realm more than any other, advocates confidently reframe market justice values. Public health advocates working to reduce the harm from alcohol, guns, motor vehicles, lead, fast food, and a myriad of other issues will accelerate their progress as they strengthen their social change strategies and how they make the case for them.

By adopting these lessons, health educators will not create perfect messages that will stop the opposition in its tracks. Instead, better equipped to target their solutions and frame their messages, public health advocates will have renewed vigor for answering the frequent and forceful challenges they will receive any time they want to confront market justice norms and advance social justice values.

Conclusion

Many public health advocates share a fundamental worldview that reflects their values. They might not always agree on every issue or strategy, but they agree that the population's health is dependent not only on the choices individuals make but also the environments in which they make those choices. They recognize the interconnection between individual actions and the settings and circumstances surrounding those actions. They acknowledge that policy is an important tool for creating healthy environments.

Those who oppose public health policies see the world differently. The primary reason for society's progress, they believe, is personal initiative. Consequently, anything that inhibits that initiative is bad, and anything that fosters it is good. Public health advocates certainly do not eschew personal initiative, but they understand that it is constrained, or bolstered, by the world around it.

The discussion of values we have presented here may seem foreign to some in the field, particularly because another widely shared value in public health is objective science. Public health educators rightly search for evidence-based strategies that can guide their practice. But the reality is that epidemiology is limited; it is simply not as robust as we would like it to be in all situations. This means that sometimes health educators are making choices based on values, not science. Being clear about what those values are becomes crucial. When public health educators can articulate their values and balance market justice with social justice values, they will be able to transmit coherent, consistent, and compelling messages inside and outside the field.

Beauchamp's (1976) insights about public health as social justice have motivated a generation of health educators who have found themselves struggling against increasingly dominant market justice values. How the debate is framed, especially how it is framed in news stories, has had a profound effect on how Americans understand and relate to public problems. These analyses now can be used to reinforce and make tangible Beauchamp's notions of public health as social justice in the context of framing specific public health battles.

References

Bagdikian, B. H. (2004). *The new media monopoly.* Boston: Beacon Press.

Barboza, D. (2003, July 10). A warning in expanding waistlines, food markets trim fast as lawsuits and new regulations loom. *The New York Times,* p. C1.

Beauchamp, D. E. (1976). Public health as social justice. *Inquiry, 13,* 3–14.

Bellah, R. N., Madsen, R., Sullivan, W. M., Swidler, A., & Tipton, S. M. (1985). *Habits of the heart: Individualism and commitment in American life.* Berkeley: University of California Press.

Bellows, J. (1998). *Newspaper frames of childhood lead poisoning.* Berkeley, CA: Berkeley Media Studies Group.

Chapman, S. (2001). Advocacy in public health: Roles and challenges. *International Journal of Epidemiology, 30,* 1226–1232.

Chapman, S., & Lupton, D. (1994). *The fight for public health: Principles and practices of media advocacy.* London: British Medical Journal Publishing.

Chávez, V., & Dorfman, L. (1996). Youth and violence on local Spanish language television news. *International Quarterly of Community Health Education, 7,* 121–138.

Dorfman, L., Ervice, J., & Woodruff, K. (2002, November). *Voices for change: A taxonomy of public communications campaigns and their evaluation challenges.* Paper presented at the Communications Consortium Media Center, Media Evaluation Project, Washington, DC.

Dorfman, L., & Schiraldi, V. (2001). Off balance: Media coverage of youth crime. *Guild Practitioner, 58,* 75–78.

Dorfman, L., & Wallack, L. (1998). Alcohol in the news: The role for researchers. *Contemporary Drug Problems, 25,* 65–84.

Dorfman, L., Woodruff, K., Chávez, V., & Wallack, L. (1997). Youth and violence on local television news in California. *American Journal of Public Health, 87,* 1311–1316.

Entman, R. (1993). Framing: Toward clarification of a fractured paradigm. *Journal of Communication, 43,* 51–58.

Gamson, W. A. (1992). *Talking politics.* New York: Cambridge University Press.

Gilliam, F. D., Jr. (2003, December 19). Right for the wrong reasons. *Frame Works Institute Ezine, 26.* Retrieved June 16, 2004, from http://www.frameworksinstitute.org/products/issue26framing.shtml

Gitlin, T. (1980). *The whole world is watching: Mass media in the making and unmaking of the New Left.* Berkeley: University of California Press.

Harrington, M. (1999). *Care and equality: Inventing a new family politics.* New York: Routledge.

Iyengar, S. (1991). *Is anyone responsible? How television frames political issues.* Chicago: University of Chicago Press.

Jernigan, D., & Dorfman, L. (1996). Visualizing America's drug problems: An ethnographic content analysis of illegal drug stories on the nightly news. *Contemporary Drug Problems, 23,* 169–196.

Lakoff, G. (1996). *Moral politics: What conservatives know that liberals don't.* Chicago: University of Chicago Press.

Lakoff, G., & Morgan, P. (2001, June). Framing social issues: Does "the working poor" work? In Institute for Government Innovation, *Public obligations: Giving kids a chance* (pp. 16–38). Cambridge, MA: Harvard University Press.

Lawrence, R. (2002). *American values and the news about children's health.* Berkeley, CA: Berkeley Media Studies Group.

Lippmann, W. (1922). *Public opinion.* New York: Macmillan.

McBride, S. (2003, November 15). Are soft drinks responsible for the obesity epidemic? *Beverage World,* p. 23.

McManus, J., & Dorfman, L. (2005). Functional truth or sexist distortion? Assessing a feminist critique of intimate violence reporting. *Journalism, 6,* 43–65.

Novello, A. C. (1992). Underage drinking: A report from the surgeon general. *Journal of the American Medical Association, 268,* 961.

Pew Research Center for the People and the Press. (2002, December 4). *What the world thinks in 2002: How global publics view their lives, their countries, the world, America.* Retrieved October 26, 2004, from http://people-press.org/reports/display.php3?ReportID=165

Public Health Institute. (2000). *2000 California High School Fast Food Survey: Findings and recommendations.* Sacramento, CA: Author.

Pynchon, T. (1973). *Gravity's rainbow.* New York: Viking.

Reich, R. (Ed.). (1990). *The power of public ideas.* Cambridge, MA: Harvard University Press.

Rovner, J. (2004, July 18). Health care fails to register in campaigns. *All things considered.* National Public Radio.

Smith, A. (2000). *The wealth of nations.* New York: Modern Library. (Originally published 1776)

Themba, M. (1999). *Making policy making change: How communities are taking the law into their own hands.* Berkeley, CA: Chardon.

Tronto, J. (1994). *Moral boundaries: A political argument for an ethic of care.* New York: Routledge.

Wallack, L., Dorfman, L., Jernigan, D., & Themba, M. (1993). *Media advocacy and public health: Power for prevention.* Thousand Oaks, CA: Sage.

Wallack, L., & Lawrence, R. (2005). Talking about public health: Developing America's "second language." *American Journal of Public Health, 95,* 567–570.

Wallack, L., Woodruff, K., Dorfman, L., & Diaz, I. (1999). *News for a change: An advocate's guide to working with the media.* Thousand Oaks, CA: Sage.

Wintemute, G., Teret, S., Kraus, J., Wright, M., & Bradfield, G. (1987). When children shoot children: 88 unintended deaths in California. *Journal of the American Medical Association, 257,* 3107–3109.

Woodruff, K., Dorfman, L., Berends, V., & Agron, P. (2003). Coverage of childhood nutrition policies in California newspapers. *Journal of Public Health Policy, 24,* 150–158.

Woodruff, K., & Villamin, E. (1997). *Junk gun bans in California newspapers.* Berkeley, CA: Berkeley Media Studies Group.

CHAPTER SEVEN

WORKING COLLABORATIVELY TO ADVANCE PREVENTION

Larry Cohen, Ashby Wolfe

From the civil rights movement to women's health organizing to environmental justice advances, history is full of examples of the power of collaboration. Collaboration is useful for accomplishing a broad range of goals that reach beyond the capacity of any one individual or organization. This chapter focuses on coalition building, one of the more common forms of collaborative work for achieving preventive health success. A coalition is a union of people and organizations working to influence outcomes on a specific issue (see Exhibit 7.1).

As noted by Butterfoss and Francisco (2004), "The pooling of resources and the mobilization of talents and diverse approaches inherent in a successful coalition approach make it a logical strategy for . . . prevention" (p. 108). Sometimes, people assume it's "natural" to lead coalitions and take for granted that they have the skills needed. But even though coalitions are a common and a logical approach to solving a problem, creating a successful coalition can be much more difficult than it may seem. Often groups fail or, perhaps worse, flounder, given the inherent challenges present in alliances between organizations and individuals. To avoid

Portions of this chapter are adapted from *Developing Effective Coalitions: An Eight-Step Guide* by Larry Cohen, Nancy Baer, and Pam Satterwhite, available at http://www.preventioninstitute.org/eight step.html

EXHIBIT 7.1. COLLABORATIVES AND COALITIONS.

Coalitions are affiliations of people or groups with a shared purpose. They are one of various types of group processes. The following are working definitions of other types of collaborative efforts. However, people may use the terms interchangeably for various types of collaborative partnerships. In this article, the word *coalition* is used in a general sense to represent a broad variety of organizational forms that might be adopted, including any of the following.

- **Advisory committees** generally provide suggestions and technical assistance to an individual or institution but do not make final decisions.
- **Alliances and consortia** tend to be semiofficial membership organizations. They typically have broad policy-oriented goals and may span large geographical areas. They usually consist of organizations and coalitions as opposed to individuals.
- **Commissions** usually consist of citizens appointed by official bodies.
- **Networks** are generally loose-knit groups formed primarily for the purpose of sharing resources and information.
- **Task forces** most often come together to accomplish a specific series of activities, often at the request of an overseeing body.
- **Associations** are generally formed by professionals or people that have common interests and tend to have a more formal structure.

this type of experience, which only erodes faith in collaborative efforts, people need to sharpen the skills that are necessary to make partnership building more efficient and purposeful.

This chapter addresses ways to build and maintain an effective partnership and common challenges of working in coalitions, including how to engage a diverse and effective membership, how to focus joint efforts on accomplishments, how to create an effective structure, how to develop and strengthen interdisciplinary partnerships, and how to resolve problems, including turf struggles, that can make coalitions ineffective. The information presented here is equally applicable to practitioners and organizations considering initiating and leading a coalition and to anyone participating in—and eager to strengthen—an established coalition.

Collaborating to Improve Community Health:
Smoking Education Coalition Achieves a Multi-City Policy

In 1984, the Contra Costa County, California, board of supervisors and all eighteen city councils in the county adopted uniform multi-city tobacco laws, becoming the first multijurisdictional region in the nation to do so. The legislation, restricting smoking in restaurants, workplaces, and public spaces, was a powerful victory against the tobacco industry and set the stage for other antismoking landmarks. The victory was achieved through the intricate web of resources that only a powerful coalition could secure. Larry Cohen walks us through the process.

While working as director of prevention for the Contra Costa County Health Services Department, I was involved in forming a coalition that brought together local chapters of the American Cancer Society, the American Heart Association, and the American Lung Association, as well as the county health department. In creating the coalition, it became clear that there was a lot to learn about how collaboration could be most effective in improving community health.

Since smoking contributes greatly to cancer and to heart and lung diseases, I assumed that the aforementioned organizations would be eager to collaborate with one another. I also assumed that they would identify policy as a key arena for changing tobacco norms and thus improving health. However, the organizations were not at first the natural partners that I imagined they would be. Instead of seeing potential partners and a common goal, each organization viewed the others as competition for the donations it depended on to maintain its staff and services. And when it came to prevention approaches, most of the organizations' notions of prevention were limited to information and education.

Fortunately, organization leaders, reminding one another of the values that brought them to careers in health, were able to set competition aside and find common ground. The basis for our alliance was the need to support a policy proposal that would confront smoking and its deadly health effects. In addition to the policy goal, part of what enabled member organizations to set their competitive fundraising hats aside was the notion that promoting a powerful policy agenda could expand the financial pie instead of leaving only crumbs to fight over. Thus by understanding the objectives of each coalition member organization and appealing to the organizations' fundraising goals and interest in addressing an alarming health problem, we were able to create the glue of shared interest. Because the county was not interested in fundraising, it was seen as impartial in that sense and thus could play a neutral facilitative role with credibility.

We formed the Contra Costa County Smoking Education Coalition. Together we proposed legislation that addressed the dangers of secondhand smoke exposure. One of the first challenges we faced was that a countywide policy doesn't have standing within the boundaries of the cities in that county. Contra Costa County had eighteen cities, some near one another, some contiguous, with many businesses operating in more than one. We agreed that without a multijurisdictional policy, smoking laws would become hard for both consumers and business owners to comply with. Different policies, or a patchwork with some cities having policies and some not, wouldn't work; countywide success was the key to creating a policy that could be successfully implemented. We began to strategize ways to build support for our initiative.

(Continued)

My naiveté was again revealed by my belief that as a county health official, I would be able to call on city managers to influence their city councils to pass our proposed legislation. I did not know, however, that the apparently common friction between cities and counties over issues like property tax allocations was thriving in Contra Costa County. Further, most cities in the United States (except those that also comprise counties) do not see health as a key issue for them. They don't have staff with responsibility for health and are apt to say "that's the county's responsibility—talk to the county health department." People involved with policy development in the county advised me that my calls to city managers would not have been returned, and even calls from the directors of the cancer, heart, and lung associations might well have been ignored, as such organizations have little influence on city government.

We set out in search of leverage and found that we already had it within our coalition. Board members of the Cancer Society, the Heart Association, and the Lung Association included influential and involved community members who in many cases also contributed to local politicians' campaigns. Doctors involved in the associations treated local politicians and their families and knew other local politicians through social networks. By taking an inventory of board members and volunteers and their contacts, we were able to widen our support network.

Rather than looking at cities as a whole, the coalition began looking one by one at every member of each city council and considering who would most likely influence them. We identified who on each city council would be most likely to sympathize with our legislation and approached that member first. We figured that a city council member might ignore a call from me, but a call from his or her number-one contributor or his or her father's heart surgeon would almost certainly be returned. And when local media received op-ed pieces and letters to the editor written by local health practitioners or could interview these practitioners, the media were apt to print their ideas.

Also, we identified the relevant skills and resources of each member organization. One was particularly adept at dealing with the media, another had strong ties to the business community, and some were able to rally their members and volunteers to show up at city halls and support the proposed legislation. As the initiative attracted attention, we received offers of funds and of volunteers, and these were funneled to the three nonprofits. In this way, we maximized our resources and quickly broadened our coalition to include business members, government officers, and other influential members of the community that would have seemed unlikely partners had we not fully appreciated the potential of our member organizations.

Media attention in the cities where legislation was proposed resulted in far more community education than might have been achieved through the use of brochures and also helped perpetuate volunteer involvement. Coordinators dispersed volunteers to various cities. They recruited citizens to sign onto the legislation or attend their local city council meetings in support of it. Involved community members, including members of the business community who helped counteract the notion that tobacco legislation was anti business and would damage bottom-line revenues, bolstered our argument. Our coalition was able to garner widespread support. Each city became an ad hoc strategy group. Coalition participants in each city figured out what the most important elements were in order to garner support and marshaled those forces.

Such momentum did not go unnoticed by the tobacco industry. In fact, shortly after our coalition's first meeting, the tobacco industry approached me through its lobbying arm, the Tobacco Institute. The institute's lead lobbyist for the state tried to persuade me over lunch that our coalition should use an educational instead of a policy approach. "We're not opposed to prevention," he said; "just prevention . . . *policy.*" In fact, the lobbyist offered a lot—resources for other prevention issues, educational materials with my name as the author—and implied that the institute would be happy to give me another job if we stayed away from policy. This was evidence that we were on the right track. As we continued to pursue legislation, the Tobacco Institute opposed it in every jurisdiction, attempting to organize business owners against it, questioning the veracity of our concerns about secondhand smoke, and flying in experts from across the country for media appearances and testimony. We identified clients who lived in the local communities and could speak about the impact of secondhand smoke to them. The industry efforts to parry our coalition failed.

Following the 1984 success, the local cancer, heart, and lung associations brought the collaborative approach to each organization's national offices. The national offices then joined with Americans for Non-Smokers' Rights to end smoking on airlines. Local coalitions prospered across the country, gradually upping their policy goals. In retrospect, it's clear that these ordinances had a ripple effect, leading to ever more smoking regulations by all levels of government, changing smoking norms, and ultimately improving health.

Advantages of Coalitions

Coalitions provide the opportunity to generate broad-based support to improve prevention efforts. They can serve as a forum to share information and resources, to consider a problem from different angles, and to combine forces to resolve it. By bringing together people who may be struggling to achieve the same solution, coalitions minimize duplication of effort and can accomplish objectives beyond the scope of any single organization. They are particularly useful for resolving complex problems. In fact, as the prevention strategist Marshall Kreuter and his colleagues point out, in attempting to solve complex community problems, prevention researchers and public health practitioners must understand that the process involves social, environmental, political, and scientific collaboration (Kreuter, De Rosa, Howze, & Baldwin, 2004). By working together, community and systemwide changes, such as policy victories that no group could achieve alone, can be made. Given that quality prevention requires creating these changes, this unique ability of coalitions is of particular importance.

Coalitions can be very beneficial for neighborhood groups. Because coalitions are comprised of a number of organizations, they tend to be taken more seriously and are often viewed as more credible than individuals when asking for community services or change in government or corporate practices. For example, if a city were to slate a local bicycle path for removal, a neighborhood association would be more successful than a lone individual in getting politicians' attention and preventing the path from being removed.

Coalitions can be particularly helpful for disenfranchised communities, which too often have no voice in decisions affecting them. In cases where these communities face the financial and lobbying power of corporations or address government institutions that maintain a bureaucratic "business as usual" approach of government in ignoring neighborhoods with the least clout, collaboration is essential in securing change. As has been shown through environmental justice organizing, collaborations can bring to light the inequities of environmental health decisions, such as the siting of toxic wastes and the placement of factories in neighborhoods where, without organizing, residents would have neither the wealth nor the clout to stop them.

One of the most powerful differences coalitions have made for disfranchised communities is the emergence of community-based participatory research, the concept that the community should have input into the conditions of how research is conducted and shared and the benefits given back to the community in exchange for allowing the research to be done. Traditionally, academic research institutions and government agencies perform studies in low-income communities, eliciting the support of grassroots organizations and other community members. Until residents organized effectively, these opportunities tended to benefit the institutions far more than the communities. Once communities organized into coalitions and began working together, they ensured that community needs were considered and that research done in a community would benefit it.

Coalitions can be valuable to government agencies. Coalitions between agencies allow governmental efforts to be aligned. Different departments of government tend to work in "silos" and have differing backgrounds, beliefs, and objectives. Sometimes this means that government agencies can be duplicating efforts or working at cross purposes. But from the broader community perspective, we expect and need our government agencies to operate as one entity working toward a common goal. For example, in violence prevention, health education and justice agencies need to work together. For nutrition-related chronic disease, health education and agriculture must combine efforts. And traffic safety improvements require input from health education, justice, zoning, and planning agencies. The tool known as Collaboration Math (Prevention Institute, 2002) can be particularly helpful in understanding how to meld the objectives and approaches of different disciplines. Partnerships with community groups can help agencies, especially health and human service organizations, better understand community needs and more effectively achieve them.

Eight Steps to Building and Maintaining an Effective Coalition

Although collaboration is a strategic and beneficial method for prevention efforts, successfully achieving it is a challenge. The eight-step guide presented in Figure 7.1 provides a framework for acknowledging and addressing difficult issues.

These steps are not necessarily meant to be undertaken consecutively or sequentially. Sometimes a situation necessitates that steps be conducted in a different order or even simultaneously. And there isn't always one right direction at each step. The key to an effective approach to coalition design lies in considering each step and having clear reasoning related to each decision.

FIGURE 7.1. DEVELOPING EFFECTIVE COALITIONS: THE EIGHT-STEP PROCESS.

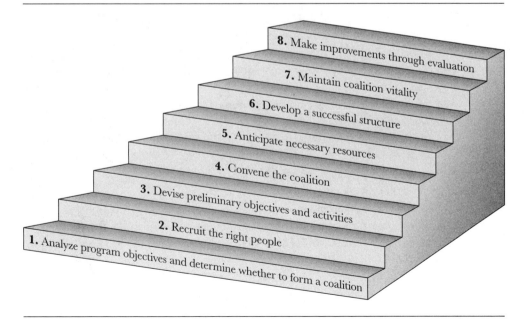

8. Make improvements through evaluation
7. Maintain coalition vitality
6. Develop a successful structure
5. Anticipate necessary resources
4. Convene the coalition
3. Devise preliminary objectives and activities
2. Recruit the right people
1. Analyze program objectives and determine whether to form a coalition

Most coalitions are developed by, or in any case require, a lead agency to work effectively. This paper is written from the perspective of the lead agency, although *every member of a collaborative has responsibility for leadership in helping shape its success.* The lead agency convenes the coalition and assumes significant responsibility for its operation. However, the lead agency does not control the coalition. A lead agency should consider carefully the responsibilities of developing and coordinating a coalition, including recognizing the amount of resources necessary to initiate and maintain it and the importance of respecting the differences between the coalition's and the lead agency's perspectives.

Step 1: Analyze Program Objectives and Determine Whether to Form a Coalition

Typically, three different situations may cause an organization to consider forming a coalition: the organization recognizes a community need or responds to community leaders' requests to facilitate an effort, the organization recognizes that a coalition will help it fulfill its own goals, or the process of building a coalition is required, for example, by a grant mandate. When deciding whether to form a coalition, a lead agency must first consider whether a coalition is the appropriate tool to serve the organization's needs and if the agency has the resources necessary to support the coalition.

First, the lead agency must clarify the objectives and appropriate activities. A coalition is one of a number of potential tools to get things done. Some tasks are inappropriate for coalitions because they may require quick responses that are unwieldy for coalitions or an intensity of focus that is difficult to attain with a large group. Coalitions are best used when broad support is needed, a diversity of views is beneficial, or multiple activities are needed to achieve a solution. If improving well-being requires changes in organizational practice, policies, or norms, a coalition is probably essential.

Obviously, it is important to clarify a coalition's purpose, directions, and general methods before approaching potential members. One tool for doing so is the Spectrum of Prevention, described in Chapter One, which is particularly useful for delineating the elements of broad-scale change.

Also, the agency should assess community strengths. In determining the coalition's efforts, it is important to fully assess current activities within the community. This clarifies the viability of the approach. It also generates knowledge about other groups working in similar arenas and locates crossovers or commonalities among interest groups (Action for Healthy Kids, 2003). Before initiating a coalition, it is important to determine if related partnerships already exist within the community. There are times when it will be far more effective to participate in an existing group with compatible goals than to form a new coalition.

It is valuable to determine the costs and benefits to the lead agency. Lead agencies tend to underestimate the requirements needed to keep coalitions functioning well, especially the commitment of substantial staff time. And coalitions also require significant commitment from the members, who must frequently weigh coalition membership against other important work.

Step 2: Recruit the Right People

"The main factor in unproductive business meetings is . . . having the wrong people present," says Lynn Oppenheim (as cited in Goleman, 1988). The makeup of a coalition's membership should be determined on the basis of its overall goals. Most coalitions should have members representing multiple sectors and points of view; however, coalitions with less diverse membership may communicate and work more quickly because members' objectives may be more alike. These coalitions, though, may be weaker in their ability to comprehend factors that contribute to the problem that lay beyond the purview of their member organizations. When coalitions are performing community-oriented work, it is important that the coalition's membership reflect the community that it serves. "Meaningful local-level engagement ensures the greatest relevance and appropriateness of programs for people affected and establishes essential ingredients for sustained collaboration" (Kreuter et al., 2004, p. 448). Those with the greatest stake in the community outcomes are likely to be highly effective in ensuring that collaboration serves the goals of the community rather than the interests of one discipline or constituency.

As discussed previously, coalitions are one of the premier ways that disfranchised groups, largely ignored by interest groups and elected officials, can have a voice. Not only is the input of these groups valuable to advocates not from the community, but it also provides a sense of ownership and involvement for the community.

Of course, not all coalitions are community-focused. For example, a statewide or national group might come together to develop a plan to address inequities in health. But if a coalition isn't diverse in every way—ethnicity, class, types of discipline—it should at minimum have considered the value of such diversity and be clear about the reasons it is taking another path.

The following are matters a lead agency should consider in recruiting coalition members.

Organizations. Start by identifying organizations that already work on the identified issue, and look broadly for other organizations that should be involved. Consider those who have influence, those who will be supportive, and even those who may put obstacles in the coalition's path.

Individual Members. Many coalitions welcome individuals who aren't affiliated with organizations. These individuals may be community members, community leaders, or people who have directly experienced the problem. Unless there is a reason not to, it is a good idea to include individual members because they can perform functions that other coalition members may not easily be able to perform. Since they are speaking for themselves and not for a larger organization, individual members may be perceived by the media as having less of a vested interest and therefore more credibility. In addition, individual members can provide advice and outreach from a different and perhaps more personal perspective. In one adolescent health coalition, a woman who had herself become pregnant as a teen was the best spokesperson for legislative hearings and meetings with the press.

Competitors and Adversaries. Whether to include potential competitors and adversaries should be based on the sincerity of their commitment to the coalition's goals, how willing they might be to reconsider some of their positions, and whether they will be more of an impediment to the coalition if excluded. For example, one violence prevention coalition did not allow a gun manufacturing company to join its coalition because the work of the company directly opposed the objectives of the coalition to reduce firearm use. However, the coalition did allow a toy company to join the coalition in the hopes that the coalition's efforts would encourage the company to produce alternatives to toy guns.

Keep in mind that a coalition must *get things done*—it isn't just a forum for discussion. Although engaging adversaries seems appealing, it can result in a very rapid drop-off of current members.

Representatives of Organizations. Having identified key organizations, consider who will best represent each organization on the coalition. Agency directors are often more effective at making policy decisions and establishing credibility as coalition representatives. On the other hand, line staff might be more committed, enthusiastic, and available than top leaders and are often more in touch with the issues related to "hands-on" service delivery. Often participation by a mix of top leadership and line staff is best for achieving coalition goals. Of course, organizations must make their own decisions about who represents them but are often responsive to suggestions.

Membership Size. Consider the desired number of organizations and the diversity of membership when selecting organizations to approach about joining the coalition. The coalition's goals and objectives are an important consideration in deciding membership size. As size gets larger (beyond about fourteen members), approaches to the work need to become more structured (as through the creation of subcommittees), less formalized, and facilitation of meetings requires greater skill.

Step 3: Devise Preliminary Objectives and Activities

In Step 1, the lead agency's objectives were examined in determining whether a collaborative was needed. It is important to meld these objectives with the objectives of other members and with the interests of stakeholders in the community whose goals generally fit with coalition objectives. Defining coalition goals and objectives and determining how to implement them require the inclusion of all coalition members in discussions. Therefore, the lead agency will need to broaden and modify its objectives. A written mission statement can be a useful tool to achieve clarity about coalition goals. However, it is important to avoid getting too bogged down in semantics early in the life of a coalition.

In some cases, coalition objectives or activities may be at cross purposes with those of an individual organization. Based on these cross purposes, one or another organization may elect not to participate in the coalition. It is important to anticipate these issues before they arise and try to design win-win situations.

Melding Objectives of Member Groups. Although some coalitions arise with a number of commonalities among the member organizations, each member organization usually has its own varying goals. It is important to create options that satisfy the goals of other coalition members and community partners and to structure both objectives and activities in such a way that other coalition members feel included in the decision-making process. The central mission of the coalition must fit both its own primary objectives and the overall community goals (Action for Healthy Kids, 2003). An example of this is the Harm Reduction Coalition, a group of individuals and agencies concerned with the lack of effective and respectful services for active drug users, particularly those underserved by traditional social and medical services: youth, women, people of color, and people living in poverty. While members may vary in their ultimate goals, they share a belief in *harm reduction,* a set of practical strategies that reduce the negative consequences of drug use, ranging from safer use to managed use to abstinence.

Coalition Goals, Objectives, and Activities. When dealing with long-term objectives over time, it is important to set some objectives and activities that can be addressed by all member organizations more immediately. Activities that parallel stakeholder interests will reinforce commitment to the coalition and may garner further community support. These activities increase members' motivation and pride while enhancing coalition visibility and credibility. However, always keep the long-range objectives clearly in mind. "Far too often . . . the effectiveness of a coalition decreases as the breadth of its agenda increases" (Black, 1983, p. 266). Activities should be well defined and meet the needs of participating organizations and make use of the skills of coalition representatives.

In some cases, broad goals can be accomplished best by joint activities with other coalitions rather than by a single coalition. For example, a traffic safety coalition, a sexual violence prevention coalition, and an alcoholism prevention forum could join together on a media campaign focusing on the norms promoted through alcohol billboards. While regular meetings of all of the coalitions in one broad group might prove unwieldy to the members, it can be in everyone's interest to work cooperatively on a specific issue.

Bear in mind that what keeps a coalition going is the commitment of the individual representatives and the support of the organizations they represent. Coalition members come to meetings with their own perspectives, interests, and approaches, and generally, the more directly coalition activities relate to and resonate with the specific values and objectives of the participants and the more each member is able to enjoy and be proud of his or her individual participation and contributions, the more the coalition will flourish.

Step 4: Convene the Coalition

Before convening the coalition for the first time, carefully select and talk with potential members to determine their individual goals and goals for the coalition. This way, conveners will have a good idea beforehand of how the first meeting will turn out. At the first meeting, the lead agency should clearly define the purpose of the coalition. In addition, the invited organizations and their representatives should have a chance to introduce themselves, state what they see as their role in the coalition, and consider what their organization's interest is in participating in the coalition. Potential members should be given an opportunity to define what they perceive as the purpose and goals of the coalition and to recommend others who they think should be involved. Of course, not all potential members will find the coalition worth their time and energy. Two determinants will be the specific activities the coalition chooses to undertake and the worth of the coalition as seen by the management of the member organizations.

Step 5: Anticipate Necessary Resources

Effective collaboratives generally require minimal financial outlay for materials and supplies but substantial time commitments from people. The most successful coalitions "take the time to build relationships, mobilize the community and personally visit the key players." (Wolff, 2001, p. 176). The ability to allocate considerable staffing to these and additional pursuits is one of the most important considerations for organizations providing coalition leadership.

Some of the specific resources that coalition leaders should anticipate include clerical needs; meeting planning, preparation, and facilitation; member recruitment, orientation, and encouragement; research and data collection; and participation in activities and projects.

It is important to recognize that coalition members' time is their most valuable contribution. Commitments are sometimes made in response to the enthusiasm of the meeting and seem less realistic when members return to their regular jobs. At other times, coalition members will fulfill their commitments but may resent the extra work. Periodic discussions about members' resources, support, and time limitations can minimize potential problems. Members should never be pressured to do more than they are comfortable doing. The more the coalition's objectives complement those of its member agencies, the less member time will seem like "extra" work.

Step 6: Develop a Successful Structure

The technical details, or "anatomy," of the coalition's structure are vital to achieving success. As with other coalition considerations, it is important to have well-developed ideas, as well as the flexibility to allow for input and modifications by coalition members. Six key structural issues are coalition life expectancy; meeting location, frequency, and length; membership parameters; decision-making processes; meeting agendas; and participation between meetings. There are no set rules about how a coalition should be structured, but each of these six elements should be dealt with thoughtfully. In all areas of coalition "anatomy," the same rules apply: minimize complications, maximize relevance to the objectives of the group, and encourage participation.

Coalition Life Expectancy. The coalition's goals should dictate its longevity. Although an open-ended time frame may seem attractive to the lead agency, member organizations and their representatives often prefer coalitions with a specific life expectancy. And such coalitions achieve more, more quickly. When long-standing credibility is a vital goal, an ongoing coalition might be needed.

Meeting Location, Frequency, and Length. To promote an atmosphere of equal contribution, consider holding coalition meetings on neutral territory, such as the local library. Rotating the meeting to different members' sites can add interest, although meetings may be delayed if people get lost or confused by ever-changing locations. The geography of the room—setting up conditions for thoughtful discussion and comfort and ensuring that people face one another—are essential conditions for achieving success.

Meeting frequency can affect the commitment of the membership as well. Other than an ad hoc emergency situation—such as a legislative deadline—coalitions typically should not meet more frequently than once a month.

Membership Parameters. Coalition members must play a role in decisions about the extent to which new members will be invited and how defined or open the membership should be. In many cases, a compromise solution in which certain people are recruited and encouraged but virtually no one is excluded is best. More formalized membership procedures may become an issue when and if the coalition wishes to make public statements or endorse policy measures; otherwise, less formal procedures are preferable.

Decision-Making Processes. Miller (1983) identifies good decision-making procedures as key to coalition success. He recommends establishing a specific decision-making process before problems occur. "You cannot count on stamina," he writes. "Make clear early in the life of the coalition . . . how decisions are going to be made" (p. 49). Decisions can be made by consensus. Research on community-based coalitions has suggested that this process reduces impulsive decision making and improves stakeholder participation (Snell-Johns, Imm, & Wandersman, 2003). However, this process can become unmanageable. To avoid this, define consensus as an approach that the majority supports and others can live with. Health-based coalitions are usually happy to relinquish some of the detailed decision making in exchange for simplicity and reasonable results. There will be cases in which consensus cannot be reached and the group must either vote or accept that there will be no action on a certain issue. Sometimes having the group clarify in advance the kinds of issues that are charged (grants, turf, or legislation, for example) will help avoid problems later.

Meeting Agendas. One of the most important ingredients for an effective coalition is a good meeting agenda. It gives participants, especially new ones, a road map and lets them know where they can best fit in. A clear and reasonably consistent agenda, which may be modified by those present at the beginning of the meeting, can reinforce the coalition's purpose and foster collaboration. The skill of keeping to the agenda but being flexible and open to new ideas is a vital one in maximizing meeting success.

Participation Between Meetings. Successful coalitions often have subcommittees, which carry out coalition activities. Unless coalition objectives are closely related to the objectives of the membership, it is not wise to expect more than a few hours of additional commitment between meetings. It may be helpful to encourage the most active and strategic participants in the coalition to form a steering committee, which provides leadership by discussing long-range goals and the tactics to achieve them. A steering committee often works well as an informal open body.

Step 7: Maintain Coalition Vitality

Building an effective coalition includes articulating a vision, establishing adequate structure, developing leadership opportunities, and making significant commitment to community diversity (Bandeh, Kaye, Wolff, Trasolini, & Cassidy, 2003). Leadership in coalition building requires knowing not only how to create a coalition structure but also how to recognize the warning signs of problems that may arise. It is important for leaders to work hard at maintaining the vitality and enthusiasm of the coalition. By dealing with potential problems as they emerge, however, the vitality of the coalition can be maintained. The following activities are important for maximizing coalition vitality.

Addressing Coalition Difficulties. One clear indication that a coalition is having difficulties is a decline in coalition membership. This may be due to multiple factors, including conflicts of interest, overlapping efforts, and role confusion, all of which may lead to the loss of collective voice within a coalition (Weed, n.d.). Although earlier warning signs are less obvious, they might appear as repetitious meetings or meetings that consist primarily of announcements and reports, meetings that become bogged down in procedures, significant failures in follow-through, ongoing challenges of authority or battles between members, lack of member enthusiasm, or an unacceptable drain on lead agency resources. Turf struggles are perhaps the most commonly identified explanation when vitality sags.

Tension over Turf

Turf struggles are a common threat to coalition vitality and success. Peck and Hague (2003) have defined "turfism" as noncooperation or conflict between organizations with seemingly common goals or interests. There are three types of turf struggles:

- *Coalition member versus coalition member:* Conflict between coalition members can reflect historical tensions between their organizations.
- *Coalition member versus coalition:* As a coalition gains visibility and starts to apply for funding, conflict can develop between individual coalition members and the coalition as a whole because of the increased competition for resources.
- *Members versus lead agency:* Lead agencies can sometimes benefit most from the work of the coalition, leading to tension among the members who see the lead agency acquiring the resources and recognition that result from the contribution of all coalition members.

(Continued)

Too often we expect self-sacrifice from individuals and organizations as they move toward coalition solutions. Instead of instructing members to "leave turf at the door," a more realistic approach acknowledges that turf issues will challenge the group and blends the pursuit of individual interests with the greater goals of the coalition. Coalition leadership can sometimes anticipate turf battles and make preemptive moves to avoid them. The following are suggestions that coalition leaders can use to illuminate turf struggles by bringing attention to some of the problems with the coalition and to limit the negative impact of turf squabbles.

1. Acknowledge potential turf issues. Choose coalition representatives whose job descriptions and personalities make them less influenced by the past.
2. Talk details. Encourage coalition members to openly discuss their reasons for being at the table and share information about their respective organizations at the initial coalition meeting.
3. Shape collective identity. Develop opportunities to fulfill the needs for recognition among members and foster a sense of collectivity.
4. Make fair decisions. Create a clearly stated decision-making policy in conjunction with coalition members to develop consensus when possible and ensure fairness.
5. Seek funding for coalition coordination. Secure outside funding to help alleviate internal pressure for resources, and develop a plan for how resourced needs will be shared, acquired, and distributed.
6. Reward members and celebrate successes. Acknowledge the accomplishments of the coalition to inspire and motivate members.
7. Build bridges. Maintain an environment fostering trust, respect, and amicability among coalition members through a friendly tone, small workgroups, and after-meeting socializing.
8. Remind participants of the big picture. If turf issues arise, make space in a meeting where an objective coalition member dedicated to the coalition's cause, such as a survivor, youth, or faith leader, can remotivate coalition members.
9. Make struggles overt. Acknowledge that conflict exists, and discuss potential causes so that it does not fester and drain the vitality of a coalition.
10. Encourage flexibility. Create an open environment where members feel comfortable with diverse perspectives and with conflict.

Source: Adapted from Cohen & Gould (2003).

Kreuter and colleagues note that a high failure rate of coalitions suggests that problems are not well anticipated, nor are they skillfully resolved once they occur (Kreuter, Lezin, & Young, 2000, p. 60). Therefore, it is crucial to maintain open communication among the members so that problems surface quickly. Although the lead agency will not always be able to overcome coalition challenges, effective management of the problem is an essential first step. In fact, all that may be needed is a decomposition of current activities into smaller, more achievable tasks. It may be necessary to revisit the original objectives of the coalition and modify them to more accurately reflect the current atmosphere (Action for Healthy Kids, 2003). It is the lead agency's responsibility to bring identified problems to the attention of coalition members and to encourage collaborative solutions. The most valuable source of information about negative coalition conditions is input from the coalition members themselves. People who are no longer attending or who have left the coalition are important sources of input as well.

Sharing Power and Leadership. Many coalition members will readily defer power to the lead agency to facilitate smooth functioning. However, if the coalition solidifies as an independent entity and develops a body of work that it performs or creates collectively, members will expect greater involvement in decision making. It is at this point that the coalition becomes a more independent group and requires less guidance from the lead agency. Ironically, the characteristics that indicate a strong coalition—a heightened sense of collective identity and a high degree of interest in and commitment to work that is developed collaboratively—can also exacerbate tensions in defining the direction of the coalition. It is important to deal with these issues directly. Negotiating issues of a power imbalance in decision making, especially when a coalition has achieved this state of maturity, calls for sensitivity and may require setting aside extra time to clarify.

New energy is often needed to restore a coalition. One way to achieve this is to recruit new members. Membership changes are to be expected. New members add energy and enthusiasm to the coalition's ongoing activities. Attention must be paid to ensure that they are welcomed and oriented to fulfill vital coalition functions. Another way to promote renewal is by providing training and by bringing challenging, new ideas to a group.

Celebrating and sharing successes may be the most important step in maintaining morale. Everyone needs a sense—and reminders—that the coalition is playing a vital role in addressing the problem. Acknowledgment of success, however small, is a key to maintaining the vitality and motivation of the coalition (Action for Healthy Kids, 2003). Keys to boosting coalition morale can include implementing effective activities that result in tangible outcomes, giving coalition members credit for coalition successes, and celebrating short-term successes with publicity or awards.

Step 8: Make Improvements Through Evaluation

Evaluation should be an ongoing process throughout the life of a coalition. Indeed, the success of the coalition itself can hinge on the evaluation process: "evaluation must be performed [to demonstrate] a sustainable infrastructure and purpose, programs that accomplish their goals, and measurable community impacts" (Butterfoss & Francisco, 2004, p. 113). Evaluating a coalition can lead to changes in the coalition's approach. In addition, evaluation can increase the coalition's effectiveness and can ensure that the community and participants benefit from the coalition's activities. Taking the time to evaluate the effectiveness of coalition efforts is a way of acknowledging that the skills and contributions of coalition members are important. Honest reflection also ensures that the coalition grows from its experiences, regardless of the programmatic outcome. The results, if positive, can also help the coalition improve its reputation in the community and can be included in future resource development proposals. Furthermore, when a coalition modifies its efforts to eliminate problems pinpointed by an evaluation, the coalition's credibility can improve significantly.

Coalitions can employ two basic types of evaluations: formative and summative. Formative evaluations focus specifically on the coalition's process objectives. For example, a coalition may want to encourage the media to promote a particular goal. A formative evaluation would analyze the process by which the coalition attempted to achieve this goal. The results of formative evaluations help staff and members improve the functioning of the coalition.

Summative evaluations help coalition members determine whether or not the coalition's strategies resulted in the desired consequences. The answers to summative evaluation questions help coalition members make strategic decisions about strengthening promising interventions and discontinuing ineffective ones. Coalitions often move in unexpected directions, and it is important to recognize that what may at first have been unintended consequences are in fact significant outcomes. Also, there is a tendency to just evaluate what the coalition as a whole has accomplished, but often there are new initiatives and new partnerships that emerge from different dyads and triads whose relationships become more solidified through the coalition.

Coalition evaluation is an emerging field and is much more demanding than simply determining if a program is effective. Because coalitions aim in many cases to achieve multifaceted environmental change, changes are harder to see and the coalition's role in them is difficult to measure. To ensure that evaluators advance the important work that collaboratives are engaged in requires melding existing evaluation skills with a new way of thinking.

Conclusion

Widespread and lasting change is difficult for any organization to achieve alone. Major improvements require a variety of resources and perspectives, and health leaders increasingly recognize that improving community health requires a new way of working, not only giving direction but also being able to engage in and facilitate partnership.

Virtually every carefully crafted coalition will have an impact. "An effort may fail, then partially succeed, then falter, and so on. Since mutual trust is built up over a period of time, coalition organizers should avoid getting so caught up in any one effort as to view it as 'make or break.' Every effort (at cooperation among groups) prepares the way for greater and more sustained efforts in the future" (Brown, 1984).

References

Action for Healthy Kids. (2003). *Coalition building: Tips and techniques.* Skokie, IL: Action for Healthy Kids. Available in hard copy from Action for Healthy Kids at (800) 416-5736.

Bandeh, J. G., Kaye, T., Wolff, S., Trasolini, A., & Cassidy, A. (2003). Developing community capacity. Module 1: Sustaining community-based initiatives. Battle Creek, MI: W. K. Kellogg Foundation/The Healthcare Forum.

Black, T. R. (1983). Coalition building: Some suggestions. *Child Welfare, 62,* 263–268.

Brown, C. R. (1984). The art of coalition building: A guide for community leaders. New York: American Jewish Committee.

Butterfoss, F. D., & Francisco, V. T. (2004). Evaluating community partnerships and coalitions with practitioners in mind. *Health Promotion Practice, 5,* 108–114.

Cohen, L., & Gould, J. (2003). *The tension of turf: Making it work for the coalition.* Oakland, CA: Prevention Institute. Retrieved October 12, 2006, from http://www.preventioninstitute.org/pdf/TURF_1S.pdf

Goleman, D. (1988, June 7). Why meetings sometimes don't work. *The New York Times,* p. B1.

Kreuter, M. W., De Rosa, C., Howze, E. H., & Baldwin, G. T. (2004). Understanding wicked problems: A key to advancing environmental health promotion. *Health Education and Behavior, 31,* 441–454.

Kreuter, M. W., Lezin, N. A., & Young, L. A. (2000). Evaluating community-based collaborative mechanisms: Implications for practitioners. *Health Promotion Practice, 1,* 49–63.

Miller, S. M. (1983). Coalition etiquette: Ground rules for building unity. *Social Policy, 4*(2), 47–49.

Peck, G. P., & Hague, C. E. (2003). *Ohio State fact sheet: turf issues.* Retrieved April 13, 2003, from phttp://ohioline.osu.edu/bc-fact/0012.html

Prevention Institute. (2002). *Collaboration math.* Oakland, CA: Author. Retrieved October 12, 2006, from http://www.preventioninstitute.org/collmath.html

Snell-Johns, J., Imm, P., & Wandersman, A. (2003). Roles assumed by a community coalition when creating environmental and policy-level changes. *Journal of Community Psychology, 31,* 661–670.

Weed, D. (n.d.). When coalitions collide: Managing multiple coalitions. Amherst, MA: AEHC/Community Partners. Retrieved October 12, 2006, from http://www.compartners.org/stacks/archive/hcm/cb_collide.pdf

Wolff, T. (2001). A practitioner's guide to successful coalitions. *American Journal of Community Psychology, 29,* 173–191.

CHAPTER EIGHT

MAKING CHANGE

The Power of Local Communities to Foster Policy
Makani Themba-Nixon

Prevention advocates increasingly find that if they are interested in shifting norms, traditional health education approaches are not enough. More and more, advocates are looking to the domain of law and other forms of social policy where many norms are forged. In tobacco control, for example, policies that raised the price of tobacco products and prohibited smoking in certain public spaces contributed significantly to the drop in prevalence for youth smoking as well as increased the number of smokers that quit (Chaloupka & Wechsler, 1997). Policies that regulate gun safety have contributed to decreasing gun-related death and injury (Sugarmann & Rand, 1998), and laws mandating seat belt use have contributed significantly to decreasing death and injury as a result of auto crashes (National Highway Traffic Safety Administration [NHTSA], 1997). These are some of the many examples of the importance of policy as a tool for primary prevention.

Policy is more than law. It is any agreement (formal or informal) on how an institution, governing body, or community will address shared problems or attain shared goals. It spells out the terms and the consequences of these agreements and is the codification of the body's values as represented by those present in the policymaking process.

Prevention advocates need to be present in the policymaking process as policy formation can be an effective tool for prevention. Policy initiatives—concerted campaigns to advance specific policies—can affect a community in at least two ways. First, enactment of the policy itself can address problems that put communities at risk and help improve quality of life. For example, policies to reduce access to tobacco have resulted in decreased use and mortality. Successful campaigns to raise local wages and benefits have meant increased access to health care and stabilized nutrition for affected families. Second, the act of organizing a community to engage in the policy initiative can increase social networks and reduce isolation and alienation, which can be as effective in reducing problems as the policy itself. For example, research shows that participation in local community institutions and organizations is considered vital for effective crime and drug abuse prevention. Efforts that engage community residents and give them a sense of their own power can make a real difference in their ability to solve problems as well as strengthen individual members' sense of community. Community-based efforts to change policy not only address problems through the policy changes they achieve but also aid communities in addressing the factors that put them at risk in the first place (Curtis, 1987; Florin, 1989; Mayer, 1984; McMillan & Chavis, 1986).

The best kind of policy initiative engages the community that shares the problem and ensures that it is a part of the solution. These initiatives take into account the kind of advocacy efforts required to make policy changes and look to expanding the base of support for public policy for future efforts. This chapter provides policymaking strategies on the local level from the perspective of historically disfranchised communities. Many times these communities have had experiences leading to a well-deserved mistrust of government and industry. Therefore, this chapter includes strategies of policymaking that can be used when government or industry is either unsupportive of or opposed to proposed policies.

Common Stages in the Development of a Policy Initiative

Most initiatives go through a development process characterized by seven stages (see Figure 8.1). Initiatives usually begin with some kind of testing the waters to help identify key issues and concerns to shape the second stage, where advocates take the relevant issues and form them into a clear policy initiative. In the third stage, advocates engage in strategy and analysis to assess public and policymaker support as well as mechanisms for building support and influence to advance the initiative. Implementing the strategy takes place throughout stages 4 and 5 as advocates engage in direct issue organizing to build support around the specific initiative as a way to effectively address issues of concern while often simultaneously working "in the belly of the beast" to steer the initiative through the appropriate

Policy Case Study: Mandatory Child Safety Restraints

"I walked out on the balcony alone and had a few tears well up. I said, 'By golly, it's happened, and if this works, it may happen all over the United States!'" That is how Dr. Robert Sanders, a soft-spoken Tennessee pediatrician and catalyst for groundbreaking injury prevention legislation, described his victory after a historic 1978 vote in the Tennessee senate over mandatory car seat use.

Today, few parents question the benefits of using child safety seats in cars. In fact, 99 percent of infants and 94 percent of toddlers nationally are restrained using child safety seats while riding in automobiles (NHTSA, 2004). Yet behaviors that are now norms were once anomalies. During the early 1970s, car crash injuries were the leading cause of death among children in Tennessee and in many other states, and car seat use was less than 15 percent nationally (Kahane, 2001). At that time, many legislators and citizens saw car seat use as an issue of personal freedom and civil liberties rather than a matter of injury prevention (Solomon, Leaf, & Nissen, 2001).

When Sanders became chair of the Tennessee chapter of the Accident Prevention Committee of the American Academy of Pediatrics, he realized that he had an opportunity and responsibility to address this easily preventable cause of morbidity and mortality through state legislation. In 1976, he proposed that Tennessee enact the nation's first mandatory child restraint law, but the bill was stopped in committee. Opponents vehemently attacked the bill and Sanders, even going so far as to falsely accuse him of owning stock in a safety seat manufacturing company.

The following year, Sanders redoubled his efforts. He, his wife, and the opposing lawmakers' own family physicians began to call legislators' homes on weekends to enlist their support. An impressive cadre of health professionals distributed fact sheets throughout the state. The bill was finally approved by two votes in 1978. By 1985, all fifty states had adopted similar legislation (NHTSA, 2002).

Between 1975 and 2004, approximately 7,472 lives were saved by child safety restraints systems (safety seats or seat belts) (National Center for Statistics and Analysis, 2004). During that same time, risk of injury to children was reduced by 59 percent when compared to children who used only safety belts (New York State Department of Health, 2006). Sanders's efforts not only saved children's lives in Tennessee and beyond but also established a precedent for using policy to effect broad norm and behavior change. One person's willingness to see beyond current trends in thinking, to take on the often uncomfortable job of changing norms, and to recognize the power of legislation in altering behaviors resulted in sweeping national change and set a precedent for similar initiatives. Arguably, the successful enactment of similar policies (such as helmet laws, drinking age statutes, and tobacco control regulations) was, at least in part, due to Dr. Robert Sanders's success.

Source: Prevention Institute.

FIGURE 8.1. STAGES IN THE DEVELOPMENT OF A POLICY INITIATIVE.

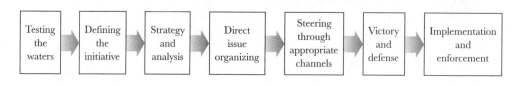

policymaking channels. If successful, advocates will move on to stage 6, victory and defense, to help solidify their policy victory and ensure that no subsequent legislation or litigation occurs to undermine the initiative. In the final stage, advocates are focused on effective enforcement and implementation of the policy so that it works as intended.

These stages are not strictly sequential but tend to overlap—more like a spectrum than a staircase. Often groups are working at more than one stage at a time once an initiative is under way. For example, groups will test the waters throughout the life of an initiative and use that feedback to refine and improve their work. Effective initiatives rarely miss any of these stages in development. Weaker initiatives often do. Sometimes groups will go ahead without much preparation because of some unique opportunity that "just wouldn't wait." It is true that the right timing can aid an initiative's success, but it is more often the case that groups wish they had waited and become better prepared. In any case, good preparation and solid organizing invariably help a group take better advantage of existing opportunities as well as create new ones.

Initiatives concerned primarily with the enactment of policy necessarily involve considerations and assessments of power. Advocates must consider what body has the power to enact the policy, where each individual member stands, and what influence members may have to help build support for the initiative. Even seemingly "win-win" initiatives such as seat belt mandates or lowering speed limits may face tough and at times unexpected opposition. Opposition can come not only from people who oppose the specific regulations but also from people concerned about regulations per se or people who feel that this regulation might become a stepping-stone or precedent for other regulations they don't want to see developed or that this might be a distraction from other efforts they regard as more important. Consequently, prevention advocates must pay attention to issues of power and take care to undertake the research, strategy development, and analysis necessary to ensure that they have not only evidence-based policy initiatives but community-based support as well.

A coalition in a small college town in Nebraska provides a poignant example of what can happen when groups try to skip the strategy development and organizing phases in the process. The group of alcohol policy advocates knew that alcohol abuse and consumption was involved in a large number of the hospital visits in their county, but the hospital did not keep track of alcohol involvement in admissions. The process of "external coding" or "E-coding" for alcohol-related injuries was beginning to catch on in hospitals in larger cities around the country, tracking additional factors in a hospital admission. The coalition surveyed the research and found clear evidence that developing a system for E-coding local data on alcohol-related admissions would be helpful in their efforts to better regulate alcohol in their town.

The chief hospital administrator, the policymaker with the power to enact the initiative, was a good friend of coalition leaders and a coalition supporter. The group took its initiative directly to the administrator without analysis or community organizing efforts because the leaders believed that the request would be swiftly granted. They were caught completely by surprise when the hospital administrator would not agree to enact the policy and in fact expressed strong opposition. The coalition partners had banked on their relationship with a decision maker without thinking through how the administrator might perceive the impact of such a policy on his institution or the risks in implementation. And without public support for the issue, the proposal was easy to dismiss.

It is a common mistake to launch policy initiatives without any preparation or prior analysis as required in the first three stages of development, before direct advocacy begins. Numerous policy initiatives skip stage 4 and therefore suffer from inadequate grassroots support because not enough attention was paid to community organizing. Advocates in this case often go directly to stage 5, working with policymakers, without grassroots support or even public awareness of their efforts in hopes that policymakers will be swayed by the "sensibleness" of their initiative. However, policy is not as much about acting sensibly as it is about negotiating interests. Advocates must never assume support based on the logic of their argument or the strength of a personal relationship.

It is also important to recognize that policy is a *process* of negotiation and compromise. When working on a policy for which there is little or no precedent, keep in mind that local governments are often afraid to be the first jurisdiction to adopt a new and untested ordinance. First ordinances are usually more conservatively written and less comprehensive than those that follow. It is always helpful to know about similar policy initiatives that have been enacted without legal challenge or upheld in court. Without some precedent, making a case for a new policy can be tough—but not impossible. In any case, it helps to decide early on what can be given up and what is nonnegotiable.

Stage 1: Testing the Waters

In the initial stage, most groups are focused on the problem and are just beginning to develop ideas for solutions. People sense that something concrete can be done about an issue, but no one is sure exactly what. It is important that a group spend time defining the specific problem or set of problems it would like to address through policy. Too often policy-related solutions to community issues are hard to find because the problems are too broadly defined. For example, a community with high rates of diet-related chronic diseases of children in local schools may need first to identify the problem it needs to address: the food being served in schools, the lack of parks and open spaces in the neighborhood for children to exercise, the prevalence of junk food advertising in the neighborhood, or something else. Once the problem is clearly and specifically defined, suitable approaches are easier to propose. Often a number of approaches are tested and screened for community support, legality, and likelihood of success. When a San Diego community group organized in the wake of the shooting death of a local youth, its first target was gun regulation. After conducting research on the legislative remedies available, the group focused on a ban on junk guns and local regulation of bullets. A key lesson: the coalition was flexible and moved in the direction that residents wanted to go.

Where to Focus. Policy development should not always focus on community problems. Sociologist John McKnight and his colleagues at Northwestern University pioneered a method of community mapping that enables neighborhoods to chart their assets and develop strategies for addressing issues based on their strengths. Used primarily in public health and community development efforts, asset mapping is a valuable tool for any group seeking to organize around any issue. The process includes detailed surveys of both institutions and individuals, building networks that help leverage both individual and institutional assets, and case studies and project ideas for implementing the project (see Kretzmann & McKnight, 1993).

Some of the best policies address a community's vision of what it would like to become instead of focusing on community problems or deficits. Usually, when a community works from a vision of itself, it manages to address a number of problems simultaneously. One example is found in the growing number of local policies to increase the amount of open parks and green space or unpaved natural areas for recreation and rest. Although these policies are a result of the residents' vision of their community as a beautiful place to live, increasing the number of parks in the community also helps address issues of blight, youth development, increasing physical activity, and negative land uses.

Community Context. Traditionally, advocates are individuals who speak on behalf of others. Advocates can be from a community affected by a particular issue or outside the community but committed to working on the issue. Sometimes advocates who are not fully familiar with a community play an important role in helping community members shape policy, and to do so, it is important that they get to know the community. Advocates often identify issues by spending time talking with neighbors, walking around observing their neighborhoods "with fresh eyes," and identifying the assets (or protective factors) and factors that put neighbors at risk.

Any behavior or activity operates within a context or an environment that shapes it. Defining problems in a social change context means shifting the focus from individual problems to the social and environmental context in which these problems occur. Identifying risk and protective factors requires attention to a community's environment, the context in which these factors exist. This shift is important because environmental factors can play a major role in proliferation *and prevention* of problems in a community. This shift from an individual to an environmental perspective is much like shifting a camera lens away from a simple portrait to capture the "big picture" or landscape that surrounds it. There are different levels and dimensions of a community landscape.

- *Physical or land use factors.* Buildings, roads, open space, institutions, and businesses (or lack of them) are all a part of the physical infrastructure that forms the foundation of a community.
- *Availability of goods and services.* What we eat, wear, and read is largely determined by what is available to us. Goods and services are more than what we can buy; they include public services like schools, hospitals, water, and recreational facilities.
- *Institutional factors.* What is the impact of institutional behavior on the community?
- *Human factors.* Who lives here? To what organizations do they belong?

Techniques for Community Assessment. Identifying risk and protective factors is important, but equally critical is knowing which factors are most important to address. As noted earlier, collecting data and conducting research are important tools that can help. Another equally important way to gather information is to listen to people in the community. Both outside advocates and locals need to have ways to understand the community better that add to their "gut instincts." Every coalition should have systems for collecting community input and feedback. Here are a few examples of community-focused methods of "listening."

Surveys. Whether completed over the phone, online, or at the door, surveys are structured ways of getting community input and identifying issues and the prevalence of problems or attitudes. One should take care not to develop long, complicated survey instruments—or instruments that focus only on a community's problems. Well-done surveys enable groups to collect data in standardized form on a wide variety of issues and at the same time encourage residents to participate in the policy process.

Canvassing. Going door to door unannounced can be a good way to reach new people who aren't on anyone's list; raise public awareness; and build name recognition in a neighborhood. It is difficult to carry on an extensive conversation for the most part, so input gathered will be limited.

Focus Groups. One can gather solid, qualitative input from a small group—especially a group of people who have something in common or are in some way demographically similar. Just listening to the exchange between participants can be very enlightening and reveal more about the interests and concerns in a community than a survey can. Of course, information collected from focus groups is harder (though not impossible) to quantify.

One-on-One Interviews with Key Players. Listening is one of the most important tools there is for building relationships. Listen actively with your whole body facing the speaker. Ask questions and probe deeper. After offering a guiding question or two, go wherever the conversation leads you. Suspend your expectations and your agenda for the time being. Just listen to learn more about the other person and his or her concerns. Take notes if you need to and if it is not too obtrusive.

Walkabout. Map out a route in an affected or representative neighborhood. The route should provide a mix of things to observe (businesses, institutions, homes, parks, and so on) and take no more than sixty minutes to walk. If much of the business district is abandoned, that is worth observing, too. It is best to do a walkabout in a small group. Encourage participants to take notes and to pay attention to both assets and challenges, and debrief the group's observations upon return.

Stage 2: Defining the Initiative

Once the primary issue or set of concerns is defined, it must be refined into a clear, practical policy initiative. The best initiatives emerge when residents articulate their "ideal" policy and then look for the best mechanisms for bringing their vision into reality. In Oakland, California, the Coalition on Alcohol Outlet Issues wanted fewer liquor stores and better regulation of those remaining. In its ideal policy, the group wanted store owners, not public funds, to pay for enforcement.

Coalition members took their idea to the city council, which then instructed staff to find a solution. The resulting ordinance requires merchants to pay higher conditional use permit fees to support an augmented regulatory structure.

The process of defining an initiative is also tied to the needs and aspirations of coalition partners. As a result, diverse representation in the process is key in order to ensure that the initiative defined is relevant to as many communities as possible, particularly communities most affected by the issues the group is hoping to address. Expanding a coalition can bring significant changes to how a coalition is defined, as in the case of a statewide coalition working to increase the tobacco excise tax in Colorado. When the coalition expanded to include Padres Unidos, a group organizing in Denver-area Latino communities, Padres Unidos's accountability to its base would not allow the group to simply bring Latinos to the tax initiative. The organization had to negotiate with the coalition about the language, impact, and reach of the ballot initiative to ensure that the initiative would be relevant to the group's base. Padres Unidos's extensive research on the impact of funding cuts to undocumented residents in Colorado helped expand the tax initiative to include the restoration of funding for health services for undocumented residents. When the ballot initiative passed in November 2004, a diverse group of Coloradans celebrated what was a victory for primary prevention and immigrant rights.

Stage 3: Strategy and Analysis

After gathering information and identifying assets and challenges, it is time to analyze all of that information and develop approaches to building policymaker and public support for the initiative. The process of developing strategy in this regard is informed by an understanding of the values and interests that undergird how decisions are made on a daily basis.

Community values and interests are the ideal visions and the down-to-earth concerns we carry in our daily lives. They range from dreams of a safe, green world for all families to fears that the "wrong kind" of neighbors will move in. Advocates must factor in community sentiment from all across the spectrum in order to determine how to make the initiative meaningful for the people with whom they will be working.

A power analysis is an assessment to identify targets or decision makers, allies, opponents, and other important actors in the campaign. It is wise to conduct a power analysis early on, as the initiative can be refined further in light of this information. For example, a coalition in favor of living-wage legislation intentionally omitted construction work from its initiative as a strategic and political consideration. By omitting construction work, much of which already paid a living

The Importance of Research

Prevention policy should have a strong research foundation that supports the initiative's particular strategy or approach toward addressing the problem. This is of particular importance in the case of progressive, regulatory policies, as they usually receive greater scrutiny than policies perceived to be probusiness. The extra scrutiny can be a good thing, as it forces proponents to make sure their policies have an effect on real-life issues that are of concern to communities.

Initiatives should start with a strong and respectable database. This can be done without starting from scratch or conducting new studies. Many studies are available that support prevention initiatives, though they may not be widely disseminated. The Internet is a good source for many of these documents, in addition to directly contacting community-based groups or think tanks. In the area of child and family services, for example, there are literally hundreds of well-crafted studies that examine the impact of poverty on children and hundreds more on drug policy, employment, race relations, and many other topics.

Data can guide the development of an initiative in at least three ways. They can direct how the policy should be targeted by providing detailed information about the problem. They can indicate the impact and severity of the problem and justify social action. Finally, by showing that some groups are disproportionately affected by the problem, the data establish that the problem is not random but linked to specific social and environmental factors.

Practically speaking, research should provide a clear analysis of the issues the policy initiative seeks to address. It is one thing to say, "We have a problem with teen pregnancy"; it is quite another to say, "We have a problem with unsafe sex among teens" or "a problem with predatory sex between teen girls and men in their twenties and thirties." Community-based research helps us understand the difference and point to policies that are more effective. Insist on more accountability and punishment for adult fathers? Ensure better access to preventive health care? Mandate counseling services and classes to bolster teen girls' sense of power in relationships? Increase alternative activities for youth? Given the many ways one can define the issue, it is important to gather as many reports, surveys, personal observations, and other resources that accurately describe the problems and the protective factors in play.

Another reason to have detailed information to substantiate policy recommendations is that all legislation must be based on findings or facts that provide a clear rationale for enacting the law. These findings are important because they constitute much of the legal case if the law is challenged in court. In addition, policymakers are more likely to support issues that have data to back them up; well-done research can legitimize an issue in the eyes of politicians, their constituents, and the media. Above all, you must have information that clearly describes the problem and your proposed solution in ways that policymakers, the community, the coalition, and the media can understand.

wage, the group was able to neutralize potential opposition and make allies out of building trade unions and other key players in the construction industry.

Every policy, no matter how benign it may seem, benefits some people more than others. A good organizer carefully dissects how key constituencies will perceive their self-interests as they relate to the proposed policy. Key questions include these:

How much power do they have over decision makers on this issue?

How strongly will they support or oppose the initiative?

What are the challenges or barriers to joining us?

What do they risk by being involved? By not being involved?

What is our relationship to each of these players?

How might we shape the initiative differently to maximize allies and divide opponents without undermining our objectives?

Stage 4: Direct Issue Organizing

Informed by the power analysis and strategic planning, organizing begins in earnest. In citywide or countywide campaigns without a neighborhood focus, organizing is usually done through outreach to other organizations. For example, much of the organizing for living-wage campaigns focused on unions, advocacy organizations, and nonunionized employees.

Neighborhood-oriented campaigns tend to conduct more block-by-block canvassing operations. In Los Angeles, the Community Coalition for Substance Abuse Prevention and Treatment has organizers go door to door and holds house parties as neighborhood meetings. The group focuses on neighborhoods with problem liquor stores in order to build a solid base of support among the people most affected by the issue.

Community organizing and mobilization are, in the main, communication strategies. They are about reaching people directly and inviting them to get involved because it is in their interest to do so. Organizers must understand and appreciate that people have many issues to contend with and that although our policy initiatives are important, community involvement almost always clashes with real-life obligations. The venerable organizer Fred Ross Sr. used to say that in order to organize, you had to find someone "who had to do something about it." Often these folk are the hardest to reach because they are dealing with a range of social problems. As professionals, many of us feel safer working with "leaders" who have much less stake in the issue and run a certain risk (of reputation, time, and so on) in being involved with us. This tendency can wreak havoc on efforts to build a strong, committed coalition with an authentic stake in the issue.

Even with the best analysis and outreach, potential allies can still be unresponsive. History can play a critical role in how groups respond to overtures for collaboration. It helps to do a "collaboration scan" by asking a few key residents about the history of relationships between your agency and similar agencies and targeted communities. Here are some guiding questions:

> How are resources allocated to support the various groups or communities with which I want to work? Have there been tensions over resources? How did these tensions evolve, and who were the key players?
>
> What is the group's experience with previous collaborations? Were they satisfying? Were their needs met? Was it a positive or negative experience overall? Why?
>
> What are the prevailing attitudes about collaboration? Are there issues (in professional training or culture, mistrust, and so on) that make collaboration difficult? Easier? What concerns the group most about getting involved with a collaborative project? How can those concerns be allayed?
>
> Who are the key opinion leaders in the group? Who is most open to collaborating? Who is least open? Do we or someone we know have a relationship with any of them? List names.
>
> What would the group need to get out of collaborating with others? What can we offer? What would the group be willing to contribute? What does it risk in joining us?
>
> What interests do we both share? Will this collaboration offer a vehicle for mutual benefit?

The answers to these questions will frame an initial recruitment plan. A recruitment plan identifies prospective partners, their probable interests, and background information to help begin the work of building relationships. It is important to choose candidates carefully because the first groups to join the coalition will send a strong signal to the rest of the community.

Candidates need not be the most prominent community members, but they must be trusted in their community, share common ground, and be concerned enough about the core issues to make a solid commitment. Although big-name affiliations can bring media attention to a cause, big names alone without any commitment will not build working relationships. They just breed resentment and reinforce the status quo. In addition, famous people have more to risk when they do get involved. Authentic collaborations require partners who are deeply concerned, have a strong personal interest in the initiative, and risk relatively little by getting involved.

When recruiting candidates to a policy initiative, identify any shared friends or colleagues who may consent to serve as go-betweens to initiate contact with the candidate. If possible, discuss any outreach with a colleague who knows the candidate well. Try role-playing certain approaches and discussing the candidate's potential responses. A good recruitment pitch comes from detailed background information and plenty of practice.

Of course, recruitment is only the beginning. Building and sustaining public support for a policy initiative requires retaining partners for the long haul by integrating them into the team. This is not a blending process where everyone ends up acting and talking the same. It's more of a salad approach in which every partner is tossed lightly until the new partner has blended in. Some organizations develop a new-partner orientation system and assign a partner to the new member to help with the transition. That partner makes the introductions, brings the new member up to speed, and works with the newcomer to identify potential areas for participation. When possible, it helps to recruit at least two people from a community to minimize feelings of isolation.

Review your organizational structure. How are decisions made? Who holds the information and resources? Will there be room for new partners to make a meaningful contribution to the initiative's direction? What steps do you have in place to make new partners feel at home with the group? What language, or level of language, is spoken at meetings and gatherings? Will it alienate or welcome new partners?

Media Advocacy. It is also during this stage that media work moves into full swing. Media advocacy is strategic use of mass media to support community organizing to advance a social or public policy initiative. Most media advocacy is focused on the initiative's target (or decision-making body) because it is the target that has the power to enact the desired change. In some cases, groups use media advocacy to mobilize supporters as a preliminary step to targeting policymakers. It's important to note that although the media can support organizing goals, they can never be a substitute for organizing. That's why most groups shape their media strategy to target policymakers.

Spend time researching how targets get their information. Most elected officials and other gatekeepers read the editorial pages of local newspapers to gauge community concerns. Television news also helps set the public agenda and affects the "public conversation" on a particular issue. In any case, identifying the target will help shape a more effective and efficient strategy.

Developing a Message. A message is not a sound bite or a slogan (although it can help shape those things). It is the overarching theme that neatly frames the initiative for key target audiences. Messages should be relatively short, easy to understand, emotive, and visual. The message should be supportive of the overall strategy.

It is best to test messages on friends and coworkers—especially those who are not familiar with the issue. Colleagues working on similar issues are another good resource. Listen carefully to feedback: Did the message convey the importance of your issue? Did the recipient of the message "get" it? Keeping key targets in mind, use the input to help shape and refine the message.

Stage 5: Steering Through Appropriate Channels

At some point in every initiative, advocates must meet with policymakers and begin the long process of getting the policy enacted. This stage is characterized by intensive work with government staff, negotiations, and accountability sessions. It is important to stay focused on the group's initial goals during this phase, as it is easy to get caught up in the politics of bureaucracy. Working with policymakers is an "inside" game, but it need not mean getting disconnected from grassroots support. As the veteran organizer Greg Akili often says, "Stay connected to your base. Always go in groups and rotate the people who attend the meetings so that you build leadership and confidence."

For prevention policy initiatives, this stage is a crucial one, as prevention-focused initiatives can be technical and complicated. Having a legislative champion (or several) can be important in negotiating this phase. At the very least, it will be critical that involved staffers understand key provisions and issues in the proposed policy. Staffers are an incredibly valuable resource because most policymakers depend heavily on their staff for making key decisions. Some technical understanding is important also because policy revisions that may seem inconsequential to a layperson can undermine the intent of the initiative. For example, ventilation options for restaurants facing clean indoor air policies might seem a reasonable compromise to address secondhand smoke. However, ventilation does not effectively address the health risks because it does not *eliminate* secondhand smoke. Advocates must be vigilant to ensure that the final policy draft reflects their intentions for the initiative and at least does no harm.

It is also valuable to understand the political process and the decision-making bodies of the locale in which the policy is to be implemented. Policies are implemented by different bodies, from city councils to boards of supervisors. And some political strategies allow community groups to rely on voters, rather than policymakers, for organizing ballot initiatives or propositions. Understanding the options available is crucial.

Administrative Rule Making. Most regulatory agencies have the power to make rules and regulations without much oversight or input from elected officials or the public at large. In fact, agency rule making—not legislation—constitutes the bulk of the policies that regulate and shape our lives. Thus it is a supplement and at times an alternative to new policy creation. How public benefits are accessed and distributed, how data are gathered and made public, job creation, most trade policy, and many other matters are all determined by a small number of people as part of their daily job. The lack of formality and access that characterizes most rule making requires that advocates get a clear sense of who has the power to make what rules in which areas of concern to their efforts. This means conducting a power analysis to assess how decisions are made and where best to affect these decisions.

Once these "power points" are identified, it all becomes a classic organizing campaign to leverage additional scrutiny (including press) to raise the level of accountability in the process. Many of these agencies are rarely exposed to direct action. As a result, organizers who have focused on the rule-making process have met with a great deal of success.

Should the policy process break down and it becomes clear that the policy is not winnable in the short term, other actions are needed to set the groundwork for regulation down the line. The three most common policy actions at this stage are moratoriums, mandated studies, and lawsuits.

Moratoriums. Sometimes it is important to stop a policy activity until there can be further study of its impact and any possible alternatives. Common moratoriums include bans on new alcohol outlets, billboards, dump sites, or office construction. It is not enough to enact a time-limited ban; moratorium time should be used to gather more information and assess policy options.

Mandated Studies. Research can be costly and time-consuming. If time and support allow, why not get local government to do the research? Through policy that mandates a study or data collection, resources can be set aside to do a thorough job of information gathering. The policy can set parameters for the kind of group or institution that can conduct the study, key questions framing the study, resident involvement and monitoring of the study, and the plan for dissemination and use of the results. A Los Angeles coalition convinced the city to conduct a study on the topic of a living wage. When it came time to discuss whether a living-wage law was needed, the data were beyond dispute because they were the city's own data.

Lawsuits and Other Complaints. Lawsuits and other court actions can be tedious and expensive. Therefore, groups should carefully consider all options before deciding to take on a lawsuit. If an organization has the resources (in staff, money, or pro bono legal support), a well-framed legal intervention can accomplish much in both the short term and the long term—even if it simply gets the other side to the table or to negotiate in better faith. Other strategies include requests for information and documents from the opponents, injunctions against the implementation of laws before they have had a chance to take effect, organizing victims with standing to sue polluters or other institutions causing damage to a community, and civil suits when an institutional action has a pattern of discrimination or damage to certain populations (such as people of color, women, or people with disabilities).

In addition to lawsuits, it also helps to file complaints about bad or illegal practices with the appropriate regulatory agencies. For example, alcohol ads that appeal to children are violations in many states. Violations of pollution, labor, and fair trade laws are other avenues that can be pursued. If one regulatory agency is notoriously slow to act, try redefining the issue so that it falls under the purview of a more active regulator. For example, redefining a violation from a bad business practice to a health issue often brings a whole new set of actors into play. In any case, find out who enforces what relevant regulations, and work accordingly.

Stage 6: Victory and Defense

Once an initiative is enacted, celebration is definitely in order. However, for most ordinances, as soon as the partying is over, the litigation begins. Prepare for the possibility of litigation at the beginning of the initiative, and be ready to play an active role in any legal action, even if the local government (and not the advocating coalition or group) is the defendant. Some organizations, like the Community Coalition and the Coalition on Alcohol Outlet Issues, got intervenor status in litigation directed toward their city's government. Baltimore's Citywide Liquor Coalition made sure its attorney worked closely with the city attorney throughout the process, carefully crafting public testimony with an eye toward building a strong public record in preparation for the inevitable litigation against the ordinance it was promoting, regulating alcohol and tobacco billboards.

Media advocacy and framing are also important in this phase of the work. Framing the victory on a group's terms can help consolidate public support and build a base for future initiatives. Strong support for an initiative after its enactment can also help prevent lawsuits challenging the policy's implementation.

Stage 7: Implementation and Enforcement

After the policy is enacted, it sometimes also needs to clear court hurdles. Then the work begins to get the new law properly implemented and enforced. One of the biggest mistakes in policy development is failing to consider implementation thoroughly, including mechanisms of funding and enforcement, before the policy is advanced. For initiatives with powerful opposition, negotiation continues around issues like the timeline for implementing the policy, interpretation of particular clauses, and fitting the new policy in with other government priorities.

Ensure that there are adequate resources for monitoring and enforcement. Build in funding, excise tax and license fee increases, and other relevant resource allocation formulas that tie the amount of the enforcement budget to the scope and objectives of enforcement. For example, tying alcohol outlet licensing fees and penalties to the cost of enforcement helps ensure that enforcement resources keep up with problems at the expense of those making a profit from the product and not forcing residents to shoulder the burden.

Develop an interagency oversight body that brings the partners together for comprehensive enforcement and monitoring. This includes community members, school and youth-serving agencies, supportive business representatives, researchers, planners, law enforcement, and health department professionals to ensure compliance and oversight of monitoring and enforcement. Clear criteria for board membership, including independence from regulated industry funding or limits on the number of representatives with industry ties, must be established in advance. The body should hold the group accountable to open meeting and documentation requirements as outlined in municipal and state law.

Ensure enforcement of the policy in areas where underserved communities are most targeted. Communities of color and the LGBT (lesbian, gay, bisexual, and transgender) community are directly targeted by key industries on which prevention regulation is focused, such as tobacco and alcohol. As a result, care must be taken to ensure that enforcement resources are equitably allocated. Some enforcement activities related to reducing disparities may include the following:

- Ensuring compliance with youth access laws
- Regular surveillance and research to monitor targeting
- Hiring enforcement staff with the appropriate cultural, language, and community competencies
- Advertising restrictions in specific neighborhoods

California-based "smoke-free bars" campaigns, promoting the health interests of Asian American communities, exemplify the promise and proven success of backing culturally specific enforcement activities. The Asian Pacific Islander Tobacco Control Network pushed a smoke-free campaign that focused on Asian American venues and cultural nights. After local bars went smoke-free, campaign activities shifted to enforcement as network members joined with local BREATH advocates (the California Smoke-Free Bars, Workplaces, and Communities Program) to monitor compliance at locales catering to Asian American patrons. This effort also provided a valuable opportunity to appraise the community impact of smoke-free laws while raising general awareness of the perils of tobacco use in these communities (Asian and Pacific Islander American Health Forum, 2004).

Work with business owners. On some issues, businesses are likely targets for prevention policy interventions. Many of the outlets (tobacco vendors, liquor stores, corner grocers, and so on) are heavily concentrated in low-income areas with large communities of color. Many business owners in these areas are themselves immigrants and racial minorities who have not received adequate training on policy enforcement or ways their businesses can be better community citizens. When ensuring compliance with newly enacted laws, it is imperative to use culturally sensitive approaches that embrace building relationships with business owners. Having outreach workers who can communicate in the appropriate ethnic or cultural language can facilitate constructive dialogue around enforcement. These outreach workers can offer on-site general education on policy enforcement. The working partnerships between community organizations and business owners can be the basis for future prevention efforts.

Ensure equitable application of enforcement activities. It is important to demonstrate even-handed application of enforcement activities, given the historically strained relationships between the criminal justice systems and diverse communities that are already overrepresented in many areas of the criminal justice system. Although higher rates of violations in a specific community may be an indicator that law enforcement officers enforce policies differently in different communities, it may also reflect the greater concentration and impact of the problem in that community—a situation that may be addressed most effectively through policy initiatives that decrease outlet concentration in communities saturated with negative uses combined with culturally competent efforts to promote compliance with prevention policies.

Conclusion

Policy is a powerful tool for prevention, especially when used in concert with community organizing and media advocacy. The evidence of its efficacy is mounting as prevention-focused policies like mandatory seat belt laws, clean indoor air ordinances, and responsible beverage service regulations are literally saving tens of thousands of lives each year. However, there is much more to be done. There is a need for better, more strategic budget policies that ensure a fair allocation of resources to communities at greater risk. Some areas of prevention policymaking, such as family planning, face extraordinarily tough opposition, although organized opposition to public health interventions is on the rise overall (Woolley & Benjamin, 2004; Yañez, 2002).

Advocates face highly organized, well-funded media attacks that frame prevention-focused policies as government interference in people's private lives. The good news is that polls continue to show widespread support for much of the prevention policy agenda, including increases in certain taxes. Our challenge is to build a broad base of active supporters committed to moving these policy initiatives forward from the bottom up. As previous work has shown, when prevention advocates help build broad-based movements focused on concrete policy change, we can help create healthier environments that engage communities in ways that traditional health education and health promotion approaches cannot.

References

Asian and Pacific Islander American Health Forum. (2004). Asian and Pacific Islander Tobacco Education Network. Retrieved October 13, 2006, from http://www.apiahf.org/programs/apiten

Chaloupka, F. J., & Wechsler, H. (1997). Price, tobacco control policies, and smoking among young adults. *Journal of Health Economics, 16,* 359–373.

Curtis, L. A. (1987). *Policies to prevent crime: Neighborhood, family, and employment strategies.* Thousand Oaks, CA: Sage.

Florin, P. (1989). *Nurturing the grassroots: Neighborhood volunteer organizations and America's cities.* New York: Citizens Committee for New York City.

Kahane, C. J. (2001). *An evaluation of child passenger safety: The effectiveness and benefits of safety seats.* Washington, DC: National Highway Traffic Safety Administration.

Kretzmann, J. P., & McKnight, J. L. (1993). *Building communities from the inside out: A path toward finding and mobilizing a community's assets.* Evanston, IL: Northwestern University, Center for Urban Affairs and Policy Research.

Mayer, N. S. (1984). *Neighborhood organizations and community development.* Washington, DC: Urban Institute Press.

McMillan, D. W., & Chavis, D. M. (1986). Sense of community: A definition and theory. *Journal of Community Psychology, 14,* 6–23.

National Center for Statistics and Analysis. (2004). Children. In *Traffic safety facts, 2004* (p. 5). Washington, DC: National Highway Traffic Safety Administration.

National Highway Traffic Safety Administration. (1997). *Traffic safety facts, 1997: Occupant protection.* Washington, DC: Author.

National Highway Traffic Safety Administration. (2002). *Traffic safety facts, 2001.* Washington, DC: Author.

National Highway Traffic Safety Administration. (2004, June). *Sixth report to Congress, fourth report to the president: The national initiative for increasing safety belt use.* Washington, DC: Author.

New York State Department of Health. (2006). *Child passenger safety.* Albany: New York State Department of Health.

Solomon, M. G., Leaf, W. A., & Nissen, W. J. (2001). *Process and outcome evaluation: The Buckle Up America initiative.* Washington, DC: National Highway Traffic Safety Administration.

Sugarmann, J., & Rand, K. (1998). *Cease fire: A comprehensive strategy to reduce firearms violence.* Washington, DC: Violence Policy Center.

Woolley, M., & Benjamin, G. (2004, November 9). *Research! America/APHA national poll on Americans' attitudes toward public health.* Paper presented at the 132nd annual meeting of the American Public Health Association, Washington, DC. Retrieved October 13, 2006, from http://www.researchamerica.org/polldata/2004/apha2004.pdf

Yañez, E. (2002). *Clean indoor air and communities of color: Challenges and opportunities.* Washington, DC: Praxis Project.

CHAPTER NINE

USING MEDIA ADVOCACY TO INFLUENCE POLICY

Lori Dorfman

The history of public health is clear: social conditions and the physical environment are important determinants of health. The primary tool available to public health for influencing social conditions and environments is policy. Policies define the structures and set the rules by which we live. If public health practitioners are going to improve social conditions and physical environments in lasting and meaningful ways, they must be involved in policy development and policy advocacy. Furthermore, being successful in policy advocacy means paying attention to the news.

The reach of the news media is intoxicating. In society, the news media largely determine what issues we collectively think about, how we think about them, and what kinds of alternatives are considered viable, which, in turn, influences key policy decisions pertaining to health. The public and policymakers do not consider issues unless they are visible, and they are not visible unless the news has brought them to light. Naturally, public health educators want to take advantage of the vast audience the news media reach.

Nonprofit organizations and community activists often are unhappy with the way their issues are presented in the news, and typically respond by criticizing

This chapter is reprinted from *Community Health Education Methods: A Practical Guide* (2nd ed.), edited by R. J. Bensley and J. Brookins-Fisher. Copyright © 2003 Jones & Bartlett Publishers, Boston.

the media, ignoring it, or even becoming hostile. These responses are nonproductive because they cede power over the public portrayal of their issues to journalists and widen the gulf between journalists and advocates. Media advocacy addresses this problem. It is an approach to health communication that differs significantly from traditional mass communication approaches. Media advocacy helps people understand the importance and reach of news coverage, the need to participate actively in shaping such coverage, and the methods to do so effectively. News portrayals of health issues are significant for how they influence policymakers and the public regarding who has responsibility for health. If public health–oriented solutions are to be given full consideration, then advocates talking to journalists, and journalists themselves, must understand how to frame issues from the perspective of shared accountability so that news coverage is not focused exclusively on individual responsibility. This shared accountability recognizes that health and social problems will only be adequately addressed when all sectors of society—not just the individual—share responsibility for solutions. Media advocacy emphasizes social accountability, which typically receives less attention from the news than individually oriented solutions.

Public health practitioners tend to overlook the power of the news media to influence change. Journalists themselves, even when committed to covering social problems, often produce stories that emphasize individual behavior and treatment rather than social factors and prevention. Despite the media's enormous reach and potential as a tool for change, public health professionals rarely use mass media to its full advantage. Rather, they tend to use it in its least effective capacity: to convey personal health information to consumers (Wallack & Dorfman, 2001). By contrast, media advocacy harnesses the power of the news to mobilize advocates and apply pressure for policy change.

Steps for Developing Effective Media Advocacy Campaigns

Before public health advocates can harness the power of the news, they have to be clear and precise about why they want to use media advocacy. Four layers of strategy organize the approach to communications campaigns. The first is the *overall strategy*—the ultimate goal of the campaign. Next is the *media strategy*—chosen based on appropriateness for the overall strategy. This chapter focuses on one media strategy: *media advocacy*. Once they have selected a media strategy, advocates need to determine the specifics of what they want to say, and to whom. That is the *message strategy*. Finally, once the other layers of strategy are in place, advocates can figure out how to attract news attention—the *access strategy*. Unfortunately, many groups begin by trying to attract journalists' attention without figuring out first why they want that attention, and what they will say after they have it. This chapter is designed to prepare readers so they know when to call on journalists and are confident about what to say once they have their attention.

Develop an Overall Strategy

The most important part of a media strategy does not concern media at all. Rather, it is the clarification, articulation, and justification of the desired change. The media advocacy *prime directive* is that "you cannot have a media strategy without an overall strategy." Advocates should begin by asking themselves, "What changes will improve the public's health?" It makes sense for advocates to develop a media strategy only after they know what needs to be accomplished overall and how it will be done. In practical terms, this usually means determining the policy that needs to be enacted, changed, or enforced. The following four questions can help guide the development of an overall strategy:

1. What is the problem or issue?
2. What is a solution or policy—the desired outcome?
3. Who has the power to make the necessary change?
4. Who must be mobilized to apply the necessary pressure?

The following subsections examine each question in detail.

What Is the Problem or Issue? Defining the problem is often not as simple as it seems. It is a process rife with social and political tension because different stakeholders will offer competing definitions of the problem. This process is exceptionally important because the ultimate definition of the problem will fundamentally determine the solution. For example, the high school shooting near Littleton, Colorado, in 1999 quickly generated competing definitions of the problem of violence among youth, including the availability of guns, the barrenness of suburban lifestyles, the failure of parents to be involved in their children's lives, the inadequacy of mental health services, and the destructive social cliques of teenagers in high school. News attention to one or the other of such competing issues helps determine the saliency of various policies and, ultimately, which will prevail.

Articulating the problem is important because it will need to be conveyed concisely to a reporter. Public health is often very problem oriented. Thus, those from health departments or social service agencies can endlessly discuss the problem. Indeed, health officials often feel they have a moral and professional obligation to tell journalists everything they know any time they are asked about the problem because they know their issue is of such vital importance. The realities of news today, however, demand that health professionals identify the most critical aspect of the problem and be able to describe it well in just a sentence or two.

Advocates must isolate the piece of the large public health problem that will be addressed specifically. For example, alcohol is related to more than 105,000 deaths a year in this country and is the number one drug choice for young people. One way advocates can narrow the problem is by focusing on how alcohol creates problems on college campuses, particularly when it is consumed in large quantities over a short period of time. The problem of binge drinking on college campuses might be narrowed further and defined in terms of price specials at bars nearby that encourage those who are drinking to get drunk. Cheap alcohol is certainly not the only factor leading to alcohol problems on campus, but it is probably an important one. It is also a problem that can be remedied by a clear policy solution that would affect the overall alcohol environment.

What Is a Solution or Policy—the Desired Outcome? Sometimes advocates are so concerned about focusing attention on the problem that they give inadequate attention to the solution. Or, they may not have identified a clear solution. Public health advocates need to identify a solution or policy—not necessarily one that will solve the entire problem, but something that can make a difference. Typical inadequate responses tend to be statements such as "This is a very complex problem with multifaceted solutions," "There is no magic bullet," "Children are our future and we must do something," or "The community needs to come together." Unfortunately, none of these responses provides any concrete direction. Public health advocates need to be clear about what they want to happen: Is a new law necessary? Is more enforcement required? Does the budget need to be changed? Does someone need to take responsibility to do something to protect the community's health? Who? What should they do? When should they do it?

In the example of problems related to alcohol on campus, one solution is to eliminate happy hour price specials that encourage quick consumption of large quantities of alcohol. Advocates might work on only one salient part of the problem or one policy solution at a time, or more, depending on what resources are available.

Who Has the Power to Make the Necessary Change? The next step is figuring out what person, group, organization, or body has the power to make the desired change. This question identifies the target audience, but reflects a fundamental change in what that term means. In this context, there is a difference between traditional use of mass media in public health as a vehicle for public information campaigns to change personal behavior and using media as an advocacy tool to change policy. In the former, the person with the problem is the one with the power to make the change—for example, the person who drinks too much, smokes, does not exercise, or has a poor diet. When using media advocacy to change, implement, or enforce policy, the target is different because the power may reside with a legislator, other elected official, regulatory agency, small business owner, or corporate officer. In addition, the locus of power—or target audience—is likely to change over time. For example, changing a regulation may require focusing on different targets depending on the stage of development of the issue.

The primary target for a media advocacy campaign to reduce alcohol problems on and around campus would not be the students who are drinking. Instead, it would be the alcohol vendors and those who regulate them. Eliminating happy hours, to use the policy example mentioned earlier, is not in the power of the students. Once happy hours are gone there will be a beneficial effect regardless of the knowledge and attitude of student drinkers: one avenue for the dangerous behavior would be closed. News coverage generated by media advocacy activities can describe the problem and articulate the demands for solutions so the city government and campus community can more easily move ahead. Advocates must articulate for reporters the reason for the policy and what it will accomplish. Thus, the public learns about the problems alcohol causes on campus via the news, which is perceived as a highly legitimate and credible source.

Who Must Be Mobilized to Apply the Necessary Pressure?   Public health–oriented policies are often hotly contested. Public health goals such as fluoridation of drinking water, distribution of condoms, reducing the speed limit, mandating bicycle or motorcycle helmets, or limiting the availability of alcohol, handguns, or tobacco bring out intense opposition. Many legislators and other policymakers are unlikely to support a controversial change unless constituency groups put pressure on them. The pressure can consist of telephone calls, letters, demonstrations, media coverage, and office visits. The role of news coverage here is twofold. First, media coverage of the issue will let the policymaker know that his or her vote or position is being watched and will be part of the public debate. Second, media coverage can help mobilize constituency groups to contact the policymaker or get involved in other ways, thus applying pressure.

Mobilizing supportive groups is important because public health policy efforts can often be prolonged struggles. The media can only provide periodic coverage, placing the spotlight on the issue at key times. Constituency groups need to apply pressure on a continuing basis. For example, students and local merchants around campus can put pressure on bar owners directly to change their policies about pricing alcohol. They can also put pressure on campus administration, city government, and alcoholic beverage regulating agencies to take actions that will reduce the problems related to alcohol use.

Paying attention to these four questions is a good start to creating an overall strategy. Once advocates have defined the problem, selected and developed a realistic and achievable policy objective, conducted an analysis to identify the locus for change, and identified and mobilized groups to apply pressure, they can then determine the media, message, and access strategies.

Develop a Media Strategy

Traditional forms of mass media interventions emphasize the "information gap" or "motivation gap," which suggests that health problems are caused by individuals with the problem or at risk for the problem, lacking either information or sufficient desire to behave in a more healthful manner. Health educators then attempt to provide information to fill the gap. When people have the information and "know the facts," it is assumed they will adopt a positive attitude toward the health behavior and act accordingly, and the problem will be solved. The role of the media, in this case, is to deliver the solution (knowledge) to the millions of individuals who need it. Media advocacy, on the other hand, focuses on the "power gap," viewing health problems as arising from a lack of power to create change in social and physical environments.

Media advocacy can be defined as the strategic use of mass media to advance public policy by applying pressure to policymakers (Wallack, Dorfman, Jernigan, & Themba, 1993). The use of media advocacy has evolved as the definition of health problems has shifted from the individual level to the policy level. What distinguishes media advocacy from traditional health promotion and educational efforts is the goal of the effort (see Figure 9.1) (Riley, 2001).

Media advocacy differs in many ways from traditional public health campaigns. It is most marked by an emphasis on the following (Wallack & Dorfman, 2001):

FIGURE 9.1. TRADITIONAL HEALTH COMMUNICATION VERSUS MEDIA ADVOCACY.

Traditional Health Communication	Media Advocacy
Problem defined at the individual level	Problem defined at the policy level
Health is a personal issue	Health is a social issue
Mass media is used to change behavior	Mass media is used to influence public policy
Short-term focus	Long-term focus

- Linking public health and social problems to inequities in social arrangements rather than to flaws in the individual
- Changing public policy rather than personal health behavior
- Focusing primarily on reaching opinion leaders and policymakers rather than on those who have the problem (the traditional audience of public health communication campaigns)
- Working with groups to increase participation and amplify their voices rather than providing health behavior change messages
- Having a primary goal of reducing the power gap rather than just filling the information gap

In practice, media advocacy uses some of the same media relations techniques that practitioners of social marketing or public information campaigns might use: sending out news releases, pitching stories to journalists, monitoring the media and keeping a list of media contacts, and paying attention to what is newsworthy. But these practices alone are not media advocacy, though they are frequently used. Because media advocacy's target is the power gap, it attempts to motivate social and political involvement rather than changes in personal health behavior (Wallack, Dorfman, & Woodruff, 1997). It is the best media strategy choice when the overall strategy involves changing policy.

Develop a Message Strategy

The message is what is said to the target. The overall strategy determines the target audience: a single person or a small group, perhaps the CEO of a company, or a legislative committee. The message is delivered to the target through the news media. Other mechanisms for delivering the message are used at the same time, of course, because media advocacy is used in combination with community organizing and policy advocacy. Media advocacy adds power and amplification to those strategies by harnessing the news media's reach. It is a mechanism for thrusting the discussion with the target into the public conversation.

Because media advocacy messages are transmitted through the news media, it is useful to examine how the news media typically interpret and represent issues. This process is called framing. Any message that media advocates have will be filtered through the news frame.

Framing: What It Is, Why It Matters. News is organized, or framed, to make sense of infinitely sided and shaded issues. Framing is the process of identifying how the issue will be depicted; it is "the package in which the main point of the story is developed, supported, and understood" (Wallack & Dorfman, 1996, p. 299).

Inevitably, some elements of a story are left out while others are included. Similarly, some arguments, metaphors, or story lines may be featured prominently, while others are relegated to the margins of the story. News frames are important because the facts, values, or images included in news coverage are accorded legitimacy, while those not emphasized or excluded are marginalized or left out of public discussion. The coverage will significantly contribute to how the issue is felt and talked about by the public.

Journalism has traditions and routines that result in consistent frames, almost like story lines or scripts that reporters gravitate toward, such as heroes and villains, overcoming adversity, and the unexpected or ironic twist of the protector causing harm. Stories have characters, characters have roles, and characters carry out their actions on location in recognizable circumstances within a range of predictable outcomes. Television, in particular, with its two-minute storytelling, uses compact symbols to tell a familiar story. By studying the patterns of news storytelling, advocates can determine the implications for public health.

Portraits Versus Landscapes: Typical News Frames and the Challenge for Framing Public Health Issues.

Most news, especially television news, tries to "put a face on the issue." The impact of an issue on an individual's life is often of more interest to news reporters than the policy implications of an issue, in part because they believe readers and viewers are more likely to identify emotionally with a particular person's plight. News stories tend to focus on specific, concrete events, using good pictures to tell a short, simple story. Unfortunately, research on television's effects has shown that when viewers see individually focused, event-oriented stories and then are asked what should be done about the problem depicted, the viewers will respond in ways that tend to blame the victim (Iyengar, 1991). Stories about isolated episodes do not help audiences understand how to deliberate about and solve social problems beyond demanding that individuals take more responsibility for themselves. "Following exposure to episodic framing," notes researcher Shanto Iyengar, "Americans describe chronic problems such as poverty and crime not in terms of deep-seated social or economic conditions, but as mere idiosyncratic outcomes" (p. 137). Alternatively, when stories are more issue-oriented, audiences respond differently—they include government and social institutions as part of the solution. That is usually the type of response sought by public health advocates.

A simple way to distinguish between the two story types is to think of the difference between a portrait and a landscape. In a news story framed as a portrait, one may learn a great deal about an individual or an event, with great drama and detail. But it is hard to see what surrounds that individual or what brought him or her to that moment in time. A landscape pulls back the lens to take a broader view. It may include people and events, but must connect them to the larger so-cial and economic forces. The challenge for media advocates is to make stories about the public health landscape as compelling and interesting as the portrait.

To focus attention on the landscape, media advocates try to frame the *content* of a news story, or the message in that story. Framing for content shifts the indi-vidual problem to a social issue. For example, there is a current trend in many state legislatures to introduce youth tobacco access laws that heavily penalize young people who are attempting to purchase tobacco and the clerks who sell to-bacco products, but not the storeowners. A way to frame this issue for content is to focus on the responsibility for marketing and promotion that the storeowners and the tobacco companies control. Highlighting the fact that tobacco companies mar-ket tobacco products to youth using images that are appealing to this age group, such as cartoon characters, men who are ruggedly independent and rebellious, and thin, independent females, can help shift the focus to the landscape in which the individual young person in that store exists. The primary responsibility for the social issue of youth sales can be shifted from the individual to tobacco industry marketing tactics (Riley, 2001). The industry role in causing the problem is then better understood, and advocates can articulate why it is reasonable to assign re-sponsibility for changing practices to the industry.

Components of a Message. The message is what is to be said to the target audi-ence—those who have the power to make the change being sought. But the mes-sage will be delivered in the context of a news story, so it must conform to the needs of journalists for clear, concise statements. Therefore, it is important to keep it simple.

Journalists are not likely to think of the public health aspects of the stories they write, but they are always eager for a new and interesting angle. Public health practitioners can offer ideas to journalists by suggesting stories directly on the top-ics on which they work and by thinking about how the public health angle fits in to the news of the day.

To improve reporting from a public health perspective, advocates need to be well versed in social factors and other contextual variables so they can inform jour-nalists of those links. They should be able to fill in the blanks in the following state-ment. Similarly, advocates should understand how typical news stories might connect to particular health issues and be able to complete the reverse of the same statement.

Every time there is a story on _____, *it should include information about* _____.

For example, asthma rates began rising in the late 1980s, and studies began to define risk factors such as outdoor pollutants and secondhand smoke (California Center for Health Improvement, 2000). Advocates working to prevent asthma need to determine whether news stories reflect this understanding. If they do not, advocates will know how to focus their discussions with journalists. Given what is now known from epidemiologists, it is reasonable to expect that whenever there is a story on children's health, it should mention rising asthma rates. Similarly, whenever there is a story on asthma, it should mention children's rates going up, prevention measures for parents, potential environmental policy protections, and the health department as a community resource. It would also be appropriate to include an angle on asthma in stories on environmental tobacco smoke or air quality. Think of it this way:

> *Every time there is a story on* asthma, *it should include information about* secondhand smoke.

> *Every time there is a story on* secondhand smoke, *it should include information about* asthma.

Advocates can use the same formula to think through other public health issues, their risk factors, and important aspects of prevention that should be included regularly in news stories. They can collect the materials that clearly and simply make their point and have them on hand to send to reporters on short notice when an article on the topic appears. Data and examples should be at the ready to explain why reporters should include this information in their story.

The message an advocate delivers is usually in the context of an answer to a journalist's question. Journalists will usually ask at least two questions: "What is the problem?" and "What is the solution?" (Dorfman, 1994). It is common for public health professionals and their community allies to spend about 80 percent of their time talking about the problem and 20 percent talking about the solution. Strategically, it is important to reverse the ratio. Advocates should identify the problem briefly, but emphasize what needs to be done to solve it.

A practical rule of thumb is that a good message uses concise, direct language to convey at least three elements (Wallack, Woodruff, Dorfman, & Diaz, 1999). One component is the clear statement of concern—for example, the fact that there are too many alcohol-related problems on campus. The second component represents the value dimension, such as the threat alcohol poses to healthy student life and a nurturing learning environment. The third component elucidates the policy objective, for example, the elimination of happy hours in bars near campuses. The components need not always fall in that order, but they are usually all present.

For example, when the latest study was released on drinking on college campuses, reporters sought comments from those who were directly concerned or affected by the problem. At the University of Iowa, a coalition had formed to try to reduce alcohol problems on and around campus. The coalition had several specific policy goals as its prime directive and had been trained in media advocacy. When the time came to respond to the study, Mary Sue Coleman, then president of the university, told reporters, "Of course, students who drink too much must be responsible for the problems that they cause. But students are not responsible for manufacturing and marketing alcoholic beverages. Students are not responsible for the excessive number of bars within walking distance of our campuses. Students are not responsible for the price specials that encourage drinking to get drunk" (Wilgoren, 2000). In that statement, Dr. Coleman was able to acknowledge the personal responsibility of students but also paint a picture of the landscape surrounding those students that helped illustrate why the policies she sought were both necessary and reasonable. She cannot say everything in one small media bite, but her example goes a long way to define the problem and effectively point to the solution.

Media advocates can develop all the story elements that reporters need to tell the public health side of the story. Media bites, like Dr. Coleman's, are essential. In addition, media advocates can prepare compelling visuals to help illustrate their point of view, calculate "social math" so large numbers can be made meaningful, identify "authentic voices"—those advocates who can effectively "put a face on the issue," as reporters might put it—and identify and use evocative symbols in their descriptions of the problem and solution. Having ready story elements that portray the public health frame will make it easier for journalists to cover the story.

Develop an Access Strategy

After advocates have determined an overall strategy, selected a media strategy, and crafted the message, they are ready to attract journalists' attention. At this point, they must think of what parts of the issue will make a good story. By emphasizing those elements, advocates will be framing the issue for access.

Monitoring the News and Building Relationships with Journalists. To work well with journalists, advocates need to understand how they define and report news. Advocates can do this by carefully watching television news, reading newspapers, and listening to the radio. Advocates should regularly scan all sections of the local newspaper for articles that directly or indirectly relate to the advocacy issue. For instance, the sports page may cover an automobile race that is tobacco-sponsored. This may provide an opportunity for a group working on a policy to ban tobacco-sponsored sporting events. Members of the group could respond to the article with a letter to the editor or an invitation to the reporter who covered the event to learn more about sponsorship. Copies of the article can be sent to other community activists and appropriate legislators (Riley, 2001).

Monitoring means listing and paying attention to the local and relevant national media outlets. For each of the outlets, advocates will have to determine how often it covers the issues that are of concern. Monitoring means noticing what the coverage says about the issue. Does it tell the whole story? Advocates need not do a detailed study of the media, but they need enough information to inform their media advocacy efforts. To do this, they should read and watch the news critically from a public health perspective. When reading the newspaper, they can ask themselves: Does the article include everything it should given the topic it covers? Are there important aspects missing? Is there a public health aspect to this story that should have been included? These questions can help advocates evaluate the comprehensiveness of a news story and determine the specifics to bring to the attention of the journalist, who may do similar stories in the future.

By carefully paying attention to news stories about an issue, advocates can identify which journalists are most interested in a specific topic, and what aspect of the topic interests them the most. Advocates will also start to see how different symbols and journalistic conventions are used to tell the story. This is the foundation from which they can approach journalists about the aspects of the story that are not receiving attention (Wallack et al., 1997).

Advocates will have greater success attracting journalists to the story if they have built a relationship with them. The first step is to compile a list of local media contacts. Each entry on the list should include (1) the name of the reporter; (2) telephone and fax numbers; (3) e-mail and mailing addresses; (4) the name of the newspaper, magazine, or television or radio station; (5) the best time to reach the reporter; (6) sections, or *beats*, for which the reporter writes or reports (e.g., sports, columnist, lifestyle, health); and (7) any notes pertaining to interactions to date. Advocates should meet with the reporters who may have an interest in their issue, or those whose beats intersect with the issue. The advocate should introduce herself or himself, explain why she or he has an interest in meeting, and get to know them. Advocates need to update the media list regularly because there is a high rate of turnover in the news business. It is therefore important to keep track of contacts as they move on to other news outlets. A relationship at a local television station today may be a relationship at a national news program tomorrow.

Newsworthiness. Framing the issue for access involves making the issue newsworthy. The following questions can help determine newsworthiness (Riley, 2001):

- Is the issue controversial (e.g., freedom of speech versus encouraging the sale of illegal products to minors)?
- Is there a milestone event (e.g., the introduction of FDA regulations)?
- Is there an anniversary (e.g., release of the Surgeon General's report on health consequences of tobacco use)?
- Can irony be used (e.g., the contrast between outrage over President Clinton's testimony to special prosecutors and the lack of interest in tobacco company executives who lied to Congress)?
- Can a local issue be connected with a larger, national event (e.g., local night spots go smoke-free for the Great American Smoke Out)?

Identifying newsworthy components can help turn an issue into a story. Stories have action, plot, and characters. What are they in relation to the topic of interest? Why is it a story *now*? Why will it matter to the people who read that newspaper or watch that television station?

General Strategies. There are four general strategies for getting in the news: creating news, piggybacking on breaking news, paying for advertisements, and using editorial strategies.

Creating News. Tobacco control advocate Russell Sciandra said, "To gain the media's attention, you can't just say something; you have to do something" (Wallack et al., 1999, p. 39). That "something" need not be elaborate, but it must be newsworthy. Creating news can be as simple as releasing new data or announcing a specific demand. The important part is that it be done publicly and that someone alert the news media, emphasizing why the story is newsworthy. For example, if advocates know that an important document will be released, they could plan a briefing for journalists so they will be prepared, or hold a news conference with the group's reaction to it.

Piggybacking on Breaking News. When advocates identify a connection between an issue and news of the day, they should make the story known to journalists. Tobacco control advocates used the occasion of President Clinton's perjury hearings to highlight the fact that tobacco company executives had lied under oath to Congress. Family planning advocates used news hype about Viagra to point out that health insurance plans were not covering contraceptives for women, though they covered Viagra. Piggybacking on breaking news can be achieved in a letter to the editor, with a news conference, or by other actions.

Paid Advertising. Buying space is sometimes the only way to be sure a message gets out unadulterated. In San Francisco, children's advocates used paid advertising to highlight a positive policy change that the news media were ignoring. The job market was tight in San Francisco in 2000, and that meant a crisis for child care. Childcare teachers, typically paid less than $7 an hour—less than parking attendants—were leaving the field for more lucrative jobs. Families that qualified for subsidized care could not get it because the childcare centers did not have the staff. Working with Coleman Advocates for Children and Youth, among others, Mayor Willie Brown took an unprecedented action: he allocated $4.1 million to increase the wages of 1,000 childcare workers serving low-income families. Never before had the city subsidized the salaries of noncity employees. The advocates were thrilled and immediately alerted the local news media. The reporters, however, refused to cover the story. They did not want to "toot the mayor's horn."

The advocates thought it was a legitimate story and were frustrated by the nonresponsive reporters. They decided to tell the story themselves in a full-page ad in the West Coast edition of the *New York Times*. The ad ran on August 7, 2000, during the Democratic national convention, which was being held in San Diego that year. It proclaimed: "Childcare History in the Making—San Francisco Mayor Willie Brown Sets National Standard for Quality, Affordable Childcare!" It suggested that readers challenge their own mayors to take the same action in their home towns. Mayor Willie Brown was still talking about the ad six months later when he signed the next budget allocations for child care.

Editorial Strategies. Letters to the editor, editorials, and op-eds (opinion editorials, or opinion pieces found opposite the editorial page) provide other opportunities for bringing attention to a policy solution. Letters are usually 200 words or less and can be written, faxed, or e-mailed to the editor of the newspaper. They are usually in response to a specific article or editorial the paper has published, offering a concise statement of support or objection.

Editorials are unsigned and written by the editorial board of the newspaper. Advocates can make an appointment to talk with the editorial board to ask them to take a position and make a statement about an issue or a pending policy. The meeting is usually attended by the newspaper staff responsible for writing the editorial and those who will make the decision about whether the newspaper will take a position on the issue. The advocates may have two or three people there who can speak to various aspects of the issue or represent different perspectives.

If the newspaper decides not to do an editorial, the advocates can ask if the paper would publish an op-ed. Op-eds are usually 600 to 800 words, written from a personal point of view. They describe the problem, solution, and its relevance to the readers. Monitoring should include reviewing op-eds, both to keep tabs on how an issue is being argued and to identify the style the news outlet prefers.

Newspapers often publish on the editorial pages the contact information and instructions for submitting letters and op-eds. Some radio stations and television news programs allow audience members to record commentaries that function like op-eds, though they are usually short (i.e., no more than a few minutes).

Tips and Techniques for Successful Media Advocacy

Several techniques can enhance media advocacy's effectiveness: calculating social math, localizing stories, cultivating authentic voices, and reusing the news.

Calculate Social Math

Social math is the art of making large numbers meaningful, usually by breaking them down and making a relevant, vivid comparison. Calculating social math can illustrate a message. Raw numbers assume that the audience already knows something about the issue and why the numbers are important or revealing. Comparisons, on the other hand, can highlight a specific point of view at the same time they deliver basic information.

To calculate social math, restate large numbers in terms of time or place, personalize numbers, or make comparisons that help bring a picture to mind. Consider these simple facts, stated with effective comparisons.

- About 950 packs of cigarettes are being sold in the United States every second of every day (Gloede, 1989).
- A children and youth advocacy group wanted to increase county spending on prevention of violence. To make their point they said, "In San Francisco, there is one police officer for every 18 young people and only one school counselor for every 500 kids" (Coleman Advocates, n.d.).
- Other violence prevention advocates wanted to make clear to the public and their policymakers that availability of firearms was a problem. They said, "Contra Costa County has 700 federally licensed firearms dealers—more than the number of schools, grocery stores and gas stations combined" ("Contra Costa County," 1995).

- Newspaper columnist Ellen Goodman (1998) noted that a worker who helps bury people makes more than one who helps them learn: the median wage for a funeral attendant is $7.16 an hour, while the median wage for a childcare worker is $6.17 an hour. Goodman feels that childcare workers are being paid based on what mothers are paid—nothing—and on what professional teachers earn.
- Public health education professor Meredith Minkler (1999) noted, "In a single year one company spent more than $30 million advertising a single sugar-coated cereal. During the same year, the amount spent by the U.S. government on nutrition education for school children was just $50,000 per state."
- A reporter in the *Wall Street Journal* illustrated the amount of chewing tobacco being consumed by writing, "Cigarette sales are down; dip sales are up. Laid out tin-to-tin, the dip sold last year would stretch between New York and Los Angeles 11 times. So there is quite a bit of furtive spitting going on" (Morse, 2000).
- A victim's rights advocate used irony to point out society's skewed priorities and illustrate the need for more resources when he said, "We have more shelters for animals than we have for human victims of abuse" (Stein, 1997).

Localize Stories

Every day there is a multitude of news from which to choose. News outlets are tuned in to satellite broadcasts from around the world that operate 24 hours daily. Assignment editors, city desk editors, reporters, and producers read several newspapers every day, listen to news radio and police scanners, and monitor wire services. One way advocates can break through that clutter is to alert their news contacts about the local relevance of a story. Questions they can consider include the following: "Why does this story matter to people who live here?" and "Why would it matter to the listeners at this radio station, the viewers of this local television news, or the readers of this newspaper?" When advocates know the answers to those questions, they will know what to tell the reporter. Every reporter has to convince his or her boss why to select one story over another. If the story has local relevance, it is much more likely to be pursued.

Cultivate Authentic Voices

Reporters populate their stories with characters. A common character in health stories is the "victim"—someone who has suffered from or has direct experience with the problem, whatever it might be. If the story is about binge drinking on college campuses, reporters will want to talk to students. If the story is about gun safety in the home, they will want to talk to a parent whose child was killed by a gun in the home. If the story is about immunizations for children, they will want to show a toddler getting a shot.

Reporters do this for two reasons. First, the reporter needs to present evidence in the story that what happened was real, that it happened to a real person. Showing someone with direct experience in the story makes that clear. Second, reporters feel that their audience will connect more with the emotion than the facts of a story. People who actually endured a trauma or other experience can be more compelling because they are speaking from experience. They qualify as a "real person," in journalists' parlance.

Besides the usual questions—"What is the problem?" and "What is the solution?"—reporters will ask victims another question: "How do you feel about the tragedy?" The problem, of course, is that if the story does not move much beyond the victim—if it is a portrait rather than a landscape—then when audiences see the story they are likely to distance themselves from the individual and say, "That won't happen to me," or, in some cases, even blame the victim. Journalists cannot tell stories without characters, and victims can be powerful spokespeople for public health. However, a better approach is to change the dynamic and think of victims as survivors or *authentic voices*. Authentic voices are survivors who have become advocates. They bring personal experience to the story, just like a victim, but they understand their role as advocates. When an authentic voice gets the question, "How do you feel about this tragedy?" he or she responds, "I feel angry because this tragedy could have been prevented," and then explains how.

Victims become authentic voices with training and experience as they move through their grief and put it to work for prevention. There are many authentic voices in public health to thank for opening up their lives to the public and becoming leaders for change regarding issues such as breast cancer, HIV/AIDS, and tobacco control. For example, in 2000 Mary Leigh Blek became the first chair of the board for the Million Mom March; she lost her son Matthew to a "Saturday night special" handgun and has been advocating for reasonable gun laws ever since. In 1980, Mothers Against Drunk Driving was created by a small group of women in California after a drunk driver killed Candy Lightner's 13-year-old daughter. Survivors have joined with public health advocates to advocate for safer baby cribs, drowning prevention, pedestrian safety, motorcycle helmets, mandatory CPR training, and auto safety, including interior trunk release latches (McLoughlin & Fennell, n.d.). All of these authentic voices have selflessly shared their stories and been willing characters in news stories to help further policies that can save lives.

Reuse the News

Media advocacy uses mass communication to reach a very small target—sometimes just one person. The power comes from the fact that a vast audience has been privy to this conversation between the advocates and the target. It is a public conversation, not a private conversation. To ensure the target understands this, advocates can reuse the news. If their op-ed is published, advocates can clip it, copy it, and send it to the target. They can have the target's constituents copy and send news stories and letters to the editor that have been published. They can also reuse the news to educate reporters who are just coming to the issue or to educate new advocates. They can share clippings and discuss them in order to become better at framing issues and anticipating the opposition's questions and challenges. News, simply by virtue of having been published, confers legitimacy and credibility on issues. Media advocates reuse the news to remind the target that the public is paying attention and knows what it wants done.

Overcoming Challenges in Media Advocacy

The biggest barrier to successful media advocacy is in the development of a clear overall strategy, even before getting access to reporters is considered. Other barriers include institutional constraints, not staying "on message," and being distracted by the opposition. This section discusses strategies for overcoming these barriers.

Avoid Having a Murky Strategy

The most important part of media advocacy is developing strategy. If the strategy is not clear and the target has not been well defined, the media advocacy effort will be diffused and ineffective. Public health advocates sometimes resist the simplification necessary to carve out a viable strategy. Public health problems are complex, and that complexity needs to be addressed. However, not everything can be done at once. Public health problems need to be prioritized into manageable chunks that can be addressed in specific time periods. The alternative—strategies that remain too large or overly vague—will be ineffective. Goals such as "raising awareness" are not specific enough for media advocacy campaigns. Instead, clear objectives must be stated that identify who must do what to create or change the rules that will ensure healthier social and physical environments.

Advocates must translate general principles into substantive demands. For example, in San Francisco, a campaign to seek justice for a man who unnecessarily died in police custody was transformed into a campaign to change police practices. Demanding justice was too vague and left the action up to others. So the advocates asked themselves: What would justice look like? They decided that the offending police officer should be fired and safeguards put in place to avoid future hires of officers with similar records. Advocates had then defined justice in tangible terms that could be put into practice, and used media advocacy to put pressure on the mayor and the police commission to enact the policy changes they desired.

Media advocacy strategies and targets can change over time. In fact, they *should* change. Targets and strategies will shift in response to circumstances and after the advocates achieve their objectives. Advocates can use the strategy development questions discussed earlier to refocus their efforts and evaluate their strategies. With every new activity, they should ask themselves: How will this help us achieve our objectives? And will this make a clear, positive change in the environment surrounding the people whose health we are concerned about? The answers to those questions can guide strategy and decisions throughout the media advocacy effort.

Alter Perceived Institutional Constraints

Media advocacy is about raising community voices to demand change. In most cases, policy change is the desired outcome. Sometimes this will require lobbying, which public agencies and some nonprofit organizations are prohibited from conducting. In most cases, however, there is a lot those in both public and nonprofit agencies can do that is not considered lobbying. Unfortunately, advocates often stop short of what is allowed and limit their effectiveness needlessly. Organizations such as the Alliance for Justice provide training and consultation to nonprofits to help them maximize their ability to participate legally in the policy process. Constraints are often not as prohibitive as some in the agency might perceive.

Still, media advocacy can be confrontational. Thus, public health practitioners in health departments or other institutions may not be comfortable being "out front" on media advocacy campaigns. Some have a preference for consensus when conflict is what is needed. In these cases, individuals can find roles for themselves in the media advocacy effort that place them more in the background than the foreground. For example, health departments can provide data, resources, meeting space, technical assistance, and other support without compromise.

Avoid Being Distracted by the Opposition

While media advocates need to construct thoughtful, succinct answers to the questions their opponents will raise, their goal is not to convince the opposition. Media advocates can be distracted by the arguments their opposition puts forward, and may be tempted to answer those arguments point by point. Sometimes that is necessary, but often it is a ploy by opponents to frame the issue on their own terms. Instead, media advocates' goal is to motivate and mobilize their supporters so those voices will be heard and attended to by policymakers. Everyone does not have to be convinced that the proposal is worth supporting—only those who have decision-making power must be convinced. Media advocacy employs the mass media to make private conversations public so that decision makers can be held accountable for their decisions and the impact of those decisions on the public's health. Media advocates need to be vigilant when defining the problem and the solution and focus their attention on the clear and consistent articulation of what they want. Thus, articulating a clear message and staying on message are extremely important.

Stay on Message

Staying on message means that whatever advocates may be asked, they do not stray from the key message they are trying to deliver. Staying on message is a skill that can be honed with practice. It is especially helpful to practice aloud, with colleagues. That way, advocates can anticipate what questions they might receive from reporters, decision makers, or the opposition and can craft answers that lead logically from the question to the outcome they seek. Practicing aloud is important because speaking is different from writing or thinking. The right words will flow more easily if they have been said before. At the same time, advocates should not memorize a script—that can sound stiff and forced. Instead, frequent practice and feedback sessions will help advocates prepare for staying on message.

Expected Outcomes

When media advocacy is done well, healthy public policy is enacted and implemented. Enacting policies that benefit the public's health is a long-term process, however, with many contributing factors. Media advocacy cannot achieve that end alone but can certainly amplify advocates' voices and accelerate the process. Properly applied, media advocacy can punctuate the advocacy process, add urgency to a campaign, and create visibility. Media advocacy does this by increasing the salience of issues for the public and policymakers through agenda setting and framing. Practicing media advocacy will also increase the capacity of local groups to influence the rules that govern their environments.

Increased Skills and Power

Because policy advocacy is usually a long-term endeavor, it is useful to identify some interim effects and outcomes of media advocacy. The most immediate interim effects of media advocacy are the increases in skills and power of the groups using it. By developing and adapting strategy, advocates can gain skills in critical thinking. By talking with journalists and others about the solutions they seek, advocates develop the confidence necessary to speak effectively in public. They become skillful at framing for content and understanding newsworthiness so they can frame for access. By participating in the policy process, either by meeting with decision makers or mobilizing supporters, advocates exercise their democratic power. These skills build on one another and transfer as advocates work together in a community setting to demand change.

Better Relationships with Journalists

An important outcome that advocates can expect from media advocacy campaigns is better relationships with journalists. This tangible benefit develops over the course of a media advocacy campaign—and from one campaign to another—because advocates bring good information and interesting stories to reporters. The mutually beneficial relationship helps reporters get what they need to do their job and eases advocates' access to and responsiveness from journalists. Stated simply, an expected outcome of media advocacy is that certain reporters and advocates end up in each other's Rolodex. For example, after their concerted media advocacy effort to generate news that reframed alcohol as a policy issue, staff at the Marin Institute for the Prevention of Alcohol and Other Drug Problems, located in California, were frequent sources for journalists. Eventually, reporters would call the Marin Institute for comments on stories that had been generated elsewhere. The Marin Institute was now a required source on alcohol policy issues.

Increased Visibility and Influence

Advocates' increased skills and power, along with their better relationships with reporters, lead to increased visibility for the issue and more influence from the advocates on how that issue is interpreted. If they are successful, advocates will have generated news that put their issue and solution on the policymakers' agenda. Advocates can expect to see their examples used in debate by themselves and eventually by others, shifting the debate toward the advocates' desired outcomes.

Advocates' influence will increase with the increased visibility because news coverage confers legitimacy and credibility.

Conclusion

Public health educators can harness the power of the news media to advance healthy public policy. They can increase their effectiveness by developing an overall strategy, learning about how the news media operate, developing a specific media strategy, developing a message that frames the issue from a public health perspective, and understanding how to attract journalists' attention. The news media are too important a resource to ignore. If health educators are serious about serving the public and improving its health, they need to be serious about the news and about learning how to better integrate it into prevention efforts.

Media advocacy, however, is not appropriate in every instance. The strategy requires a clear and precise plan for policy change and a constituency that can carry it out. It is a public strategy—on the record. Media advocates bring public attention to specific individuals. At times they may need to be confrontational and adversarial, depending on the situation. The policies being advocated for are usually controversial. If they were not, there would be no need for a pressure tool and publicity via media advocacy. Advocates should be clear with themselves and their colleagues about what is at stake when choosing to use media advocacy.

Media advocacy is the right choice when public demands must be made and pressure brought to bear on decision makers to protect and promote the public's health.

References

California Center for Health Improvement. (2000, December). Joining forces to fight childhood asthma: A Prop 10 opportunity. *Field Lessons*, pp. 1–8.

Coleman Advocates for Children and Youth (2000, August 7). Childcare history in the making—San Francisco Mayor Willie Brown sets national standard for quality, affordable childcare! [Advertisement]. *The New York Times*, West Coast ed., p. A19.

Coleman Advocates for Children and Youth. (n.d.). *Youth time* [Brochure]. San Francisco: Author.

Contra Costa County offers advice on reducing gun use. (1995, July). *The Nation's Health*, p. 11.

Dorfman, L. (1994). *News operations: How television reports on health.* Unpublished doctoral dissertation, University of California-Berkeley.

Gloede, W. F. (1989). Agency execs feel at home in Marlboro country. In E. Thorson (Ed.), *Advertising age: The principles of advertising at work* (pp. 103–105). Lincolnwood, IL: NTC Business Books.

Goodman, E. (1998, January 15). No easy fix for child care. *San Francisco Chronicle,* p. A23.

Iyengar, S. (1991). *Is anyone responsible?* Chicago: University of Chicago Press.

McLoughlin, E., & Fennell, J. (n.d.). Channeling grief into policy change: Survivor advocacy for injury prevention. *Injury Prevention Newsletter,* Vol. 13. San Francisco: The Trauma Foundation. Retrieved October 14, 2006, from http://www.traumaf.org/images/IPNweb.pdf

Minkler, M. (1999). Personal responsibility for health? A review of the arguments and the evidence at century's end. *Health Education and Behavior, 26,* 121–140.

Morse, D. (2000, February 11). If you can't smoke in the office, snuff can be a secret vice. *The Wall Street Journal,* p. A1.

Riley, B. A. (2001). Media advocacy. In R. J. Bensley & J. Brookins-Fisher (Eds.), *Community health education methods: A practitioner's guide* (pp. 383–409). Sudbury, MA: Jones & Bartlett.

Stein, J., deputy director of the National Organization for Victim Assistance, quoted in J. Shiver Jr. (1997, August 25). Home violence underreported, U.S. study says. *Los Angeles Times,* p. A1.

Wallack, L., & Dorfman, L. (1996). Media advocacy: A strategy for advancing policy and promoting health. *Health Education Quarterly, 23,* 293–317.

Wallack, L., & Dorfman, L. (2001). Putting policy into health communication: The role of media advocacy. In R. E. Rice & C. K. Atkin (Eds.), *Public communication campaigns* (3rd ed., pp. 389–401). Thousand Oaks, CA: Sage.

Wallack, L., Dorfman, L., Jernigan, D., & Themba, M. (1993). *Media advocacy and public health: Power for prevention.* Thousand Oaks, CA: Sage.

Wallack, L., Dorfman, L., & Woodruff, K. (1997). Communications and public health. In F. D. Scutchfield & C. W. Keck (Eds.), *Principles of public health practice* (pp. 183–194). Albany, NY: Delmar.

Wallack, L., Woodruff, K., Dorfman, L., & Diaz, I. (1999). *News for a change: An advocate's guide to working with the media.* Thousand Oaks, CA: Sage.

Wilgoren, J. (2000, March 15). Effort to curb binge drinking in college falls short. *The New York Times,* p. A16.

CHAPTER TEN

PRIMARY PREVENTION AND PROGRAM EVALUATION

Daniel Perales

E valuation is a necessary element for documenting the success of prevention efforts. This chapter is written to illustrate how primary prevention efforts can be evaluated. In fact, because quality primary prevention aims to have an impact on large populations, its effects *can* be measured by looking at overall population changes over time. In this chapter, the term *program* is defined broadly as a systematic effort to achieve multiple purposes including changing attitudes, knowledge, behaviors, organizational practices, and policies that can help create healthy environments and healthy people. Programs can occur in differing geographical and political settings and with varying purposes and structures (Fink, 2005). Primary prevention programs, specifically, are defined as those that are designed to forestall or completely prevent the onset of disease or the occurrence of injuries.

Whether programs are designed for primary prevention (for example, child immunization programs), secondary prevention (such as breast cancer screening), or tertiary prevention (as in drug rehabilitation), the programs themselves and the populations they serve benefit greatly from a well-designed and systematically implemented formal evaluation. Therefore, a critical component of any effort that is intended to effect individual- or community-level change is a systematic method for gathering information about the prevention activities and the effectiveness of those activities on the priority population. Program evaluation can be defined succinctly as ". . . the diligent investigation of a program's characteristics and merits"

(Fink, 2005, p. 4). A more comprehensive definition is ". . . a systematic process for an organization to obtain information on its activities, its impacts, and the effectiveness of its work, so that it can improve its activities and describe its accomplishments" (Mattessich, 2003, p. 3).

It is not uncommon for critics to state that primary prevention efforts are not cost-effective and that evaluation of lifestyle behavior change, in particular, is difficult at best (Russell, 1986). However, beginning with the 1979 landmark publication *Healthy People*, (U.S. Department of Health, Education and Welfare, 1979), the value of implementing population-based prevention programs has been resoundingly endorsed by the Institute of Medicine (2003) of the National Academy of Sciences and more recently by a study by the Health Partners Research Foundation (Maciosek et al., 2006) sponsored by the Centers for Disease Control and Prevention (CDC). Commenting on the study's findings, the former director of the CDC's Division of Prevention Research and Analytic Methods, Steven Teutsch (2006), stated that ". . . many of the most effective interventions occur at the population level. These include things such as systems to assure access to healthcare, laws and regulations to limit access to tobacco and assure clean air, programs to reduce toxic exposures, interventions to reduce risky behaviors, health education programs and messages, and creation of healthy environments and the availability of healthy foods."

Evaluation is considered so important to public health that the CDC lists evaluation as one of the ten essential public health services (Harrell et al., 1994). Indeed, both the Institute of Medicine and the CDC recognize that evaluation is needed in order to develop evidenced-based prevention programs. In effect, evaluation makes it possible to understand how and why programs work or do not work. This is especially important for primary prevention efforts because of the potential broad-scale social and economic impact of such programs on community health.

Although prevention efforts are commonly perceived as focusing primarily on creating small-scope individual or group behavioral change, primary prevention efforts typically reach statewide and national audiences, especially through policies that can produce communitywide norm changes. For example, in 1988, California voters passed Proposition 99 (the California Tobacco Health Protection Act), which increased the state cigarette tax by 25 cents per pack. The funds were used for health education, a statewide media campaign, and tobacco-related research. These funds were also used to create the statewide California Tobacco Control Program (CTCP). The CTCP uses a comprehensive approach to create social norms around tobacco use by ". . . indirectly influencing current and potential future tobacco users by creating a social milieu and legal climate in which tobacco becomes less desirable, less acceptable, and less accessible" (California

Department of Health Services, 1998, p. 3). In this chapter, I will provide several examples of how primary prevention efforts can be evaluated.

The Benefits of Evaluation

There are numerous reasons for evaluating a program, including acquiring answers to questions such as those posed by Rossi, Lipsey, and Freeman (2004, p. 3):

Is a particular intervention reaching its target population?

Is the intervention being implemented well?

Are the intended services being provided?

Is the intervention effective in attaining the desired goals or benefits?

In addition, program evaluation can identify a program's strengths and weaknesses; modify a program's goals, objectives, and intervention activities based on quantitative or qualitative evaluation feedback or both; validate the program's worth among constituents and stakeholders; and allow program managers to use evaluation findings to improve chances for the program's future funding and sustainability.

Evaluation is increasingly identified by program managers as an important part of their management responsibility. In addition, it is rapidly becoming an expectation of program grant funding by foundations, nonprofit organizations, and local, state, and federal government agencies. Over the past ten or fifteen years, many private and publicly funding organizations and agencies have incorporated formal evaluation into their requests for proposals. For example, the United Way of America, which raised over $3.8 billion for social and prevention programs in 2004 (United Way of America, 2006), has been a leader among organizations that fund such programs in promoting and adopting the use of program evaluation, especially outcome evaluation, among its grant recipients. This evaluation emphasis has received surprisingly appreciative responses from program managers (United Way of America, 2000).

The Evaluation Process

Evaluators often use various frameworks to conceptualize and develop their evaluation plans. This section of the chapter highlights a few of those frameworks and illustrates how they are linked to the evaluation of primary prevention.

The CDC Evaluation Framework

The Centers for Disease Control and Prevention's evaluation framework (see Figure 10.1), developed in 1999, is an excellent way for evaluators and program managers to conceptualize and plan a primary prevention evaluation.

The framework has six steps: engage stakeholders, describe the program, focus the evaluation design, gather credible evidence, justify conclusions, and ensure use and share lessons learned.

Step 1: Engage stakeholders. Stakeholders are defined as ". . . persons or organizations having an investment in what will be learned from an evaluation and what will be done with the knowledge" (CDC, 1999, p. 5). They include those involved in program operations, those served or affected by the program, and primary users of the evaluation. Engaging stakeholders in the evaluation ensures that their viewpoints are respected and that the next five steps are more easily implemented.

Step 2: Describe the program. A program description is critical to developing the evaluation design and should describe the problem or need, the expected outcomes, the intervention strategies, the resources and community assets that will be used to implement the activities, how the evaluation will assess the program,

FIGURE 10.1. THE CDC EVALUATION FRAMEWORK.

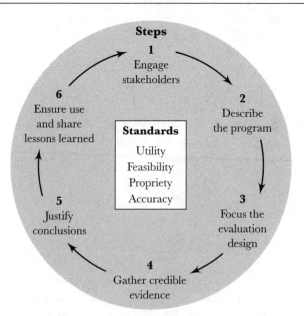

Source: Centers for Disease Control and Prevention (1999).

the social ecological context; and a logic model flowchart that sets forth the key steps that can achieve the desired outcomes.

Step 3: Focus the evaluation design. An evaluation must be systematic and focused. Focusing the evaluation design includes establishing a purpose for the evaluation (for example, to assess effects on participants, to assess policy compliance, or to assess program practices), deciding how the evaluation results will be used, and determining a specific evaluation design (experimental, quasi-experimental, or nonexperimental).

Step 4: Gather credible evidence. This step begins with gathering information on indicators that can serve as specific measures for program success. Gathering credible evidence requires that multiple information sources—including people, extant data, and primary data such as surveys—are gathered in sufficient quantity to allow for precise conclusions. Data-gathering approaches should also take cultural preferences into account and ensure privacy and confidentiality.

Step 5: Justify conclusions. Evaluation conclusions are justified when they are linked to the evidence gathered and judged against agreed values or standards set by the stakeholders. Stakeholders must have confidence that the conclusions are justified before they are used for decision making.

Step 6: Ensure use and share lessons learned. Deliberate effort is needed to ensure that the evaluation processes and findings are used and disseminated appropriately; particularly to the community stakeholders.

Involving Stakeholders: Asset Mapping and Evaluation

The CDC evaluation framework is distinctive because of the emphasis it places on involving stakeholders. Stakeholder involvement in evaluation is even more critical today as federal, state, and foundation funding increasingly requires community-based coalition involvement in program planning, implementation, and evaluation (Wallerstein, Polascek, & Maltrud, 2002). For example, the W. K. Kellogg Foundation (1998) has an evaluation framework that includes a participatory process that values multiple perspectives and involves people who care about the project. A participatory process also prepares organizations to use evaluation as an ongoing function of management and leadership.

In recent years, participatory evaluation processes such as empowerment evaluation (Fetterman, Kafterian, & Wandersman, 1996) and the more recent emergence of community-based participatory research (CBPR, discussed in greater detail in Chapter Eleven) have emphasized the importance of collaborative evaluation approaches that incorporate stakeholder participation from beginning to end. Community-based participatory research is defined by Minkler and Wallerstein (2003) as a "collaborative approach to research" that "equitably involves all partners in the research process and recognizes the unique strengths that each brings. CBPR begins with a research topic of importance to the community with the aim of combining knowledge and action for social change to improve community health and eliminate health disparities" (p. 4). The significance of CBPR in evaluation research was recently emphasized by the Institute of Medicine (2003), which stated that public health professionals must understand the major concepts and principles underlying CBPR, and achieve competency in this area, in order to engage more effectively in research and practice.

Participatory approaches are not without their difficulties for evaluators. However, evaluators who have learned from their participatory research experiences leave us with sage advice. Wallerstein and Duran (2006) believe that "in CBPR work, we suggest that the most important values are integrity coupled with humility. These values underlie our process with communities, in the science and how we present ourselves, and support our goals in doing this work" (p. 10). Roe and colleagues, in their work with a CDC-funded HIV Planning Council, were even more explicit:

> Empowerment evaluation requires an additional set of professional skills. Evaluators must be flexible, quick-thinking, self-critical, optimistic, and truly interested in the groups they work with and the potential of the community. Collecting this type of data requires the ability to engender trust, coax out stories, process qualitative information, and represent heartfelt experiences. This takes time, energy, and a keen eye for the phrase or the moment that may move a group forward. Evaluators must have an affection for the communities they work with while always maintaining an internal distance from which to observe process and explore empowering strategies. [Roe, Berenstein, Goette, & Roe, 1997, p. 321]

Involving stakeholders implies that the evaluator knows the community well. Understanding a program and its community setting is critical to evaluation. This may begin by conducting a needs assessment as part of a formative evaluation. Kretzmann and McKnight (1993) make convincing arguments for conducting assessments that go beyond the traditional focus on needs and problems because such approaches label communities as needy, deficient, and populated by problematic and deficient people whose needs must be met by outsiders. Their asset-mapping approach recognizes that all communities have the capacity to address their own problems and that external assistance should be requested by the community itself.

Mapping community capacity through a participatory process can identify key stakeholders and resources that can be used for program development, implementation, and evaluation. The accompanying case example of a primary prevention program describes a participatory asset-mapping process and its implications for evaluation.

Case Example: Evaluating the
North Philadelphia Firearms Reduction Initiative

Hausman and Becker (2000) used a participatory assessment approach, called Rapid Participatory Appraisal (RPA), to address the reduction of youth firearm violence in North Philadelphia and subsequently identify evaluation indicators of success. They developed a key informant questionnaire that incorporated key dimensions of community capacity as previously defined by Kretzmann and McKnight (1993). The questionnaire was reviewed by members of the Community Advisory Board (CAB) of the Firearm Connection: North Philadelphia Firearms Reduction Initiative (NPFRI), a collaboration of health organizations, law enforcement officials, social service agencies, and local residents. Questionnaire wording changes were made on the CAB's recommendations.

Beginning with the CAB and using a snowball technique, the evaluators identified 111 people, 33 of whom were successfully interviewed over a six-month period. After analyzing the results, all interviewees were invited to review the analysis and interpretations, a participatory method that resulted in the interviewees' confirming that their comments had been "heard well." The results showed that although firearm violence was a community concern, the most serious problem identified was drugs. Interviewees also cited unemployment, welfare reform, abandoned buildings, trash, and lack of alternative activities for youth as major issues.

The neighborhoods were mapped, and resources and activities were identified. However, the data also showed that there was a lack of coordination and visibility of those resources. This information resulted in an organizational expansion of the CAB to promote communication and intervention development that resulted in health, law enforcement, and social service partnerships. In addition, the assessment report documenting assets, agencies, and neighborhood information was offered and eagerly accepted by all of the interviewees.

The project funder had specified that reducing firearm violence was to be the purpose for the NPFRI. However, the compelling evidence produced by RPA helped the project and the evaluator convince the funder to support a project and an evaluation that both addressed the funder's primary prevention interest in reducing firearm violence and the community's concern about drugs and opportunities for youth. In effect, the researchers had defined the *real* problem, especially from the community's perspective, and developed capacity-based strategies for overcoming it.

In collaboration with the NPFRI, the evaluator developed indicators of success that were meaningful to the funder and the community stakeholders (see Table 10.1).

Overall, the evaluator felt that by understanding the community through a participatory assessment process, in collaboration with the NPFRI, he was able to develop evaluation indicators that reflected success in ways that were important to the various stakeholders, allowed for the development of strategies for gathering evaluation data from multiple sources with several methods, and used a socioecological perspective to address the identified problems and resources across several levels.

TABLE 10.1. EVALUATION MARKERS FOR PROGRESS AND OUTCOMES, NORTH PHILADELPHIA FIREARMS REDUCTION INITIATIVE.

Outcomes	Measures	Evaluation Tools or Methods
Community Capacity Outcomes		
Increased participation of youth and community in specifying key firearm issues and solutions	Participation rates of youth, parents, and community organizations in committee defined activities	Event logs; attendance records
Increased youth involvement and leadership on gun violence prevention	Youth leadership training participation; youth leadership activities	Attendance records; event logs; youth logs
Increased linkages among community-based organizations and other prevention resources	Numbers of collaborative efforts; increased use of technical assistance resources	Attendance records; event logs; network maps; committee reports
Increased number of community interventions for safety and control	Number and nature of new intervention activities; new partnerships with police, courts, and health care providers	Event logs; committee reports
Increased intergenerational communication on firearm attitudes, beliefs, and risk behaviors	Number and nature of youth and adult activities	Event logs; satisfaction surveys
Increased awareness and involvement of medical providers	Provider use of monitoring and intervention protocols; number of new links with community organizations	Event logs; health provider survey; committee reports
Community-Indicated Outcomes		
Increased sense of community safety and control	Community residents' sense of safety and control; increased civic involvement	Citywide household survey; repeat interviews; environmental observations
Increased understanding of firearm risks among youth and adults	Changes in community norms	Health provider survey; youth survey; repeat interviews

TABLE 10.1. EVALUATION MARKERS FOR PROGRESS AND OUTCOMES, NORTH PHILADELPHIA FIREARMS REDUCTION INITIATIVE, Cont'd.

Outcomes	Measures	Evaluation Tools or Methods
Health-Related Outcomes		
Reduction of illegal firearm possession among youth	Indications of a downward trend	Data derived from city-wide police gun-tracing efforts
Reduction in unintentional and intentional firearm injury among youth	Indications of a downward trend	Data derived from city-wide emergency room surveillance

Logic Models

Logic models can also be considered planning and evaluation frameworks, since they describe a process from beginning to end. Rossi, Lipsey, and Freeman (2004) note that "simply laying out the logic of the program in this form makes it relatively easy to identify questions the evaluation might appropriately address" (p. 94).

Goldman and Schmalz (2006) believe that logic models can help the evaluation do all of the following:

- Identify differences between the ideal program and its real operation
- Frame questions about attribution and contribution
- Specify the nature of questions being asked
- Determine which indicators will (and will not) be measured
- Document accomplishments
- Organize evidence about the program
- Prepare reports and other media
- Tell the program's story

A good primary prevention example of a logic model is the one used by the CDC's VERB Youth Media Campaign (CDC, 2006b). Directed at "tweeners" (youth aged nine to twelve), VERB is designed to promote physical activity among young people and prevent overweight. The CDC uses the logic model to identify the outcomes for the campaign and link them to each other and to specific activities. The VERB logic model also demonstrates that prevention outcomes are often long-term and hence take time. Table 10.2 shows the basic elements of the VERB logic model.

TABLE 10.2. ELEMENTS OF THE CDC'S VERB CAMPAIGN LOGIC MODEL.

Inputs	Activities	Outcomes
Consultants	Advertising	*Short term:* Awareness of campaign brand messages
Staff	Promotions	
Research and evaluation	Web	*Medium term:* Changes in subjective norms, beliefs, self-efficacy, and perceived behavioral control
Contractors	Public relations	
Community infrastructure	National and community outreach	
Partnerships		*Long term:* Engaging in and maintaining physical activity

Prevention Planning and Evaluation: The PRECEDE-PROCEED Model

The PRECEDE-PROCEED model is widely recognized for its program planning uses, but it also provides an excellent framework for evaluating primary prevention programs because of its comprehensiveness. In some respects, the PRECEDE-PROCEED model can also be considered a specialized logic model in that it can be used to visualize the expected sequence of program steps from program development to the evaluation of long-term outcomes.

PRECEDE-PROCEED is probably the most widely used planning model in the field of health promotion and health education and has nearly a thousand published applications (Green, 2005). PRECEDE is an acronym for Predisposing, Reinforcing, and Enabling Causes in Educational Diagnosis and Evaluation, and PROCEED is an acronym for Policy, Regulatory, Organizational Constructs in Educational and Environmental Development. The PRECEDE portion was developed by Lawrence W. Green during the late 1970s from his research and public health experiences in the areas of cost-benefit evaluation, family planning, social factors in health behavior, diffusion and adoption theory, and other models of change (Green, 2005). In 1992, Marshall Kreuter's participation helped create the full PRECEDE-PROCEED model. Kreuter and colleagues note that "from its earliest applications in the late 1970s, the model has evolved from a largely linear, causal-chain planning model to an ecological one accounting for a wide range of factors that include social, economic, and environmental determinants of health" (Kreuter, De Rosa, Howze, & Baldwin, 2004, p. 448). The latest version of the model (Green & Kreuter, 2005) is presented in Figure 10.2.

As shown in Table 10.3, the model begins with formative evaluation of the first four PRECEDE phases and uses process, impact, and outcome evaluation components of PROCEED to measure and document change on people and their environments.

FIGURE 10.2. THE PRECEDE-PROCEED MODEL.

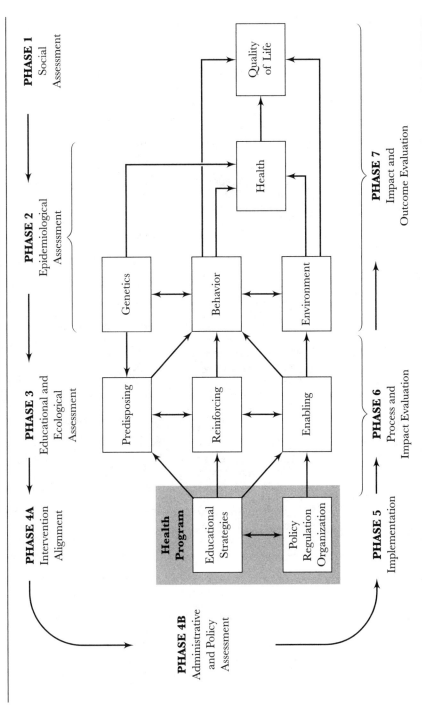

Source: Adapted from Green & Kreuter (2005), fig. 2.1.

TABLE 10.3. EVALUATION PHASES OF THE PRECEDE-PROCEED MODEL.

	Phases 1–4: Formative Evaluation	Phases 6 and 7: Process, Impact, and Outcome Evaluation
Phase 1: Social Assessment Quality of life	Assess and document feelings, needs, concerns, assets, and community capacity that describe quality of life.	*Phase 7: Outcome Evaluation* Measure the factors that describe overall changes in the quality of life.
Phase 2: Epidemiological Assessment Health conditions	Assess and document health conditions including morbidity, mortality, disability, and risk factors.	*Phase 7: Outcome Evaluation* Measure and describe the epidemiological indicators that evidence changes in health conditions.
Phase 2: Epidemiological Assessment Genetics Behavior Environment	Assess and document indicators of health including genetic, behavioral, and environmental factors that affect quality of life.	*Phase 6: Impact Evaluation* Measure and describe the epidemiological and social indicators that evidence changes in behavior and environments that affect health status.
Phase 3: Educational and Ecological Assessment Predisposing Reinforcing Enabling	Assess and document the cognitive and social antecedents that influence behaviors that in turn affect health.	*Phase 6: Impact Evaluation* Measure changes in the impact objectives that reflect the predisposing, reinforcing, and enabling factors that promote healthy behaviors and environments.
Phase 4A: Intervention Alignment Health Program: Educational strategies Policy Regulation Organization *Phase 4B: Administrative and Policy Assessment*	Assess and document administrative resources, regulations, and policies that can affect educational and environment factors and shape program implementation.	*Phase 6: Process Evaluation* Document and measure process objectives that address program capacity, the activities and strategies that comprise the intervention, and the response of practitioners and participants to the intervention's activities.
Phase 5: Implementation	Implement activities that deploy program resources, implement policy and organizational changes, and coordinate the program's interventions.	*Phase 6: Process Evaluation* Document and measure program capacity, the activities that comprise the intervention, and the response of practitioners and participants to the intervention's processes.

Some of the applications of the PRECEDE model in the evaluation of successful primary prevention programs include a one-year smoking prevention, exercise, and nutrition educational program that showed a significant decrease in chronic-disease risk factors among 2,283 fourth-graders in New York (Walter, Hofman, Connelly, Barrett, & Kost, 1985); a six-year study by Walter (1989) that showed a significant decrease in cholesterol levels, dietary fat intake, and initiation of smoking in children; and a major study of primary and secondary prevention services in a large HMO that showed that a synthesis of clinical medicine and public health population-based approaches to the development and provision of clinical preventive services resulted in decreases in late-stage breast cancer in adult smokers, in addition to increases in child immunization levels and use of bicycle helmets by children (Thompson, Taplin, McAfee, Mandelson, & Smith, 1995).

Developing Evaluation Questions

Evaluation methods are grounded in efforts to answer evaluation questions. Ideally, the questions are derived from the goals and objectives that were collaboratively developed with stakeholders. Rossi, Lipsey, and Freeman (2004) note that good evaluation questions must be reasonable and appropriate. Appropriate and reasonable questions are founded on detailed descriptions that illustrate program structure and activities, priority population characteristics, and knowledge about the problems, needs, and assets. Since many prevention programs operate from finite funding, appropriateness also means that the program should be able to answer the questions within the funding time frame and budget. The evaluation questions should also be answerable through the identification of variables that, ideally, can be measured.

Depending on the type of prevention program implemented, the evaluation questions can focus on the program's processes, the intermediate effect of those processes, or the program's final impact or outcomes. Perhaps more important, the evaluation questions can help program managers, stakeholders, and evaluators decide what data should be collected, where they should be collected, and how to collect, analyze, and interpret the data.

Evaluation Data

Evaluations are grounded in data. Most adherents of evidence-based designs view collecting quantitative data ("hard data") as the most appropriate way to measure change. A method of evaluation whereby individual cases, situations, or events are studied to formulate a general principle involves the gathering of qualitative data. This method produces what is often called "soft data," such as descriptions and opinions.

Prevention researchers (Rimer, Glanz, & Rasband, 2001; Steckler, McLeroy, Goodman, Bird, & McCormick, 1992) recognize that there has been an ongoing debate about the role of qualitative versus quantitative prevention research but advocate for the inclusion of both types of data into the definition of evaluation evidence. Indeed, qualitative research is valuable because it can ". . . provide insight not only into *what* happened but *why* it happened" (Rimer et al., 2001, p. 234). Table 10.4 describes the advantages and disadvantages of quantitative and qualitative methods.

TABLE 10.4. THE PROS AND CONS OF QUANTITATIVE AND QUALITATIVE APPROACHES TO DATA COLLECTION.

Quantitative Evaluation	Qualitative Evaluation
Larger numbers—generalizable to a broader population	Smaller number of people or cases
Deductive generalizations—objectivity; strength of the scientific method; experimental and quasi-experimental designs; statistical analysis	Inductive process—phenomenological inquiring; naturalistic, holistic; understanding the experience in context; content or case analysis
Valid, reliable instrument used to gather data; specific administration protocol	Researcher is the instrument; less rigid protocol
Use of standardized measures; predetermined response categories	Able to study selected issues in depth and detail
Rigor	Flexibility, insight
Results easily aggregated for analysis and easily presented	Understanding of what individual variation means; deepening understanding, insights
Can be perceived as biased, predictable, or rigged to obtain certain result	Offers credibility of an outsider making assessment
Results easily aggregated for analysis and easily presented	Results are longer, detailed, variable in content; difficult to analyze
Data include actual numbers; frequencies or counts of people, events, systems changes, passage of policy and legislation, trends	Data include group or individual opinions or perceptions; relationships, anecdotal comments, assessment of quality; descriptions; case studies; unanticipated outcomes
Experimental conditions and designs to control or reduce variation in extraneous variables; focus on limited number of predetermined measures	Openness to variation and multiple directions

Source: Adapted from Francisco, Butterfoss, & Capwell (2001).

Measuring and Evaluating Primary Prevention Programs

Primary prevention efforts, especially those requiring significant behavior change (such as smoking cessation), have often been viewed as difficult to measure and evaluate. This is particularly true of efforts that require long-term assessment of effect, such as the reduction in diabetes prevalence rates as a result of primary prevention efforts. The following examples will provide some insight into how primary prevention programs can be measured and evaluated.

When evaluators, stakeholders, and program managers are deciding on which type of data they will need to answer their evaluation questions and show the effects of their prevention efforts, they need to consider *what* they want to measure. This requires an understanding of the program's purpose. Some programs, especially those that are addressing new health issues, will want to know if their intervention activities are affecting the awareness, knowledge, and even attitudes of people. For example, during the early stages of the HIV/AIDS outbreak, it was very important to conduct evaluations that assessed the public's knowledge of how HIV was transmitted (DiClemente, Zorn, & Temoshok, 1986), in order to shape prevention strategies. Nearly two decades later, additional evaluation research proved that many of the HIV primary prevention strategies that were developed had been effective in the United States (CDC, 2006a).

As shown in Table 10.5, awareness, knowledge, and attitudes can be measured to only a minimal extent with interviews and surveys. These measures can be indicators that a primary prevention message is at least increasing knowledge. However, much more desirable measures of the effectiveness of prevention program interventions are ones that indicate behavior change. These not only include measures of desired behavior change, such as smoking cessation and increased exercise, but also measuring knowledge-induced behavior change such as practicing new low-fat food preparation skills or compliance with car seat belt laws via observations of drivers. Measures of health status change can provide even greater evidence of a primary prevention program's effectiveness. For example, a program designed to reduce risk for diabetes among diagnosed prediabetics will likely incorporate an educational component, a social support component, and a clinical management component. The educational component will include information about diabetes, food preparation, and exercise, all of which can be evaluated with instruments that can measure knowledge, food skills, and self-reported changes in attitudes about preventing diabetes. The social support component can be assessed through qualitative and quantitative measures of self-esteem and increased self-efficacy in managing healthier behaviors. However, the clinical component can provide quantitative health status measures such as a decrease in weight loss and normal blood tests that can showcase the biological changes resulting from the knowledge, social support, and behavior change.

TABLE 10.5. USEFUL EVALUATION MEASURES, BY DATA COLLECTION METHOD.

Focus of Measurement	Measures Yielding Quantitative Data	Measures Yielding Qualitative Data
Awareness, knowledge, attitudes	Written instruments (true-or-false items), telephone surveys	Interviews, focus groups
Behavior	Written self-reports with scaled responses	Interviews, focus groups, observations
Skills	Skills tests	Observations
Health status	Medical tests screenings, health risk or hazard appraisals	Interviews, clinical observations
Policy changes	Public records	Observations of compliance
Environmental changes	Written self-reports, public records	Observations, public records
Organizational changes	Public records	Observations, written self-reports
Quality of life	Proxy measures (absenteeism, discrimination, violence rates, clean air, socioeconomic status)	Interviews, focus groups

Tables 10.6 and 10.7, adapted from materials in the *Local Program Evaluation Planning Guide* issued by the California Department of Health Services' Tobacco Control Section (TCS) (2004), provide a synopsis of evaluation designs and data collection methods for evaluating TCS-funded prevention programs. Programs funded through the TCS are required to conduct formal evaluations (California Department of Health Services, 2005). As shown in the tables, the interventions place a strong emphasis on developing policies that can create new social norms (such as smoke-free apartments and parks), compliance with existing policies (for example, no smoking in bars and restaurants), and activities that combat the tobacco industry's marketing messages. The evaluation of these interventions use various evaluation designs and data collections methods.

Primary prevention programs often require that evaluators identify measures that are proxy indicators of long-term impact. For example, studies of the laws prohibiting smoking in bars can be used to show the effectiveness of primary prevention public health policies that are designed to create healthy environments.

TABLE 10.6. SUMMARY OF EVALUATION DESIGNS AND MEASURES FOR BEHAVIOR CHANGE AND OTHER INTERVENTIONS.

Tobacco Program Plan Type	Individual Behavior Change	Other Change with a Measurable Outcome	Other Change with No Measurable Outcome
Outcome objective	Between July 1, 2005, and June 30, 2008, one hundred high-risk smokers will participate in behavior modification–based tobacco cessation services in the community, with at least 50% of the participants who complete the cessation services quitting smoking and of those, 25% will be smoke-free at one-, three-, and six-month follow-up.	Between July 1, 2005, and June 30, 2008, the mean number of tobacco advertising signs in the one hundred convenience stores in River City will decrease from 10.6 items per store to no more than 5.0 items per store.	Between July 1, 2005, and June 30, 2006, the California Tobacco-Free Youth project will recruit and form a statewide youth coalition that will develop a statewide youth-focused antitobacco social marketing campaign.
Evaluation design	Quasi-experimental: multiple measures of the same participants over time.	Experimental: simple random sample of the three hundred tobacco retail stores in River City into seventy-five intervention group stores and seventy-five control group stores.	Nonexperimental
Process data collection	Focus group of high-risk smokers and other relevant community members to identify barriers and facilitators to cessation class recruitment and retention. End-of-cessation-class survey of remaining participants to assess satisfaction with content and willingness to quit.	Focus group of tobacco merchants to find out tobacco industry incentives for advertising. Assessment of training provided to the tobacco sign observers. Documentation of the merchant education intervention.	Focus group with selected youth coalition members to identify barriers and facilitators to the development and maintenance of the youth coalition. Review of coalition meeting minutes and other documents that describe the development of the social marketing campaign.
Outcome data collection	Telephone interview assessment of smoking status at one-month, three-month, and six-month follow-up.	Pre- and postintervention observations of store signage in the intervention and control groups.	

TABLE 10.7. SUMMARY OF EVALUATION DESIGNS AND MEASURES FOR POLICY ADOPTION AND IMPLEMENTATION.

Tobacco Program Plan Type	Policy Adoption Only	Implementation Only	Policy Adoption and Implementation	Multiple Policies, Adoption Only
Outcome objective	Between July 1, 2005, and June 30, 2008, at least three low-income housing complexes in San Antonio County will adopt a written cigarette-related fire pre-vention policy that prohibits smoking in a minimum of 25% of the housing units.	Between July 1, 2005, and June 30, 2008, 100% of all stand-alone bars and bar-restaurants in San Antonio County will maintain compliance with Labor Code 6404.5 prohibiting smoking in bars and restaurants in the incor-porated and unincorporated areas of the county.	Between July 1, 2005, and June 30, 2008, a policy will be adopted in San Antonio County that requires all to-bacco retailers to obtain a license in order to sell tobac-co products and includes a minimum fee of $100 per year per retailer to conduct compliance checks of retail-ers at least twice a year.	Between July 1, 2005, and June 30, 2008, San Antonio County will adopt a to-bacco retail licensing policy that prohibits tobacco self-service displays and bans the distribution of tobacco gear such as T-shirts and hats with tobacco logos.
Evaluation design	Process	Quasi-experimental; outcome via multiple observations of the same bars and restaurants over time.	Process, quasi-experimental; outcome via multiple observations of the same retailers.	Process
Process data collection	Review of county records related to policy adoption. Key informant interviews with policy county supervisors.		Review of county records related to policy adoption.	Review of county records related to policy adoption. Key informant interviews with policy county supervisors.
Outcome data collection		Semiannual observational surveys of smoking in bars and restaurants.	Semiannual observational surveys of youths' attempts to purchase tobacco.	

Such laws are important because they can help prevent the unnecessary workplace deaths of employees such as bartenders, who not long ago had rates of lung cancer higher than firefighters, miners, duct workers, and dry cleaners (California Department of Health Services, 1981). Weber, Bagwell, Fielding, and Glantz (2003) used observational methods to gather primary data on the long-term compliance with the California Smoke-Free Workplace Law in Los Angeles County in freestanding bars and bar-restaurants. Their observations provided clear evidence that the law has been effective at reducing patron and employee smoking in Los Angeles County bars and restaurants. It is therefore likely that this compliance will ultimately result in far fewer bar employees developing lung diseases associated with environmental tobacco smoke.

Evaluating policies can also show that the primary prevention programs will not harm business. Cowling and Bond (2005) used California state tax revenue data to assess whether the California smoke-free restaurant and bar laws of 1995 and 1998 negatively affected the distribution of revenues between bars and restaurants, since protobacco forces claimed that a prohibition on smoking would reduce bar and restaurant revenues. Review of the data revealed that between 1990 and 2002, the effect was just the opposite: passage of both laws was associated with an *increase* in bar and restaurant revenues. In addition, Eisner, Smith, and Blanc (1998) found that the respiratory health of bartenders improved shortly after the law was implemented.

Ethical and Legal Considerations

When conducting any kind of evaluation research, evaluators and program managers must be cognizant of several ethical and legal considerations, including the following:

- Anonymity involves protecting the identity of participants. The Health Insurance Portability and Accountability Act (HIPAA) of 1996 provides significant privacy protection for individually acquired health information (U.S. Department of Health and Human Services, 1996).
- Confidentiality is necessary when gathering information on "sensitive issues," such as substance use. Care should be taken to protect the confidentiality of information gathered from participants.
- Informed consent means advising clients about the nature of the data collection (research) and obtaining their approval to participate.
- Institutional review boards (IRBs) are administrative bodies that review research and evaluation plans in order to protect the privacy and other rights of participants. Human subject reviews are often required by U.S. government–supported

programs, universities, and some state and local agencies. The *Belmont Report* is the "textbook" for ethical standards in research (National Commission, 1979).

Multicultural and Culturally Competent Evaluation

Our increasingly diverse communities require that evaluators develop evaluation plans that acknowledge and respect the differences found in those communities. This is known as cultural competence. During a major meeting of evaluators discussing multicultural evaluation, Hanh Cao Yu stated that cultural competence "encompasses the whole evaluation process—from the evaluator's role, to the design and planning, through the reporting and application of findings. Multicultural evaluation also encompasses new approaches to evaluation—approaches that take into account power differentials, culture and systems analyses, and reciprocal relationships between the evaluators and the stakeholders" (quoted in Endo & Job, 2003, p. 12). Multicultural evaluation is essential, if the needs of community stakeholders are to be met.

Choosing an External Evaluator

Few programs have the internal expertise or time to conduct a formal evaluation and may therefore seek an outside evaluator. However, finding and selecting an evaluator is often difficult. Here are some tips for hiring an evaluator adapted from Atkinson and Ashton (2002).

Indicators of a Good Evaluator

A good evaluator

- Speaks your language and will not talk to you in puzzling "insider's" jargon.
- Wants to know your program and will ask questions about your program's history, purpose, and the priority population served by the program.
- Has experience evaluating your type of program and will know the terms and acronyms used in such programs. He or she will also know the evaluation designs commonly used for your type of program.
- Has experience and knowledge of your program's priority population and will consider the population's characteristics when designing the evaluation.
- Has experience in using qualitative and quantitative methods, including a good grasp of basic descriptive and inferential statistical methods, and understands

how to both gather and analyze qualitative information, such as that based on key informant interviews.

- Has experience in developing data collection instruments for measuring processes and outcomes and will provide you with examples of data collection forms developed for previous program evaluations.
- Is willing to evaluate your program's goals and objectives and make recommendations for altering objectives that cannot be properly evaluated within the program's budget. However, a good evaluator recognizes that it is the *program* that guides the evaluation and not the reverse.
- Is willing to develop a flexible evaluation design that can change as the prevention program is implemented.
- Is willing to spend time with the program, including observing the program in action, visiting program intervention sites, and scheduling periodic conference calls or face-to-face meetings with program staff to review progress on both the program scope of work and the evaluation plan.
- Is willing to produce periodic evaluation reports that are necessary for program monitoring and often required by funding agencies.
- Is willing to write the final evaluation report that meets the needs of the program manager, the community stakeholders, and the funding agency and that can be used to seek future funding.

Working with Your Evaluator

A good working relationship with an evaluator is fostered by a clear understanding of roles. However, the program managers also have important evaluation responsibilities, especially to the constituents and funding agencies. Program managers should do all of the following:

- Collaborate with the evaluator to design an evaluation plan that is consistent with the objectives and the program's resources
- Ensure that the evaluation is conducted within the terms of the evaluation plan, scope of work, and ethical considerations
- Coordinate with the evaluator and supervise the data collection
- Coordinate monthly meetings or conference calls with the evaluator and program staff
- Review and respond to the evaluator's reports
- Ensure that information for required progress reports is collected from the evaluator in a timely manner
- Ensure that the final evaluation report meets the contracted expectations

Conclusion

Despite the complex socioecological environments in which they often operate, primary prevention programs *can* be evaluated. Indeed, there is increasing recognition that consideration for the social determinants of health (including socioeconomic status, access to services, and public policies) must be incorporated into program evaluation designs for primary prevention programs.

Recognition of the many factors that influence individual *and* organizational behaviors is a major reason why program evaluation methods have evolved over the past few decades from ones in which researchers controlled the evaluation, with minimal involvement of stakeholders, to participatory evaluation methods, such as CBPR and empowerment evaluation, that engage community stakeholders in evaluation decisions.

The complexities of primary prevention efforts should not deter evaluation efforts. Program managers and evaluators should strive to develop interventions that can, within ethical and resource considerations, be evaluated with rigorous evaluation designs to show impact. This rigor is critical, even though prevention scientists recognize that new evaluation designs and statistical techniques are needed in order to measure the true complexity of primary prevention interventions (Rimer et al., 2001). In addition, such designs can counter the argument that primary prevention programs cannot be evaluated scientifically. Indeed, as illustrated in this chapter, well-designed primary prevention evaluations can show proximate outcomes, such as behavior change, organizational change, and policy compliance, that are likely indicators of long-term impact. In order to move toward *more* evidence-based primary prevention interventions, program managers and evaluators must take several actions. First, evaluators must continuously increase their prevention program evaluation skills by reading the latest evaluation literature, attending evaluation workshops and conferences, and networking with other prevention evaluators. Second, program managers must recognize that evaluation is not an additional burden but a *necessity* of responsible program management. Third, both evaluators and program managers should join with funding agencies in seeking increases in both the financial and technical assistance resources necessary for rigorous evaluation. I have too often seen funding agencies require evaluation designs that are not supported by the evaluation funds. These resources should extend not just to program managers and evaluators but also to community stakeholders. Such support will allow prevention practitioners to unequivocally show the effectiveness of their efforts and continue to add to the growing body of primary prevention knowledge.

References

Atkinson, A. J., & Ashton, C. (2002). *Planning for results: The safe and drug-free schools and communities program planning and evaluation handbook.* Richmond: Virginia Department of Education.

California Department of Health Services. (1981). *California Occupational Mortality Study, 1979–1981.* Sacramento: Author.

California Department of Health Services, Tobacco Control Section. (1998). *A model for change: The California experience in tobacco control.* Sacramento: Author.

California Department of Health Services, Tobacco Control Section. (2004). *Local program evaluation planning guide.* Sacramento: Author. Retrieved June 6, 2004, from http://www.dhs.ca.gov/ps/cdic/tcs/documents/eval/LPEPlanningGuide.pdf

California Department of Health Services, Tobacco Control Section. (2005). *Local tobacco control interventions.* Sacramento: Author. Retrieved December 30, 2005, from http://www.dhs.ca.gov/tobacco/documents/rfps/RFA05-101.pdf

Centers for Disease Control and Prevention. (1999, September 17). Framework for program evaluation in public health. *Morbidity and Mortality Weekly Report, 48* (RR11), 1–40.

Centers for Disease Control and Prevention. (2006a). Evolution of HIV/AIDS prevention programs, United States, 1981–2006. *Morbidity and Mortality Weekly Report, 55,* 597–603.

Centers for Disease Control and Prevention. (2006b). *Youth media campaign: Logic model.* Atlanta: Author. Retrieved May 28, 2006, from http://www.cdc.gov/youthcampaign/research/logic.htm

Cowling, D. W., & Bond, P. (2005). Smoke-free laws and bar revenues in California: The last call. *Health Economics, 14,* 1273–1281.

DiClemente, R. J., Zorn, J., & Temoshok, L. (1986). Adolescents and AIDS: A survey of knowledge, attitudes, and beliefs about AIDS in San Francisco. *American Journal of Public Health, 76,* 1443–1445.

Eisner, M. D., Smith, A. K., & Blanc, R. D. (1998). Bartenders' respiratory health after establishment of smoke-free bars and taverns. *Journal of the American Medical Association, 280*(22), 1909–1914.

Endo, T., & Job, C. (2003). *Shifting our thinking: Moving from traditional to multicultural evaluation in health: Proceedings from a roundtable discussion.* Woodland Hills: The California Endowment.

Fetterman, D. M., Kafterian, S. J., & Wandersman, A. (1996). *Empowerment evaluation: Knowledge and tools for self-assessment and accountability.* Thousand Oaks, CA: Sage.

Fink, A. (2005). *Evaluation fundamentals: Insights into the outcomes, effectiveness, and quality of health programs* (2nd ed.). Thousand Oaks, CA: Sage.

Francisco, V. T., Butterfoss, F. D., & Capwell, E. M. (2001). Key issues in evaluation: Quantitative and qualitative methods and research design. *Health Promotion Practice, 2*(1), 20–23.

Goldman, K. D., & Schmalz, K. J. (2006). Logic models: The picture worth ten thousand words. *Health Promotion Practice, 7*(1), 8–12.

Green, L. W. (2005). *A resource for instructors, students, health practitioners, and researchers using . . . the PRECEDE-PROCEED model for health program planning and evaluation.* Retrieved January 5, 2006, from http://lgreen.net/index.html

Green, L. W., & Kreuter, M. W. (2005). *Health program planning: An educational and ecological approach* (4th ed.). New York: McGraw-Hill.

Harrell, J. A., et al. (1994). *The essential services of public health.* Washington, DC: American Public Health Association. Retrieved June 5, 2006, from http://www.apha.org/ppp/science/10ES.htm

Hausman, A. J., & Becker, J. (2000). Using participatory research to plan evaluation in violence prevention. *Health Promotion Practice, 1*(4), 331–340.

Institute of Medicine. (2003). *Who will keep the public healthy? Educating public health professionals for the 21st century.* Washington, DC: National Academies Press.

Kretzmann, J. P., & McKnight, J. L. (1993). *Building communities from the inside out: A path toward finding and mobilizing a community's assets.* Evanston, IL: Institute for Policy Research, Northwestern University.

Kreuter, M. W., De Rosa, C., Howze, E. H., & Baldwin, G. T. (2004). Understanding wicked problems: A key to advancing environmental health promotion. *Health Education and Behavior, 31,* 441–454.

Maciosek, M. V., Coffield, A. B., Edwards, N. M., Flottemesch, T. J., Goodman, M. J., & Solberg, L. I. (2006). Priorities among effective clinical preventive services. Results of a systematic review and analysis. *American Journal of Preventive Medicine, 31,* 90–96.

Mattessich, P. (2003). *Manager's guide to program evaluation: Planning, contracting, and managing for useful results.* Saint Paul, MN: Fieldstone Alliance.

Minkler, M., & Wallerstein, N. (2003). Introduction to community-based participatory research. In M. Minkler & N. Wallerstein (Eds.), *Community-based participatory research for health* (pp. 3–26). San Francisco: Jossey-Bass.

National Commission for the Protection of Human Subjects of Biomedical and Behavioral Research. (1979). *The Belmont Report: Ethical principles and guidelines for the protection of human subjects of research.* Washington, DC: National Institutes of Health. Retrieved July 26, 2006, from http://ohsr.od.nih.gov/guidelines/belmont.html

Rimer, B. K., Glanz, K., & Rasband, G. (2001). Searching for evidence about health education and health behavior interventions. *Health Education and Behavior, 28,* 231–248.

Roe, K. M., Berenstein, C., Goette, C., & Roe, K. (1997). Community building through empowerment: A case study of HIV prevention community planning. In M. Minkler (Ed.), *Community organizing and community building for health* (pp. 308–322). New Brunswick, NJ: Rutgers University Press.

Rossi, P. H., Lipsey, M. W., & Freeman, H. E. (2004). *Evaluation: A systematic approach* (7th ed.). Thousand Oaks, CA: Sage.

Russell, L. B. (1986). *Is prevention better than cure?* Washington, DC: Brookings Institution.

Steckler, A., McLeroy, K. R., Goodman, R. M., Bird, S. T., & McCormick, L. (1992). Toward integrating qualitative and quantitative methods: An introduction. *Health Education Quarterly, 19,* 1–8.

Teutsch, S. (2006). Cost-effectiveness of prevention. *Medscape Today: Perspectives in Prevention from the American College of Preventive Medicine.* Retrieved July 13, 2006, from http://www.medscape.com/viewarticle/540199

Thompson, R. S., Taplin, S. H., McAfee, T. A., Mandelson, M. T., & Smith, A. E. (1995). Primary and secondary prevention services in clinical practice: Twenty years' experience in development, implementation, and evaluation. *Journal of the American Medical Association, 273,* 1130–1135.

U.S. Department of Health, Education and Welfare. (1979). *Healthy people: The surgeon general's report on health promotion and disease prevention.* Washington, DC: Government Printing Office.

U.S. Department of Health and Human Services, Office for Civil Rights. (1996). *Health Insurance Portability and Accountability Act (HIPAA)*. Retrieved July 26, 2006, from http://www.hhs.gov/ocr/hipaa

United Way of America. (2000). *Agency experiences with outcome measurement*. Retrieved January 20, 2006, from http://national.unitedway.org/files/pdf/outcomes/AgencyOM.pdf

United Way of America. (2006). *America's number 1 charity: A snapshot of resources raised for 2004–2005*. Retrieved January 20, 2006, from http://national.unitedway.org/files/pdf/200405RDExecutive.pdf

Wallerstein, N., & Duran, B. (2006). Using community-based participatory research to address health disparities. *Health Promotion Practice, 7*(3), 1–12.

Wallerstein, N., Polascek, M., & Maltrud, K. (2002). Participatory evaluation model for coalitions: The development of systems indicators. *Health Promotion Practice, 3*(3), 361–373.

Walter, H. J. (1989). Primary prevention of chronic disease among children: The school-based Know Your Body intervention trials. *Health Education Quarterly, 16*, 201–214.

Walter, H. J., Hofman, A., Connelly, P. A., Barrett, L. T., & Kost, K. L. (1985). Primary prevention of chronic disease in childhood: Changes in risk factors after one year of intervention. *American Journal of Epidemiology, 122*, 772–781.

Weber, M. D., Bagwell, D. A., Fielding, J. E., & Glantz, S. A. (2003). Long-term compliance with California's Smoke-Free Workplace Law among bars and restaurants in Los Angeles County. *Tobacco Control, 12*, 269–273.

W. K. Kellogg Foundation. (1998). *Evaluation handbook: Philosophy and expectations*. Battle Creek, MI: Author. Retrieved January 17, 2006, from http://www.wkkf.org/pubs/Tools/Evaluation/Pub770.pdf

PART THREE

PREVENTION IN CONTEXT

Part Three explores the application of prevention efforts over a range of contemporary health issues. Each chapter puts the current practice of prevention into context through specific examples and emphasizes the role of prevention as integral to improving community environments and changing social norms. In addition, each notes how improving norms and environments will be reflected in improved health.

The links between environmental exposures and health outcomes are well documented among conditions including cancer, asthma, and developmental disabilities. Environmental exposures are preventable and disproportionately affect disfranchised communities. In Chapter Eleven, "Preventing Injustices in Environmental Health and Exposures," Stephanie Farquhar, Neha Patel, and Molly Chidsey first describe environmental health and explain how it can be approached from a prevention perspective and then focus on injustices in environmental exposures and how they can be redressed. Traditional risk assessment for environmental exposure does not focus on prevention but rather responds to crises of illness or injury. The authors propose two critical prevention approaches to achieving environmental justice. The *precautionary principle* borrows from the medical oath to "do no harm" in placing the burden of demonstrating safety prior to public exposure on those who produce chemicals and other substances. Community-based *participatory research* is a vital primary prevention strategy that addresses the need for community capacity building and involvement of key stakeholders in decisions that affect community health.

The physical environment in which we live, work, and play has a fundamental impact on both health itself and behaviors that affect it. Health outcomes are affected directly by the environment when, for instance, the siting of a truck depot increases diesel emissions in a neighborhood, resulting in higher asthma rates. Health outcomes are also affected through the impact of environment on behavior when, for example, a community without sidewalks results in people walking less and therefore being at risk of increased rates of chronic disease.

However, the specific decisions around how the environment is built, such as street design, are generally made without considering their impact on health. In Chapter Twelve, "Health and the Built Environment: Opportunities for Prevention," Howard Frumkin and Andrew Dannenberg describe the developing emphasis on the "built environment" and its emerging links with health. They make a compelling case for the critical role that changes to the physical environment can have in preventing our most serious health problems. The authors explain why health leaders need to work with new partners and new disciplines and influence those who make built environment decisions, including city planners and traffic engineers, broadening their health and prevention perspective.

Our choices about what and how much to eat are made in the context of our social, physical, and cultural environment. The accessibility and availability of food, coupled with advertising and pricing, form the food environment. Leslie Mikkelsen, Catherine Erickson, and Marion Nestle, in Chapter Thirteen, "Creating Healthy Food Environments and Preventing Chronic Disease," link the current U.S. food environment to a range of nutrition-related chronic diseases that are resulting in significant increases in illness and death. They describe the need to prevent these diseases by transforming the food environment and discuss several primary prevention strategies that hold great promise for improving nutrition and therefore health outcomes at the community level. The authors also present new approaches that address policy areas, including access to healthy food, affordability, and advertising.

Violence can affect every family and community, and disfranchised communities are more at risk than any others. The public is generally skeptical about violence, assuming that it is natural and that nothing can be done about it. Yet violence is a learned behavior and is therefore preventable—it can be unlearned or not learned in the first place. Deborah Prothrow-Stith, the author of Chapter Fourteen, "Strengthening the Collaboration Between Public Health and Criminal Justice to Prevent Violence," was one of the first prevention advocates in the country to frame violence as a public health issue and to propose the application of public health solutions. She contrasts this approach with the criminal justice approach to violence. Like other health issues, understanding what underlies violence gives one the capacity to prevent it.

For the past quarter-century, HIV has been a high-profile public health issue, and prevention efforts have focused primarily on addressing individual behavior change. In Chapter Fifteen, "The Limits of Behavioral Interventions for HIV Prevention," Dan Wohlfeiler and Jonathan Ellen suggest that this focus on behavior change is necessary but insufficient to achieve sustainable change. Instead, the authors recommend that HIV advocates take their cues from primary prevention successes and focus on structural-level solutions that address the social, economic, and political systems in which we live and in which sexual decisions are made. They describe the need to target the sexual networks that lead to increased risk-taking behavior and point out that the ultimate outcome of HIV prevention efforts is not merely a reduction in risk-taking behavior but also a sustained decrease in the rate of new infections.

Both the editors and the authors note that reducing the number of African American men who are incarcerated could decrease HIV rates in black communities. There is a correlation, for instance, between prisons and rates of HIV. From the editors' perspective, addressing discriminatory sentencing practices, including California's "three strikes" law, would help preserve the fabric of communities and result in increased community resilience and a decrease in HIV rates.

CHAPTER ELEVEN

PREVENTING INJUSTICES IN ENVIRONMENTAL HEALTH AND EXPOSURES

Stephanie Ann Farquhar, Neha Patel, Molly Chidsey

Environment matters. The same environmental problems that contribute to poor air and water quality and to blight and neighborhood deterioration also contribute to negative mental and physical health outcomes. Cancer, asthma, birth defects, developmental disabilities, infertility, and Parkinson's disease are on the rise, and they are linked to chemical exposures from air, water, food, and products and practices used in our schools, homes, neighborhoods, and workplaces. These health problems are widespread, affecting nearly one of every two Americans (Pew Environmental Health Commission, 2001).

Health problems related to environmental exposures are also very expensive, costing $325 billion yearly in health care costs, loss of productivity, and special education programs (Pew Environmental Health Commission, 2001). An estimated $54.9 billion is spent annually on pediatric diseases linked to environmental pollutants alone (Landrigan, Schechter, Lipton, Fahs, & Schwartz, 2002).

If environmental health is the assessment and control of the environment and related health outcomes (a more complete definition will be given in the section "Environmental Health"), environmental justice provides one way to examine and discuss the unequal nature of exposures and health outcomes. Environmental justice as a framework and a practice acknowledges that pollution and related health effects fall disproportionately on residents living in economically and politically disadvantaged communities (Bryant, 1995). And there are clear patterns, in that low-income people and people of color are typically the most affected. Furthermore, these same residents are often excluded from the very decisions and environmental policies that threaten their communities' health and often face a multitude of environmental threats.

The traditional environmental risk assessments that are widely used to evaluate exposure and related health outcomes frequently fail to examine exposures among the most vulnerable residents, the synergistic effect of exposure to multiple environmental health problems, or the social or political aspects associated with exposure and risk decisions. Traditional risk assessment evaluates new technologies and products by calculating the mathematical likelihood that exposure will threaten our health and requires that we must prove that a product, practice, or chemical is harmful before discontinuing its manufacture or use.

This chapter presents two approaches that can be used to augment the types of information and solutions obtained using the more traditional risk assessment approach. These two supplemental methods—the precautionary principle and community-based participatory research—explicitly involve residents and other stakeholders and consider the social and political aspects of environmental exposure. Two case studies from Portland, Oregon, illustrate the potential power of local resident and government involvement and a preventive framework that seeks equity in environmental health burden and benefit.

Environmental Health

The *Journal of Environmental Health Perspectives* defines environmental health as "those aspects of human disease and injury that are determined or influenced by factors in the environment," . . . including "direct pathological effects of various chemical, physical, and biological agents, as well as the effects on health of the broad physical and social environment, which includes housing, urban development, land-use and transportation, industry, and agriculture" (Environmental Health Perspectives, n.d.). It should be noted that when using the terms *environment* and *environmental health,* we are drawing from this broader definition, which considers the built and social environments in addition to chemical and other exposures in the physical environment.

The environmental health movement developed in response to an increased awareness of the effects of toxic chemicals on the environment and human health. Significant dates and benchmark achievements associated with the environmental health movement are presented in Exhibit 11.1.

EXHIBIT 11.1. BENCHMARK ACHIEVEMENTS
IN ENVIRONMENTAL HEALTH.

1960s

Rachel Carson's *Silent Spring* exposes the hazards of the pesticide DDT and brings a new public awareness to the impact of widely released chemicals on health and the environment.

1970s

Twenty million people celebrate the first Earth Day.

President Nixon creates the Environmental Protection Agency.

Congress amends the Clean Air Act, restricts use of lead-based paint, bans DDT, and phases out PCB production.

1980s

Congress creates the Superfund to clean up hazardous waste sites.

Safer disposal of nuclear waste becomes a priority.

1990s

The Toxics Release Inventory is created, designed to track emissions from certain industry groups.

The Pollution Prevention Act changes the focus of pollution policies to preventive source reduction.

An executive order protects children from health risks associated with environmental factors, including asthma and lead poisoning.

The Impact of Environmental Exposure

Despite some limited progress in the past decades, pollution continues to threaten our health, and some communities are more exposed than others. Hundreds of contaminants accumulate in our bodies through exposure to cleaning products, plastics, fuels, pesticides, and cosmetics. A study conducted by researchers at Mount Sinai School of Medicine in New York and the Environmental Working Group found a total of 167 industrial compounds, pollutants, and other chemicals in the blood and urine of nine volunteers, none of whom had worked with or had any significant exposure to chemicals (Thornton, McCally, & Houlihan, 2002). Of the 167 chemicals found, 76 are known to cause cancer in humans or animals, 94 are toxic to the brain and nervous system, and 79 cause birth defects or abnormal development. The Centers for Disease Control and Prevention

(CDC) recently issued its third report on body burden and measured 148 chemicals or their breakdown products in the blood or urine of approximately 2,400 people who participated in the National Health and Nutrition Examination Survey (NHANES) from 1999 to 2002 (CDC, 2005). Other biomonitoring studies have detected high concentrations of certain classes of flame retardants in wildlife and human blood, milk, and tissues (Hites, 2004). It should also be noted that although exposure regulations are based on the assessment of single products or practices, we are exposed to a multitude of chemicals, and the potential synergistic effect of these exposures is typically not evaluated and can be more damaging to health than any one single exposure.

Many chronic and acute diseases are strongly associated with products and practices used in our schools, homes, parks, and workplaces. The incidence of asthma has nearly doubled in the past twenty-five years, and certain communities are disproportionately affected by this disease, particularly children and the urban poor (Solomon, 2002). Incidences of breast, thyroid, kidney, liver, skin, lung (in females), testicular, brain, esophageal, and bladder cancer and non-Hodgkin's lymphoma have all increased over the past twenty-five years (Houlihan, Wiles, Thayer, & Gray, 2003; Schettler, 2002). Nervous system disorders such as autism, learning impairments, and Parkinson's disease are also on the rise (Blaxill, 2004; Houlihan et al., 2003). In a study of twenty autistic children, Edelson and Cantor (1999) found that all subjects had liver detoxification profiles outside of normal. Development of Parkinson's disease is strongly associated with exposure to pesticides and other toxic agents (Liou et al., 1997; Seidler et al., 1996).

Campaign for Safe Cosmetics

The family of industrial chemicals known as phthalates, or phthalate esters, is used to soften plastics in a large variety of consumer products, including many leading beauty care products. Studies have shown that phthalates can damage the lungs, kidneys, liver, and reproductive organs, especially the developing testes. Phthalates have also been shown to cause hormone disruption, reduced fertility, and birth defects in developing fetuses, including genital feminization in baby boys (Not Too Pretty, 2003).

In 2002, a study of the phthalate content of seventy-two name-brand, off-the-shelf beauty products in the United States was commissioned by a coalition of environmental and public health organizations, including the Breast Cancer Fund, the Environmental Working Group, and Health Care Without Harm. The study revealed phthalates in almost three-quarters of the products tested. Yet phthalates were not listed on any of the product labels. The study results were published in a report called *Not Too Pretty: Phthalates, Beauty Products and the FDA* (Houlihan, Brody, & Schwan, 2002). At the same time,

Health Care Without Harm released a study called *Aggregate Exposures to Phthalates in Humans* (2002a) documenting that people are exposed to phthalates from a number of different sources—including cosmetics—whose sum effects may be causing us harm. The study also showed that women of reproductive age are most at risk for high exposure and that there were no government actions being taken to protect people from these multiple exposures. Later in 2002, a report similar to *Not Too Pretty* called *Pretty Nasty: Phthalates in European Cosmetic Products* (Health Care Without Harm, 2002b) documented phthalate levels among products in the European Union that were comparable to those in the United States. Soon after, in January 2003, the European Parliament passed an amendment prohibiting the use of known or suspected carcinogens or mutagens or toxins impairing fertility or harmful to developing humans—including phthalates—in the manufacturing of cosmetics. At that time, American lawmakers had yet to take similar action to reduce the harmful effects of phthalates on American cosmetics users.

The Campaign for Safe Cosmetics was launched in 2002 as a response to these findings. The campaign is a coalition of public health, educational, religious, labor, women's, environmental, and consumer groups working to protect the health of cosmetics consumers and workers. It asks manufacturers of personal care products and cosmetics to sign the Compact for Safe Cosmetics, pledging to meet the same standards and deadlines set by the European Union cosmetics directive. In addition, signers of the compact agree to make safe, nontoxic, reformulated products readily available in every market they serve; to determine multiple effects of potential chemicals of concern in products (or by-products), including toxicity to living things, persistence in the environment, ability to increase in concentration up the food chain, and contamination of bodies; and to develop an aggressive substitution plan and timeline to replace emerging chemicals of concern with safe alternatives (Campaign for Safe Cosmetics, n.d.-a). As of August 2006, four hundred companies had signed the compact, including The Body Shop, Aveda, and Burt's Bees.

The campaign platform also calls on the Food and Drug Administration to prohibit the marketing of all cosmetics and personal care products containing known or probable human carcinogens, mutagens, or reproductive toxins (Campaign for Safe Cosmetics, n.d.-b). The FDA does not review the safety of new cosmetic ingredients before they come to market, nor does it have the authority to recall hazardous products (Campaign for Safe Cosmetics, 2005). Rather than testing products before they hit the market, the FDA regulates these products only after they are sold, investigating health concerns only when and if complaints are filed (Campaign for Safe Cosmetics, 2005).

In October 2005, the Campaign for Safe Cosmetics celebrated success in California with the signing of SB 484, the California Safe Cosmetics Act of 2005, now considered the strongest bill in the nation to protect consumers of cosmetics. In addition, as of August 2006, five other states—Washington, Oregon, Massachusetts, New York, and Maryland—were in the process of pursuing similar legislation.

For more information, visit http://www.safecosmetics.com.

Source: Prevention Institute.

Disparities in Health Outcomes

Given the high average levels of toxic exposures and increases in related disease, it is especially distressing that exposure-related health outcomes disproportionately burden low-income communities and communities of color. For example, as noted earlier, asthma rates are increasing (Solomon, 2002). This chronic disease alone costs Americans $14 billion annually and accounts for more than 14 million lost school days and 1.8 million emergency room visits each year (Smart, 2004). But the burden of this disease that is linked to indoor and outdoor air quality is not evenly distributed. Disproportionate numbers of people of color and people from low-income households live in nonattainment areas (areas that persistently fail to meet the federally established ambient air quality standards) and may be exposed to higher than average levels of indoor and outdoor pollution. Approximately three times as many African Americans as whites die from complications related to asthma, and the hospitalization rate for African Americans and Latinos is three to four times the rate for whites (Grant, Lyttle, & Weiss, 2000). Asthma also affects children disproportionately. Although they make up only 25 percent of the population, children account for 40 percent of all asthma cases (Solomon, 2002), and five times more children than adults die from asthma each year.

Lead poisoning is another environmental health threat that disproportionately affects poor inner-city African American children. Lead poisoning affects an estimated 890,000 American preschoolers, or 4.4 percent of the under-five age group, yet African American children are five times more likely to be poisoned by lead than white children (Pirkle et al., 1998). Over 22 percent of African American children living in pre-1946 housing have high blood lead levels, compared with 5.6 percent of white children and 13 percent of Mexican American children living in older homes. Effects of exposure on behavior are potentially devastating. Even very low levels of exposure can result in reduced IQ, and an estimated 16 percent of juvenile delinquent behavior in the United States is attributable to high lead exposure (Wakefield, 2002).

There is also a "double injustice" in terms of unequal exposure and unequal access to prevention and treatment. Populations that are at a higher risk of exposure to environmental contaminants are also more likely to have little or no access to adequate health care. This lack of access makes it more difficult for certain groups to seek early detection, preventive care, and care after becoming sick. Over 45 million Americans, including 10 million children, are without health insurance today, and the cumulative effect of increased risk and less care is potentially devastating (Institute of Medicine, 2002). A 2001 Commonwealth Fund survey revealed that Hispanics and African Americans were most likely to be uninsured, as 46 percent of working-age Hispanics and 33 percent of working-age African Americans lacked insurance for all or part of the twelve months prior to the survey. In comparison, only 20 percent of both whites and Asian Americans aged eighteen to sixty-four lacked health coverage for all or part of the previous twelve months (Collins et al., 2002).

Furthermore, as evidenced by Hurricanes Katrina and Rita in 2005, natural disasters are another aspect of the environment that tends to disproportionately affect poor communities and residents of color. This exposure occurs through both subsequent toxic exposures (such as contaminated floodwater) and a more general inability to flee unsafe conditions. A community's potential for exposure to hazards such as asbestos and lead and contaminated soil and water is determined in part by its ability to access resources in the wake of a disaster. Furthermore, the conditions of people's lives before the disaster occurs—their employment status, education, social support system, housing situation, and access to health care, financial credit, and legal services—contributes to their level of vulnerability or security in terms of risks of exposure and in the recovery process (Blaikie, Cannon, Davis, & Wisner, 1994; Bolin & Stanford, 1998; Farquhar & Wing, 2003).

In a review of research studies, Fothergill, Maestas, and Darlington DeRouen (1999) documented differences in disaster experiences between racial and ethnic groups. Minority populations experience longer recoveries from natural disasters, have limited access to insurance, and use aid and relief organizations differently than majority populations (Natural Hazards Research and Applications Information Center, 2001). Furthermore, cultural marginalization and political vulnerability can exclude certain groups from disaster recovery efforts (Bolin & Stanford, 1998). For example, Farquhar and Wing (2002) documented that many of the poorer and more marginalized residents of North Carolina displaced by Hurricane Floyd in 1999 were turned down for financial assistance, received misinformation about opportunities for recovery aid, were unable to secure affordable and decent housing due to a lack of affordable rental units, and were excluded from recovery decisions.

Environmental Justice

The environmental justice movement emerged in response to the recognition that environmental exposure falls disproportionately on the economically and politically disadvantaged and out of frustration with the exclusion of affected populations in environmental health decisions. The Environmental Protection Agency (EPA) defines environmental justice as "the fair treatment and meaningful involvement of all people regardless of race, color, national origin, or income with respect to the development, implementation, and enforcement of environmental laws, regulations, and policies" (1992, p. 2). As mentioned previously, if environmental health is the science and control of environmental threats to health, environmental justice provides us with the tools, language, and framework to examine inequity in environmental exposure and decision making.

The environmental justice movement is marked by several landmark events, presented in Exhibit 11.2. Warren County, North Carolina, is widely recognized as the birthplace of the environmental justice movement. In 1982, this predominantly African American county, with more industry than any other North Carolina county, held demonstrations against the siting of a hazardous waste landfill. The following year, a study of several southern states by the General Accounting Office found that three out of four landfills were sited near communities with a nonwhite majority. In 1987, the United Church of Christ's Commission on Racial Justice issued a report that showed race to be the most significant factor nationally in determining the location of hazardous waste facility sites, with three out of every five African Americans and Hispanics living in a community in close proximity to unregulated toxic waste sites (EPA, 2003). Other studies corroborate that a greater number of environmentally hazardous waste sites and polluting industries are located in low-income communities and communities of color (Faber & Krieg, 2002) and a higher risk of cancer is associated with airborne toxics in socioeconomically disadvantaged communities and African American communities (Apelberg, Buckley, & White, 2005; Lopez, 2002).

The results of these and other studies, paired with effective local organizing efforts that challenged the government to respond to disproportionate exposure, led to the establishment of the EPA's Office of Environmental Justice in 1992 and the 1994 Executive Order No. 12898, whereby President Clinton directed eleven federal agencies to incorporate environmental justice into their policies (EPA, 2003).

One of the common responses to the issue of disproportionate exposure and unhealthy neighborhoods is the suggestion that people simply move from health-threatening neighborhoods. What is frequently underappreciated is that the same residents who bear the burden of environmental exposures are also less likely to have the means to move away from a stressful physical environment (Greenberg, Schneider, & Choi, 1994). And if residents are able to relocate, others may simply move in and take their place, leaving the new residents vulnerable to the same set of health problems. A population's location may determine its exposure, but a lack of access to resources, including education, employment, and social mobility, can also limit health-protective options (Williams, 1990). As noted by Bullard and Wright (1993), impoverished communities are not only frequently burdened with a substandard physical environment, but they are also challenged by a deteriorating infrastructure, economic disinvestment, inadequate schools, chronic unemployment, and overburdened health care systems.

EXHIBIT 11.2. LANDMARK EVENTS
IN ENVIRONMENTAL JUSTICE.

1964

Congress passes the Civil Rights Act, Title VI of which prohibits the use of federal funds to discriminate on the basis of race, color, or national origin.

1971

The Council on Environmental Quality's annual report acknowledges that racial discrimination adversely affects the urban poor and the quality of their environment.

1979

Linda McKeever Bullard files a lawsuit, *Bean v. Southwestern Waste Management,* on behalf of Houston's Northeast Community Action Group, challenging the siting of a waste facility.

1982

Warren County residents protest the siting of a PCB landfill in Warren County, North Carolina.

1983

The General Accounting Office publishes *Siting of Hazardous Landfills and Their Correlation with Racial and Economic Status of Surrounding Communities,* which found that three-quarters of all off-site commercial hazardous waste facilities in EPA Region IV were located in African American communities.

1987

The United Church of Christ Commission for Racial Justice (UCCCRJ) issues *Toxic Wastes and Race in the United States,* a report that correlated waste facility siting and race.

1991

The first National People of Color Environmental Leadership Summit was held in Washington, D.C., with over one thousand participants.

1998

The UCCCRJ convenes grassroots environmental justice, civil rights, and academic leaders to challenge the chemical company Shintech's permit application, halting the company's efforts to build a PVC plant in Louisiana.

2001

The National Black Environmental Justice Network coordinates the Congressional Black Caucus Hearing on environmental justice in Washington, D.C.

Dr. Robert Bullard

The year 1978 witnessed the largest PCB spill ever recorded in the United States. Oil laced with PCB (polychlorinated biphenyl) was illegally dumped along 210 miles of roadway in North Carolina (Bullard, Glenn, & Torres, 2004). Four years later, in 1982, Warren County, a poor and mostly African American county, was selected for disposal of the contaminated soil. Protests erupted over the decision, and although opponents were not able to block the siting of the PCB landfill, the battle that ensued in Warren County brought environmental justice into public view (Bullard & Johnson, 1997).

Robert Bullard, sociology professor at Clark Atlanta University and director of the Environmental Justice Resource Center, has been instrumental in the quest for environmental justice. When Bullard's wife, Linda McKeever Bullard, filed a lawsuit (*Bean* v. *Southwestern Waste Management*) that opposed the placement of a landfill in the middle of a predominantly black, middle-class, homeowning suburban neighborhood (Dicum, 2006), her husband collected data to support her case.

His research revealed that 100 percent of the city-owned landfills in Houston were in black neighborhoods, even though blacks made up only 25 percent of the population. Similarly, six out of eight of the city-owned incinerators were in predominantly black neighborhoods. Of the privately owned landfills, three out of four were located in predominantly black neighborhoods. Bullard concluded that in the absence of zoning in Houston, these decisions had to have been made by government officials (Dicum, 2006).

The United Church of Christ's Commission for Racial Justice responded by publishing a study in 1987, *Toxic Waste and Race* (Bullard & Johnson, 1997). It documented that three in five African Americans lived in communities with abandoned toxic waste sites, three in five lived in communities with one or more active waste sites, and three of the five largest commercial hazardous waste landfills were located in predominantly African American or Latino communities, accounting for 40 percent of the nation's total hazardous waste landfill capacity in 1987. Among other publications documenting environmental injustice, *Dumping in Dixie: Race, Class, and Environmental Quality* (Bullard, 1990) chronicled environmental justice struggles in the South. Grassroots organizations began to spring up in reaction to such findings.

Bullard helped plan the first National People of Color Environmental Leadership Summit in 1991, which generated the organizing principles of the environmental justice movement. He went on to help the Clinton administration write the executive order that required federal agencies to consider environmental justice in their programs (Motavalli, 1998), and he served on the Environmental Protection Agency's National Advisory Council for Environmental

Policy and Technology, offering direction on complaints filed under the antidiscriminatory Title VI of the Civil Rights Act of 1964 (Motavalli, 1998).

According to Bullard, "The environmental justice movement has basically redefined what environmentalism is all about. It basically says that the environment is everything: where we live, work, play, go to school, as well as the physical and natural world. And so we can't separate the physical environment from the cultural environment" (Schweizer, 1999, p. 1).

Source: Prevention Institute.

Two Preventive Approaches to Environmental Health

So how do we measure exposure, determine health effects, quantify risk, and inform policy and practice? For the last several decades, environmental public health and the study of exposure and related health outcomes has been guided by the risk analysis model. This model assesses new technologies and products by calculating the mathematical likelihood that they will threaten our health and typically includes four steps: hazard identification, dose-response evaluation, exposure assessment, and risk characterization. The quantitative risk assessment model allows commercial and industrial interests to require that harm be "scientifically" proved before discontinuing a process or product (Myers & Raffensperger, 2005). The primary deficit of quantitative risk assessment is that it frequently fails to consider most social, cultural, or broader environmental factors or costs to the environment or future generations. Furthermore, assessing risk based on a single exposure to a single chemical does not take into account the combinations of chemicals that people are exposed to daily or other individual differences such as nutrition, immune system health, and age.

We propose two approaches that can be integrated with traditional risk assessment in an effort to obtain more complete information about what types of exposures communities are facing. The precautionary principle is based on a precautionary approach to local policy and decision making around environmental exposures and health outcomes, while community-based participatory research is based on the meaningful and significant participation of community residents in assessing environmental health problems and seeking solutions to them. Both approaches offer methodologies for public health practitioners and researchers working with affected communities and are guided by principles of equality, justice, and prevention, and both can be used to augment the types and quality of information we obtain using more traditional approaches for assessing risk.

Precautionary Principle

Today, over eighty-five thousand industrial chemicals are registered for use in the United States, and an average of twenty-three hundred more are added each year. Unfortunately, toxicological data exist for only 7 percent of the registered chemicals, meaning that tens of thousand of chemicals are not registered (Goldman & Koduru, 2000). This makes it difficult for us to know definitively which products or toxic contaminants threaten our health and environment. In fact, the U.S. Toxic Substance Control Act does not require chemical companies to perform basic health and safety tests on their products (Goldman & Koduru, 2000; Schettler, 2002; Thornton et al., 2002). The responsibility falls to the federal government and the public to demonstrate that a chemical poses an "unreasonable risk" to society. In the current regulatory system, a chemical is generally considered safe until proven harmful—in other words, innocent until proven guilty. This can mean that by the time the evidence of harm is apparent, many people (most of them typically low-income or people of color) have already developed symptoms and health problems.

In an effort to address the limitations of a traditional risk assessment model, an international group that included scientists, government officials, lawyers, and labor and grassroots environmental activists, such as leaders from the Science and Environmental Health Network and the Center for Health, Environment and Justice, convened at the Wingspread Conference Center in Wisconsin in 1998 (Montague, 1998). In the same spirit of medicine's principle of "first do no harm," this group called for a more preventive and protective approach to environmental assessment. The Wingspread Statement on the Precautionary Principle, developed at the conference, states, "When an activity raises threats of harm to human health or the environment, precautionary measures should be taken even if some cause-and-effect relationships are not fully established scientifically. In this context the proponent of an activity, rather than the public, should bear the burden of proof. The process of applying the precautionary principle must be open, informed and democratic and must include potentially affected parties" (Myers & Raffensperger, 2005). Over the past decade, especially in European countries, the precautionary principle has emerged as one of the leading environmental health frameworks in shaping new policy that prevents harm and that allows for participation of community residents and leaders.

Although facing constant challenges by industry and manufacturers who would be asked to prove that their products are safe, the precautionary principle has produced some recent victories (Myers & Raffensperger, 2005). The U.S. Toxic Substances Control Act authorizes the EPA to halt marketing and require safety testing or other measures for any substance determined to pose an unreasonable risk (EPA, 1976). Similarly, the CDC has begun monitoring human exposure to chemicals, collecting data that can be used to inform future precautionary policies (CDC, 2003). And the White House Policy Declaration on Environment and Trade from 1999 acknowledges that a precautionary approach is an essential element of the U.S. regulatory system since regulators often have to make decisions in the absence of full scientific certainty (Wirth, 2002).

This framework provides policymakers and communities with a more comprehensive way to estimate the full costs of a product or practice. The precautionary principle considers both "seen" costs (for example, equipment purchase and hazardous waste disposal costs) and "hidden" costs (such as insurance and hazardous waste liability, employee health benefits, and impact on social and cultural well-being) associated with substance manufacture, use, and disposal. Refuting detractors who argue that the precautionary principle will be cost-prohibitive for businesses, adoption of the principle has actually been shown to initiate economic development by creating new opportunities for local businesses to provide safer products, processes, and technologies (Ackerman & Massey, 2002).

Despite a few early successes—including the adoption of a set of purchasing guidelines based on the precautionary principle by the City and County of San Francisco (San Francisco Commission on the Environment, 2003)—the approach has been underutilized by local government, businesses, and policymakers in the United States. This approach, which calls for transparency, democracy, and preventive action, requires a systematic change in the way we think as well as what we do. Rather than asking how much harm is acceptable, we must determine the least amount of harm that can be achieved. The principle can also be used to protect communities, rather than corporations, from exposure and related health outcomes, as described in the accompanying case study.

Toxics Resolution in Multnomah County and the City of Portland

In September 2004, the Portland City Council and the Multnomah County Board of Commissioners became the first government bodies in Oregon to unanimously adopt the precautionary principle as the basis for reducing toxics in city and county government operations and to protect public health. The resolution states:

Every resident of Portland and Multnomah County has an *equal right* to a healthy and safe environment. In order to achieve this goal locally, our government, residents, and businesses must work together to ensure that our air, water, soil, and food are safe. As a first

---

(Continued)

step in reaching this goal and developing the toxics reduction strategy called for by the resolution, the Sustainable Development Commission and the Oregon Center for Environmental Health recommend the city and county resolve to create a Toxics Reduction Strategy for government operations utilizing the Precautionary Principle (Multnomah County Board of Commissioners, 2004).

While Portland and Multnomah County are often perceived as having a healthy environment, particular neighborhoods were challenged with toxic threats to human health. For example, fourteen air toxics in the county exceed health-based benchmarks, with six pollutants more than ten times national health standards (Multnomah County Health Department, 2003). Similarly, a section of the lower Willamette River in Portland is listed as a Superfund site, designating it as one of the most polluted rivers in the country. Demographic data from the 2000 census indicate that while only 1.7 percent of Oregon residents are African American, they make up 60 to 95 percent of the total population living within a few blocks of the 7-mile stretch of the lower Willamette River designated as the Portland Harbor Superfund site (U.S. Census Bureau, 2000).

Work to develop the resolution began in the spring of 2003 through a collaboration between the Sustainable Development Commission of Portland and Multnomah County (SDC) and the Oregon Center for Environmental Health (OCEH). The SDC is an appointed citizen advisory board charged with making policy recommendations to the city and county to ensure a sustainable future. The OCEH is an environmental and health advocacy organization that works to protect public health and the environment by promoting alternatives to the use, manufacture, release, and disposal of toxic chemicals.

The SDC and the OCEH convened workshops and work groups with area residents and other key stakeholders, including government officials and community members, to develop a dialogue on using precaution as a basis for protective environmental and public health policy. Following the adoption of the resolution, a more formal work group was formed in 2005 of community members and city and county staff to develop a process to reduce the purchase and use of toxics in city and county operations. Although the work group has made significant steps forward, the development of the strategy has progressed slowly. However, allowing ample time for stakeholder participation and input and moving through the proper channels of city and county government during the development of the strategy will help ensure that the implementation is supported and purchasing practices are amended.

Every phase of this local effort has incorporated the tenets of the precautionary principle, including prevention of new toxic pollution and inclusion of stakeholders. A complete proposed toxics reduction strategy was presented to the county board of commissioners and the city council in May 2006 and was unanimously adopted, providing specific directives for both agencies to reduce their impact on toxic pollution for all residents.

Community-Based Participatory Research

Community-based participatory research (CBPR) creates an opportunity for the individuals and groups who are most affected by potential environmental health threats to influence policy and practice. Environmental justice advocates demand more than clean air and water and insist on the participation of all people as equal partners in decision making regardless of class, race, ethnicity, or national origin (EPA, 1998; Kuehn, 1996). Community organizations and federal agencies alike have called for the inclusion of community residents in assessing and characterizing risk assessment and establishing policy (O'Fallon & Dearry, 2002). On November 4, 2005, EPA Administrator Steve Johnson issued a memorandum that identifies national environmental justice priorities and calls for ensuring greater public participation in the agency's development and implementation of environmental regulations and policies.

Some environmental health research has united communities and researchers to challenge a few of the basic assumptions of traditional science, such as the supposition that research must maintain objectivity and remain detached from participants (Lynn, 2000; Minkler, 2000). CBPR—a collaborative approach to research that equitably and meaningfully involves all partners in every step of the research process—encourages equal partnerships between community members and academic investigators (Israel, Schulz, Parker, & Becker, 1998; Keeler et al., 2002; O'Fallon & Dearry, 2002). CBPR has its roots in the work of American researchers in the mid-twentieth century, notably the psychologist Kurt Lewin, who were frustrated by the inability of traditional research methods to understand complex phenomena and experiences. Much of the most innovative CBPR work has been conducted in developing countries by researchers, educators, and activists, such as Paolo Freire in Brazil, interested in empowerment and social change. An important step of CBPR is the shared translation and dissemination of research findings with the broader community, including residents, policymakers, and the media, so that they can be applied to future policy and practices.

The CBPR approach has been widely used by environmental justice researchers and activists and has the potential to achieve social change while creating a healthier and less polluted environment. For example, the National Institute of Environmental Health Sciences (NIEHS) has promoted and supported the use of CBPR to research environmentally related disease. One of the studies funded by NIEHS, the Southeast Halifax project, was a partnership among the University of North Carolina at Chapel Hill, Concerned Citizens of Tillery, and the North Carolina Student Rural Health Coalition. This community-academic partnership determined that corporate hog operations were more concentrated in poor non-white areas and that there was a marked increase in reported headache, runny nose, sore throat, excessive coughing, diarrhea, and burning eyes in those areas compared to communities not located near intensive livestock operations (Wing & Wolf, 2000).

Using CBPR in the Protocol for Assessing Community Excellence in Environment Health

Following a participatory model of environmental health assessment, the Mult-nomah County Health Department in Portland, Oregon, collaborated with several organizations and dozens of residents to form the PACE Coalition between 2002 and 2005. The PACE Coalition was guided by the Protocol for Assessing Community Excellence in Environmental Health (PACE EH), developed in 1995 by the National Association of County and City Health Officials (NACCHO) and the CDC as a series of thirteen steps designed to help local health officials work collaboratively with communities to identify populations at disproportionate risk of environmental exposure, to assess and prioritize environmental health concerns, and to create an action plan and evaluation. The following discussion highlights the process used to complete one of the most vital preliminaries of the thirteen PACE steps, the process of defining and characterizing the community.

The vision of members of the PACE Coalition was to create a network of individuals and local organizations who take an active role in setting an environmental health and environmental justice agenda for their Portland communities. As the initiator of the PACE Coalition, the Multnomah County Health Department (MCHD) sought to establish the department's programmatic priorities based on resident input and participation, rather than on narrowly defined and short-term federal funding opportunities (what some health department representatives referred to as the "environmental health issue du jour").

While recognizing that there was an unequal burden on certain communities in Multnomah County, the MCHD did not have the internal capacity or the public consent to address environmental justice issues. The environmental health services department in the MCHD reflected a more common approach to environmental disease diagnosis and control, such as illnesses and injuries related to swimming pools, vectors, and food safety. This more traditional mandate, paired with a general mistrust by the public of county agencies, made it difficult for the MCHD to begin to conduct a comprehensive and participatory assessment of environmental health needs. To build relationships with the broader community, the MCHD hired two community "connectors," or organizers, to reach out to residents and encourage their participation in the PACE Coalition. Hiring the community connectors demonstrated the MCHD's commitment to a different way of doing business, especially since the hiring happened during state and county budget cuts.

Community Selection. The PACE Coalition, with more than sixty members, structured meetings to develop leadership among community members and ease among agency partners who might not have been used to working with communities. An assessment team, including representatives from the health department, local residents, community-based organizations, and a local university, gathered census data and maps documenting the exposure level of dozens of indicators ranging from potential brownfields (contaminated sites) to solid-waste facilities in the county to determine which areas were most heavily affected by environmental health hazards. After a community discussion of the findings, the Inner North/Northeast area of Portland was selected as the community of greatest immediate concern.

Community Outreach. The community connectors and the assessment team began conducting extensive outreach to community leaders and residents in the affordable housing communities of Inner North/Northeast Portland to generate a top-ten list of environmental health concerns: mold and mildew, pesticides, indoor air quality, outdoor air quality, brownfields, lead, trash and garbage, lack of meeting places, water quality, and lack of green spaces. The discussions between community residents and members of the PACE assessment team included both the *physical* and the *social* environment and acknowledged their complex interplay. For example, many residents talked about feeling unsafe or the lack of community meeting places as threats to environmental health and well-being.

The coalition members, especially the staff from the MCHD, committed themselves to identifying funding that could support sustained efforts in one or more of these identified priority areas. In 2005, the MCHD and its PACE partners received a $900,000 Housing and Urban Development (HUD) Healthy Homes grant to address the issues of lead, mold, and trash—the very issues that the affected communities identified as most important.

Conclusion

To adequately address disproportionate exposure, the discipline and practice of environmental health must identify ways to involve communities, government agencies, and academic partners in eliminating and preventing injustices in environmental health and exposures. Government and local leaders should be invited to play a key role in rehabilitating our communities and planning for a healthier and safer environment. In both of the Portland case studies, the projects were largely facilitated and supported by innovative thinkers in the city and county governments. In cities and counties that lack a progressive health department or city council, however, community residents can still initiate the assessment and prioritization of environmental health needs by generating awareness and gathering a critical mass. For example, concerned residents can use community organizing tactics and hold town meetings, conduct resident surveys, or gather their own data that can then be presented to government and local leaders as evidence of environmental exposure. The citizen-led "bucket brigades" that are cropping up in towns and cities across the United States provide one example. Residents take air samples with a bucket provided by an international environmental group called the Bucket Brigade and analyze the air samples in a lab. Community residents can then present the assessment results to educate public leaders and pressure industries and governments to identify solutions.

Furthermore, with the wider acceptance of CBPR principles and methods, community residents should feel increasingly comfortable approaching academics and researchers to help them investigate environmental toxins and potential health effects. "Science shops" are one model of CBPR whereby residents and community groups work with university-based researchers to examine and address environmental health problems. Science shops were first established in the Netherlands during the 1970s. The term *science* includes the natural and social sciences and humanities; the term *shop* reflects the notion that the university should be used by community members to address research questions posed by the local community. Researchers at science shops may use existing data, collect new data, or help facilitate a new research project created and conducted by community members themselves to answer the question posed by the community.

Public health practitioners and researchers should consider ways to use the precautionary principle and CBPR in tandem to supplement traditional risk assessment methods. In fact, the two approaches share many qualities and principles that may facilitate their blending. For example, both approaches advocate for an open and democratic process of decision making. Both approaches value lay people's knowledge, in contrast to experts' knowledge, which is the primary driver of traditional risk assessment methods. In addition, each approach has inherent limitations that may be eliminated when the two approaches are combined. For example, an assessment using the precautionary principle may not clearly acknowledge disproportionate environmental exposure; CBPR tends to explicitly identify and address the causes of injustice and inequality. Conversely, CBPR may not consider the value of "precaution" or seek to prevent exposure before the health problems are manifested, whereas prevention is at the core of the precautionary principle. Implementation of these approaches, alone or together, provides the opportunity to create a dialogue with community stakeholders and local environmental health leaders that can wholly transform the assessment of environmental risks and the creation of preventive solutions.

References

Ackerman, F., & Massey, R. (2002, August). *Prospering with precaution: Employment, economics, and the precautionary principle.* Boston: Global Development and Environment Institute, Tufts University. Retrieved October 16, 2006, from http://ase.tufts.edu/gdae/policy_research/PrecautionAHTAug02.pdf

Apelberg, B. J., Buckley, T. J., & White, R. H. (2005). Socioeconomic and racial disparities in cancer risk from air toxics in Maryland. *Environmental Health Perspectives, 113,* 693–699.

Blaikie, P., Cannon, T., Davis, I., & Wisner, B. (1994). *At risk: Natural hazards, people's vulnerability, and disasters.* New York: Routledge.

Blaxill, M. F. (2004). What's going on? The question of time trends in autism. *Public Health Reports, 119,* 536–551.

Bolin, R., & Stanford, L. (1998). The Northridge earthquake: Community-based approaches to unmet recovery needs. *Disasters, 22,* 21–38.

Bryant, B. (1995). *Environmental justice, issues, policies, and solutions.* Washington, DC: Island Press.

Bullard, R. D. (1990). *Dumping in Dixie: Race, class, and environmental quality.* Boulder, CO: Westview Press.

Bullard, R. D., Glenn, S. J., & Torres, A. O. (Eds.). (2004). *Highway robbery: Transportation racism and new routes to equity.* Boston: South End Press.

Bullard, R. D., & Johnson, G. S. (1997). *Just transportation: Dismantling race and class barriers to mobility.* Stony Creek, CT: New Society.

Bullard, R. D., & Wright, B. H. (1993). Environmental justice for all: Community perspectives of health and research needs. *Toxicology and Industrial Health, 9,* 821–841.

Campaign for Safe Cosmetics. (2005, October 8). Governor signs safe cosmetics bill: New law heightens scrutiny of industry safety. Retrieved July 5, 2005, from http://www.safecosmetics.org/newsroom/press.cfm?pressReleaseID=13

Campaign for Safe Cosmetics. (n.d.-a). About us. Retrieved July 5, 2006, from http://www.safecosmetics.org/about

Campaign for Safe Cosmetics. (n.d.-b). Frequently asked questions. Retrieved June 5, 2006, from http://www.safecosmetics.org/faqs

Centers for Disease Control and Prevention. (2003). *Second national report on human exposure to environmental chemicals.* National Center for Environmental Health, Division of Laboratory Sciences. (NCEH Publ. No. 02-0716). Atlanta: Author.

Centers for Disease Control and Prevention. (2005). *Third national report on human exposure to environmental chemicals.* National Center for Environmental Health, Division of Laboratory Sciences. (NCEH Publ. No. 05-0570). Atlanta: Author.

Collins, K. S., Hughes, D., Doty, M., Ives, B., Edwards, J., & Tenney, K. (2002). *Diverse communities, common concerns: Assessing health care quality for minority Americans.* New York: Commonwealth Fund.

Dicum, G. (2006, March 14). Justice in time: Meet Robert Bullard, the father of environmental justice. *Grist Magazine*. Retrieved October 16, 2006, from http://www.grist.org/news/maindish/2006/03/14/dicum

Edelson, S. B., & Cantor, D. S. (1999). Autism: Xenobiotic influences. *Journal of Advancement in Medicine, 12,* 35–47.

Environmental Health Perspectives, Science Education. (n.d). Frequently asked questions. Retrieved July 26, 2006, from http://www.ehponline.org/science-ed/faq.html

Environmental Protection Agency. (1976). *Toxic Substances Control Act.* Retrieved January 23, 2006, from http://www.epa.gov/region5/defs/html/tsca.htm

Environmental Protection Agency. (1992). Environmental equity: Reducing risk for all communities. In R. M. Wolcott & W. A. Banks (Eds.)., *Workgroup Report to the Administrator,* Vol. 1. Rep. No. EPA 230-R-92-008. Washington, DC: Author.

Environmental Protection Agency. (1998). *Final guidance for incorporating environmental justice concerns in EPA's NEPA compliance analyses.* Washington, DC: Author.

Environmental Protection Agency. (2003, July 25). *History of environmental justice.* Retrieved January 4, 2005, from http://www.epa.gov/envjustice/History

Faber, D. R., & Krieg, E. J. (2002). Unequal exposure to ecological hazards: Environmental injustices in the Commonwealth of Massachusetts. *Environmental Health Perspectives, 110*(Suppl. 2), 277–288.

Farquhar, S. A., & Wing, S. (2003). Methodological and ethical considerations of community-driven environmental justice research: Examination of two case studies from rural North Carolina. In M. Minkler & N. Wallerstein (Eds.), *Community-based participatory research for health* (pp. 221–241). San Francisco: Jossey-Bass.

Fothergill, A., Maestas, E., & Darlington DeRouen, J. (1999). Race, ethnicity, and disasters in the United States: A review of the literature. *Disasters, 23,* 156–173.

Goldman, L. R., & Koduru, S. (2000). Environmental chemicals in the environment and developmental toxicity to children: A public health and policy perspective. *Environmental Health Perspectives, 108,* 443–448.

Grant, E. N., Lyttle, C. S., & Weiss, K. B. (2000). The relation of socioeconomic factors and racial/ethnic differences in U.S. asthma mortality. *American Journal of Public Health, 90,* 1923–1925.

Greenberg, M., Schneider, D., & Choi, D. (1994). Neighborhood quality in areas with multiple technological and behavioral hazards. *Geographical Review, 84,* 1–15.

Health Care Without Harm. (2002a). *Aggregate exposures to phthalates in humans.* Washington, DC: Author.

Health Care Without Harm (with Women's Environmental Network, UK, & Swedish Society for Nature Conservation). (2002b). *Pretty nasty: Phthalates in European cosmetic products.* Stockholm, Sweden: Author.

Hites, R. A. (2004). Polybrominated diphenyl ethers in the environment and in people: A meta-analysis of concentrations. *Environmental Science and Technology, 38,* 945–956.

Houlihan, J., Brody, C., & Schwan, B. (2002, July 8). *Not too pretty: Phthalates, beauty products, and the FDA.* Washington, DC: Environmental Working Group, Health Care Without Harm.

Houlihan, J., Wiles, R., Thayer, K., & Gray, S. (2003). *Body burden: The pollution in people.* Washington, DC: Environmental Working Group, Health Care Without Harm.

Institute of Medicine. (2002). *Unequal treatment: Confronting racial and ethnic disparities in health care.* Washington, DC: National Academies Press.

Israel, B. A., Schulz, A. J., Parker, E. A., & Becker, A. B. (1998). Review of community-based research: Assessing partnership approaches to improve public health. *Annual Review of Public Health, 19,* 173–202.

Keeler, G., Dvonch, T., Yip, F., Parker, E. A., Israel, B. A., Marsik, F. J., et al. (2002). Assessment of personal and community-level exposures to particulate matter among children with asthma in Detroit, Michigan, as part of Community Action Against Asthma (CAAA). *Environmental Health Perspectives, 110*(Suppl. 2), 173–181.

Kuehn, R. (1996). The environmental justice implications of quantitative risk assessment. *University of Illinois Law Review, 38,* 103–172.

Landrigan, P. J., Schechter, C. B., Lipton, J. M., Fahs, M. C., & Schwartz, J. (2002). Environmental pollutants and disease in American children: Estimates of morbidity, mortality, and costs for lead poisoning, asthma, cancer, and developmental disabilities. *Environmental Health Perspectives, 110,* 721–728.

Liou, H. H., Tsai, M. C., Chen, C. J., Jeng, J. S., Chang, Y. C., Chen, S. Y., et al. (1997). Environmental risk factors and Parkinson's disease: A case control study in Taiwan. *Neurology, 48,* 1583–1588.

Lopez, R. (2002). Segregation and black/white differences in exposure to air toxics in 1990. *Environmental Health Perspectives, 110*(Suppl. 2), 289–295.

Lynn, F. M. (2000). Community-scientist collaboration in environmental research. *American Behavioral Scientist, 44,* 649–663.

Minkler, M. (2000). Using participatory action to build healthy communities. *Public Health Reports, 115,* 191–198.

Montague, P. (1998, February 18). The precautionary principle. *Rachel's Environment and Health News,* #586. Retrieved October 16, 2006, from http://www.rachel.org/bulletin/pdf/Rachels_Environment_Health_News_532.pdf

Motavalli, J. (1998, July-August). Dr. Robert Bullard—Some people don't have "the complexion for protection." *E/The Environmental Magazine, 9*(4). Retrieved June 3, 2006, from http://www.emagazine.com/index.php?toc&issue=11

Multnomah County Board of Commissioners. (2004). Precautionary principal resolutions. Portland, Ore.: Author. Retrieved July 26, 2006, from http://www.besafenet.com/ppc/docs/environmental_precaution/ENV_OR_Rep.pdf

Multnomah County Health Department. (2003). *The environmental health of Multnomah County.* Portland, OR: Author.

Myers, N. J., & Raffensperger, C. (Eds.). (2005). *Precautionary tools for reshaping environmental policy.* Cambridge, MA: MIT Press.

Natural Hazards Research and Applications Information Center. (2001). *Holistic disaster recovery: Ideas for building local sustainability after a natural disaster.* Retrieved July 20, 2002, from http://www.colorado.edu/hazards/holistic_recovery

Not Too Pretty. (2003). *Poisoned cosmetics, not too pretty.* Retrieved October 15, 2006, from http://www.nottoopretty.org

O'Fallon, L., & Dearry, A. (2002). Community-based participatory research as a tool to advance environmental health sciences. *Environmental Health Perspectives, 110*(Suppl. 2), 155–159.

Pew Environmental Health Commission. (2001). *Transition report to the new administration: Strengthening our public health defense against environmental threats.* Baltimore: Pew Environmental Health Commission, Johns Hopkins School of Public Health.

Pirkle, J. L., Kaufmann, R. B., Brody, D. J., Hickman, T., Gunter, E. W., & Paschal, D. C. (1998). Exposure of the U.S. population to lead, 1991–1994. *Environmental Health Perspectives, 106,* 745–750.

San Francisco Commission on the Environment. (2003). *White paper: The precautionary principle and the City and County of San Francisco.* San Francisco. Retrieved November 15, 2006, from http://www.environmentalcommons.org/precaution-white-paper.pdf

Schettler, T. (2002). Changing patterns of disease: Human health and the environment. *San Francisco Medicine, 75*(9), 10–13.

Schweizer, E. (1999, July). Environmental justice: An interview with Robert Bullard. *Earth First! Journal,* pp. 1–5. Retrieved October 16, 2006, from http://www.ejrc.cau.edu/earthfirstinterviewrb.htm

Seidler, A., Hellenbrand, W., Robra, B. P., Vieregge, P., Nischan, P., Joerg, J., et al. (1996). Possible environmental, occupational, and other etiologic factors for Parkinson's disease: A case-control study in Germany. *Neurology, 46,* 1275–1284.

Smart, B. A. (2004, Fall). The costs of asthma and allergy. *Allergy and Asthma Advocate.* Retrieved October 16, 2006, from http://www.aaaai.org/patients/advocate/2004/fall/costs.stm

Solomon, G. M. (2002). Rare and common diseases in environmental health. *San Francisco Medicine, 75*(9).

Thornton, J. W., McCally, M., & Houlihan, J. (2002). Biomonitoring of industrial pollutants: Health and policy implications of the chemical body burden. *Public Health Reports, 117,* 315–323.

U.S. Census Bureau. (2000). *Census data for the state of Oregon.* Retrieved May 11, 2006, from http://www.census.gov/census2000/states/or.html

Wakefield, J. (2002). The lead effect? *Environmental Health Perspectives, 110,* A574–A580.

Williams, D. R. (1990). Socioeconomic differentials in health: A review and redirection. *Social Psychology Quarterly, 53,* 81–99.

Wing, S., & Wolf, S. (2000). Intensive livestock operation, health, and quality of life among eastern North Carolina residents. *Environmental Health Perspectives, 108,* 233–238.

Wirth, D. A. (2002). Precaution in international environmental policy and U.S. law and practice. *North American Environmental Law and Policy, 10,* 219–268.

CHAPTER TWELVE

HEALTH AND THE BUILT ENVIRONMENT

Opportunities for Prevention

Howard Frumkin, Andrew L. Dannenberg

The built environment refers to the many components of our surroundings formed by human acts of creation or modification. Almost all the settings in which we live, work, study, and play are parts of the built environment.

Many features of the built environment affect health, ranging in scale from the design of furniture in a room to the layout of a home or office building to the infrastructure of the neighborhood and metropolitan area in which one lives. The built environment concept includes not only fixed objects such as sidewalks but also activities that give rise to the built environment, such as architecture and urban planning, as well as functions that are embedded in and directly dependent on physical infrastructure, such as transportation and energy production. The concept of the built environment includes contact with nature, since most urban and suburban dwellers encounter nature primarily in such places as backyards and parks that are designed and built by people.

This chapter focuses on the links between health and the built environment on various scales and on strategies to help create health-promoting environments, such as parks to promote physical activity, and to reduce health-damaging environments, such as automobile-dependent communities with increased air pollution.

The Small Scale

The built environment on a small scale refers to tools and other implements that people use, wear, or occupy. Examples include computer keyboards and office furniture. The scientific study of these small-scale environments draws on both ergonomics and biomechanics. Details of the health issues related to small-scale environments are beyond the scope of this chapter.

The Intermediate Scale: Buildings

People spend much of their time in buildings—homes, schools, workplaces, stores, and places of worship—that are perhaps the most familiar examples of the built environment. Physical conditions of buildings such as noise levels, temperature, humidity, and lighting may have a major effect on comfort, productivity, and health. In addition, the design of built environments can affect injury risk. The following discussion focuses on a few of these issues.

Lighting

The level and quality of indoor lighting affect several aspects of health and well-being (Smith, 2000). Good lighting supports and restores normal circadian rhythms (Duffy & Wright, 2005). In schools and workplaces, adequate natural lighting (or "daylighting") is associated with improved subjective well-being, academic performance and behavior, and task performance, while glare is associated with diminished performance (Heschong, 2003a, 2003b; Kuller & Lindsten, 1992). Bright nighttime lighting may help shift workers adjust to schedule changes, although data are not definitive (Knauth & Hornberger, 2003). Well-designed lighting may help alleviate seasonal depression (Lewy, Kern, Rosenthal, & Wehr, 1982), speed recovery from severe depression (Beauchemin & Hays, 1996), and improve sleep patterns in people with insomnia (Lack & Wright, 1993) and with dementia (Van Someren, Kessler, Mirmirann, & Swaab, 1997).

Crowding

Crowding is both an objectively measurable condition—in terms of the density, or number of people per unit area—and a subjective experience reflecting loss of privacy, loss of control, or overstimulation (Maxwell, 2006). Crowding may occur in many indoor settings, including primary environments such as the home, school, and workplace and more transient secondary environments such as a train or a department store.

Crowding has negative effects on health and well-being. Children from crowded homes demonstrate diminished motivation and aggressive or withdrawn behavior (Aiello, Nicosia, & Thompson, 1979; Saegert, 1982). Crowding is associated with less cooperative behavior among young children (Aiello et al., 1979) and with more disruptive, aggressive, and hostile behavior (Maxwell, 2003; Saegert, 1982), inattentiveness (Evans, Saegert, & Harris, 2001), or withdrawal from classroom participation (Loo & Smetana, 1978) among older children. Crowding at home and in classrooms is associated with lower academic achievement (Evans, Lepore, Shejwal, & Palsane, 1998; Maxwell, 2003; Saegert, 1982). Similar effects—stress, psychological dysfunction, and impaired interpersonal relations—have been associated with crowding among both institutionalized adults and adults in community settings (Evans, 2003). Crowded indoor environments may also increase the risk of infectious disease transmission (Lienhardt, 2001). It appears important for built environments to offer adequate space and privacy to avoid some of the adverse aspects of crowding.

Injury Risk

Substantial numbers of unintentional injuries occur in and around buildings. The home environment is the setting for more than thirty thousand fatal injuries and thirteen million nonfatal injuries per year in the United States (National Safety Council [NSC], 2004). The majority of these injuries occur among young children, the elderly, and the poor (NSC, 2004). Two categories of injury, falls and burns, illustrate the magnitude of the problem and the potential for environmental design to reduce risk.

Falls are the leading single cause of fatal and nonfatal unintentional injuries in homes (Runyan & Casteel, 2004). Children are at risk of falls through open windows or railings, off rooftops and other elevations, and down stairs (Staunton, Frumkin, & Dannenberg, 2006). Design features that can reduce risk include window guards and window stops, limited access to rooftops and other elevations, and closely spaced posts on guard rails (American Academy of Pediatrics, 2001; Bergner, Mayer, & Harris, 1971; Istre et al., 2003). The elderly are also at risk of home falls (Cayless, 2001; Gill, Williams, Robison, & Tinetti, 1999; Sattin, Rodriguez, DeVito, & Wingo, 1998). Environmental interventions that may reduce the risk of falls in the elderly include removing tripping hazards such as throw rugs, using nonslip mats in tubs and showers, installing grab bars in bathrooms, installing handrails on both sides of stairways, and improving lighting throughout the home (Centers for Disease Control and Prevention [CDC], 2005).

Residential burns are also a leading cause of injury, accounting for about 2,200 deaths and more than 250,000 injuries in the United States each year (NSC, 2004). Most fatal burns result from home fires, while most nonfatal burns result from scalds, thermal burns, and electrical burns. Environmental interventions that reduce the risk of burns include smoke detectors (Runyan et al., 2005), indoor sprinkler systems (Cote, 1984), and reduced hot water heater temperature settings (Erdmann, Feldman, Rivara, Heimbach, & Wall, 1991; Feldman, Schaller, Feldman, & McMillon, 1978). Other strategies for reducing burn injuries include child-resistant lighters, roll-up cords for electric coffeepots, kitchens with shorter distances between the stove and the sink, and cooking pans and kettles designed to reduce the probability of tipping (Staunton et al., 2006).

The Large Scale: From Neighborhood to Metropolis

At a larger scale, the built environment consists of neighborhoods, towns, and cities. For many centuries, towns and cities were relatively dense, walkable places where people lived and worked in close quarters (Hall, 1998; Mumford, 1961). Over time, however, a combination of technical advances, cultural values, commercial opportunities, and policy initiatives led to the geographical expansion of cities in a pattern commonly known as "sprawl" (Bullard, 1990; Cervero, 1989; Fishman, 1987; Garreau, 1991; Gillham, 2002; Jackson, 1985; Whyte, 1958). As automobiles became the predominant form of transportation, transit use, walking, and bicycling declined. Automobiles enabled people to live far from their workplaces, schools, and other destinations and to travel these distances regularly.

These developments led directly to land use changes. Land development since World War II has occurred at much lower density than prevailed in traditional cities and towns. Accordingly, the distances people routinely travel are greater. Different land uses—residential, commercial, educational, recreational, and so on—are separated, a phenomenon known by planners as "low land use mix." Suburban street networks feature low "connectivity." The prototypical neighborhood is no longer a walkable grid in a small town or city, with homes located near stores, workplaces, and schools and with bus or trolley service available for longer journeys. Instead, it is a low-density suburban subdivision with poorly connected serpentine roads that requires an automobile trip for nearly every errand. There is a well-established link between land use and travel behavior: cities with low residential density, low connectivity, and related indicators are associated with less walking and bicycling and more automobile travel (Cervero & Gorham, 1995; Cervero & Kockelman, 1997; Frank & Pivo, 1995; Newman & Kenworthy, 1999; Transportation Research Board, 2005).

Features of the built environment combine with cultural preferences, public policy, and other factors to determine travel behavior. In the Netherlands, 28 percent of all trips in urban areas are on bicycles and 18 percent are on foot; in England, these figures are 4 percent and 12 percent, and in the United States, 1 percent and 6 percent, respectively (Pucher & Dijkstra, 2003). Approximately 25 percent of all trips in the United States are less than one mile, and of these, 75 percent are by car (Koplan & Dietz, 1999).

Transportation and land use patterns—key aspects of the built environment—can affect health and well-being. For example, the heavy reliance on automobiles for transportation has implications for air quality and safety. Similarly, low-density land development with separation of different land uses has implications for physical activity and for water quantity and quality. These transportation and land use patterns may also affect mental health and social capital.

Physical Activity

Sedentary lifestyles have become the norm in the United States. More than half of American adults are physically inactive on a regular basis, and just over one in four Americans reports no leisure-time physical activity at all (Macera et al., 2003). In 2000, only 26.2 percent of adults were classified as meeting recommended levels of physical activity (defined as any physical activity for at least thirty minutes a day at least five days a week or vigorous physical activity for at least twenty minutes at least three days a week). This pattern is similar among children aged nine to thirteen, 61.5 percent of whom participate in no organized physical activity outside of school (Duke, Huhman, & Heitzler, 2003).

A sedentary lifestyle, in turn, increases the risk of cardiovascular disease, stroke, and all-cause mortality, while physical activity prolongs life (Lee & Paffenbarger, 2000; U.S. Department of Health and Human Services, 1996; Wannamethee, Shaper, & Walker, 1998; Wannamethee, Shaper, Walker, & Ebrahim, 1998). Low physical fitness produces cardiovascular risk comparable to, and in some studies greater than, the risk of hypertension, high cholesterol, diabetes, and even smoking (Blair et al., 1996; Wei et al., 1999). Physical activity also appears to be protective against cancer (Bauman, 2004; Kampert, Blair, Barlow, & Kohl, 1996; Lee, 2003).

Beyond the direct effects on health, physical inactivity is also a risk factor for weight gain. Overweight and obesity are on the rise. (Overweight is defined as a body mass index, BMI, of at least 25 kg/m², and obesity as a BMI of at least 30 kg/m².) In 1960, only 24 percent of Americans were overweight, but by 1990, that proportion had increased to 33 percent (Kuczmarski, Flegal, Campbell, & Johnson, 1994). During the same interval, the prevalence of obesity nearly doubled (Flegal, Carroll, Kuczmarski, & Johnson, 1998). According to data from the CDC's Behavioral Risk Factor Surveillance System, this trend continued during the 1990s, with the prevalence of obesity rising from 12.0 percent in 1991 to 20.9 percent in 2001 (Mokdad et al., 1999, 2001, 2003).

Being overweight or obese, in turn, is a well-established risk factor for a number of diseases: ischemic heart disease, hypertension, stroke, dyslipidemia, osteoarthritis, gallbladder disease, and some cancers; obese people die at as much as 2.5 times the rate of nonobese people (Must et al., 1999; Sesso, Paffenbarger, & Lee, 1998; Shaper, Wannamethee, & Walker, 1997; Wannamethee, Shaper, & Walker, 1998; Willett, Dietz, & Colditz, 1999). Overweight people face as much as an eighteenfold increase in the risk of type-2 diabetes, and the current epidemic of type-2 diabetes tracks closely with the increase in overweight (Mokdad et al., 2001; Must et al., 1999). Obese persons have increased risks of some cancers such as colorectal, prostate, and breast (Calle, Rodriguez, Walker-Thurmond, & Thun, 2003). Obesity is also associated with depression (Stunkard, Faith, & Allison, 2003).

The built environment plays a role in sedentary lifestyles, overweight, and obesity. As noted earlier, people in suburbs and exurbs drive more and walk less than people in cities and towns. Transportation research has also focused on neighborhood "walkability" with respect to travel behavior. Highly walkable neighborhoods are characterized by high density, high land use mix, high connectivity, good walking infrastructure, pleasing aesthetics, and safety. In general, people in highly walkable neighborhoods record more walking trips per week, especially for errands and going to work (Craig, Brownson, Cragg, & Dunn, 2002; Frank & Pivo, 1995; Kockelman, 1997; Powell, Martin, & Chowdhury, 2003; Saelens, Sallis, Black, & Chen, 2003). This finding translates into a higher total amount of physical activity with its associated health benefits.

Research has started to examine the entire hypothesized causal chain, from environmental features to physical activity to health risk factors to health outcomes. Although this is a complex set of relationships, with many variables operating on many different spatial scales, emerging evidence supports the notion that certain built environments—known by some as "active living environments"—promote physical activity and good health (Frank, Andresen, & Schmid, 2004; French, Story, & Jeffery, 2001; Handy, Boarnet, Ewing, & Killingsworth, 2002; Humpel, Owen, & Leslie, 2002; Kahn & Kellert, 2002; Saelens, Sallis, & Frank, 2003; Sallis, Bauman, & Pratt, 1998; Transportation Research Board, 2005; Trost, Owen, Bauman, Sallis, & Brown, 2002).

Air Pollution and Respiratory Diseases

Motor vehicles are a leading source of air pollution, especially carbon monoxide, carbon dioxide, particulate matter, oxides of nitrogen (NOx), and hydrocarbons (Environmental Protection Agency [EPA], 2006). In the presence of sunlight, NOx and hydrocarbons form ozone. In the United States, cars and trucks account for approximately 33 percent of NOx and 30 percent of human hydrocarbon emissions (EPA, 2006). In automobile-dependent metropolitan areas, the relative contribution of mobile sources may increase substantially. These pollutants, especially NOx, hydrocarbons, ozone, and particulate matter, account for a substantial part of the air pollution burden of U.S. cities. Certain pollutants, such as carbon monoxide, reach their highest concentrations alongside roadways, raising the exposure risk for homes, schools, and other places near heavy traffic routes. Other pollutants, most notably ozone, are formed from precursors over time. As the precursors move downwind from their sources, the highest ozone levels may occur miles away. Thus vehicle-related air pollution may be a problem throughout entire regions.

The health hazards of air pollution are well established. Ozone is an airway irritant, and higher ozone levels are associated with more respiratory symptoms, worse lung function, more frequent emergency room visits and hospitalizations, more medication use, and more absenteeism from school and work (Bell & Samet, 2005). People with asthma and other respiratory diseases are especially susceptible to such adverse effects. Particulate matter is associated with many of the same respiratory effects and also with cardiovascular disease, lung cancer, and increased mortality (Brook et al., 2004; Dockery et al., 1993; Pope et al., 1995).

Motor vehicles emissions are a source of carbon dioxide and other greenhouse gases, including methane, NOx, and volatile organic compounds (VOCs). As a result, automobile traffic is a major contributor to global climate change, accounting for approximately 26 percent of U.S. greenhouse gas emissions (EPA, 2001a). During the 1990s, greenhouse gases from mobile sources increased 18 percent, primarily a reflection of an increase in vehicle-miles traveled (EPA, 2001b). Global climate change, in turn, is expected to threaten human health in several ways, including through the direct effects of heat, aggravation of some air pollutants, and increased prevalence of some infectious diseases (Epstein, 2000; Haines & Patz, 2004; National Assessment Synthesis Team, 2000).

A built environment that reinforces automobile dependence contributes to air pollution, which threatens health. This effect is mitigated by cleaner-burning, more fuel-efficient vehicles, but technical improvements are counteracted by increased vehicle-miles traveled. Conversely, a built environment that reduces travel demand by placing trip origins and destinations close together or that promotes alternatives to automobile travel may reduce air emissions.

Motor Vehicle Crashes

In the United States, automobiles claim over forty thousand lives every year (National Highway Traffic Safety Administration [NHTSA], 2004). Automobile crashes are the leading cause of death among persons between one and twenty-four years old (CDC, 1999). They account for 3.4 million nonfatal injuries each year and cost an estimated $200 billion (CDC, 1999). Thanks to safer cars and roads, laws that discourage drunk driving, and other measures, rates of automobile fatalities and injuries per driver and per mile driven have decreased substantially. Still, the absolute toll of automobile crashes remains high.

The automobile is a relatively dangerous mode of travel. Depending on the assumptions used, a mile of automobile travel is between thirty and several hundred times more likely to result in the traveler's death than a mile of bus, train, or airplane travel (Halperin, 1993). Built environments that entail more time in an automobile would be expected to increase an individual's probability of a motor vehicle crash (Lourens, Vissers, & Jessurum, 1999).

In automobile-oriented environments such as suburban and exurban communities, several additional aspects of driving add to the risk of crashes. First, suburban roads may pose a special hazard, especially major commercial thoroughfares and "feeder" roads that combine high speed, high traffic volume, and frequent "curb cuts" where drivers enter and exit stores and other destinations (Ossenbruggen, Pendharkar, & Ivan, 2001). In addition, suburban drivers often travel longer distances—commuting, transporting their children, running errands—resulting in tired, busy people. Fatigue is an important risk factor for traffic crashes (Horne & Reyner, 1995; Pack, Cucchiara, Schwab, Rodgman, & Pack, 1994). Furthermore, the increasing use of cellular phones while driving further amplifies the risk of crashes (Laberge-Nadeau et al., 2003; Redelmeier & Tibshirani, 1997).

Denser metropolitan areas that require shorter trip distances and rely more on walking and public transportation have lower automobile fatality rates for both drivers and passengers than more sprawling cities (NHTSA, 2004). In a recent study of 448 counties in the largest 101 metropolitan areas in the United States, for every 1 percent decrease in the level of sprawl (as measured by density and other factors), the traffic fatality rate fell by 1.49 percent and pedestrian fatality rates fell by 1.47 to 3.56 percent, leading to the conclusion that "urban sprawl was directly related to traffic fatalities and pedestrian fatalities" (Ewing, Schieber, & Zegeer, 2003). Reducing time spent in automobiles can therefore be considered a form of primary prevention. As noted by injury expert Ian Roberts (1993, p. 437), "Strategies which reduce the need for car travel or substitute car travel with safer forms of transport would substantially reduce population death rates."

Pedestrian Injuries and Fatalities

The implications of the built environment for pedestrian safety are more complex. Annually, automobiles cause about 5,000 fatalities and 110,000 injuries among pedestrians nationwide. In a built environment oriented more toward driving than nonmotorized travel, a mile of walking or biking is more likely to be fatal than a mile of driving. In 2001, a mile of walking was twenty-three times more likely to kill a pedestrian, and a mile of biking was twelve times more likely to kill a bicyclist than a mile of driving was likely to kill a car occupant (Ernst & McCann, 2002).

Fortunately, pedestrian and bicyclist injury and fatality rates are decreasing in most industrialized nations, including the United States (Pucher & Dijkstra, 2003). In terms of public health, this is a Pyrrhic victory, since it reflects reduced walking and bicycling. For example, data from the National Personal Transportation Survey show that half of U.S. children are driven to school in a private vehicle and approximately one-third travel by school bus, while fewer than one in seven trips to school is made on foot or bicycle, a substantial decline from a generation ago (Dellinger & Staunton, 2002). In the 1999 nationwide HealthStyles survey, the two leading reported barriers to walking or biking to school were distance and traffic. Although safety was not offered as a perceived barrier, the concern with traffic is presumably a safety concern (Dellinger & Staunton, 2002). Parental concerns about the dangers of heavy traffic are well founded. For example, a New Zealand policy that temporarily restricted automobile use resulted in a 46.4 percent decline in child pedestrian mortality (Roberts, Marshall, & Norton, 1992).

Design of the built environment helps determine traffic volume and defines another factor that affects pedestrian and bicyclist safety: physical infrastructure. Environmental modifications that help protect pedestrians and bicyclists include separating pedestrians from vehicles, making pedestrians more visible and conspicuous to drivers, and reducing vehicle speeds (Retting, Ferguson, & McCartt, 2003). Pedestrian-activated crossing signals, favorable traffic signal timing, and no-right-on-red laws can all help separate pedestrians from vehicles in time. They can be spatially separated with pedestrian overpasses, wide sidewalks on both sides of the street, and pedestrian refuge islands in the middle of wide streets. One strategy used in some European cities is the banning of motor vehicles from designated streets or entire zones. Furthermore, separate paths and other infrastructure for pedestrians and bicyclists help prevent injuries from motor vehicles (Pucher & Dijkstra, 2003). Methods to make pedestrians more conspicuous to drivers include increased roadway lighting, raised intersections and crosswalks, and "bulb-outs" that extend the sidewalk corners into the street. Vehicle speeds can be reduced with traffic circles, narrowed traffic lanes, curving or zigzag roadways, raised intersections, and speed bumps. These techniques are collectively known as "traffic calming" (Elvik, 2001; Sarkar, Nederveen, & Pols, 1997; Shaw, 1994), and there is good evidence that they help prevent pedestrian injuries and fatalities (Bunn et al., 2003; Retting et al., 2003).

The apparent trade-off between pedestrian travel and pedestrian safety is not inevitable. Under the right circumstances, higher levels of walking and bicycling are associated with *lower* rates of injuries and fatalities to pedestrians and cyclists. In the Netherlands and Germany, countries where walking and bicycling are far more common than in the United States, pedestrians and cyclists are killed at far lower rates than in the United States (Pucher & Dijkstra, 2000). In observational studies of intersections in both Sweden and Ontario, heavier pedestrian and bicycle traffic predicted lower rates of collisions with automobiles (Ekman, 1996; Leden, 2002). This relationship was confirmed in studies of California cities, Danish towns, and European countries (Jacobsen, 2003). There is therefore a paradox, one that contains an important public health opportunity: whereas lower pedestrian and bicyclist injury rates may result from built environments that *decrease* walking and bicycling, a marked *increase* in foot and bicycle trips, with associated benefits—greater awareness among drivers, better roads and paths—also decreases pedestrian and bicyclist injuries.

Water Quantity and Quality

Features of the built environment may threaten the quantity and quality of the water supply. Land converted from forest and grassland to residential and commercial buildings yields extensive impervious surfaces such as rooftops, driveways, roads, and parking lots that do not effectively absorb rainwater and replenish groundwater aquifers (Noble, 1999; Zielinski, 2000). In suburban Indianapolis over nearly twenty years, an 18 percent increase in impervious areas resulted in an estimated 80 percent increase in annual average rainwater runoff (Bhaduri, Harbor, Engel, & Grove, 2000). About half of U.S. communities depend on groundwater for their drinking water; such communities are at risk of water shortages if increased impervious surfaces prevent adequate groundwater recharge. High-density development confined to limited areas and balanced by preserved greenspace (especially along waterways) may limit the impact of impervious surfaces on a watershed. The amount of impervious surface has been suggested as a key environmental indicator, much like air pollutant levels (Arnold & Gibbons, 1996).

Features of the built environment may affect water quality by increasing water pollution that occurs when rainfall or snowmelt deposits contaminants into surface water such as lakes, rivers, wetlands, and coastal waters. Such contaminants include oil, grease, and toxic chemicals from roads, parking lots, and other surfaces, as well as sediment from improperly managed construction sites. Suburban development increases surface-water levels of contaminants such as polycyclic aromatic hydrocarbons, zinc, and organic waste (Callender & Rice, 2000; Dierberg, 1991; Van Metre, Mahler, & Furlong, 2000). Surface runoff may also carry microbial contaminants from feces of pets and wildlife (Bannerman, Owens, Dodds, & Hornewer, 1993) or in sediment. The result is that waterways downstream from developed areas may be contaminated after significant rainfalls, increasing the risk of waterborne diseases (Curriero, Patz, Rose, & Lele, 2001; Gannon & Musse, 1989). In addition, in suburban developments that rely on wells and septic tanks, well water may be contaminated if the density of septic systems overwhelms the soil's ability to accommodate the wastes.

Water quantity and quality may be threatened by land use and development patterns. Source water protection, both upstream and in residential areas, is an important aspect of health protection often overlooked in decisions about the built environment.

Nature Contact

An atrium with trees and plants, an urban park, and a grassy backyard are examples of built environments that offer opportunities for nature contact. People may find tranquillity in certain natural environments, a soothing, restorative, even healing sense. Nature contact may help through mechanisms such as attention restoration and reduced stress (Ulrich, Simons, Losito, & Fiorito, 1991).

Some built environments offer visual access to nature, such as nature views through windows. Studies suggest improved attention and decreased distractibility in apartment dwellers and in college students in dormitories who have views of nature from their windows (R. Kaplan, 2001; Tennessen & Cimprich, 1995). Other studies have found that views of nature were associated with reduced sick call visits in prisoners (E. O. Moore, 1981), fewer headaches in employees (R. Kaplan, 1992; S. Kaplan, Talbot, & Kaplan, 1988), and shorter postoperative hospital stays and less need for pain medication in cholecystectomy patients (Ulrich, 1984).

A series of studies among residents of inner-city housing projects in Chicago compared two configurations of otherwise identical buildings, some with barren surroundings and others surrounded by trees. Living in a building with nearby trees was associated with higher levels of attention and greater effectiveness in managing major life issues, lower levels of aggression and violence among women, and lower levels of reported crime (Kuo, 2001; Kuo & Sullivan, 2001a, 2001b).

Some built environments go beyond visual access and offer people the chance to work or play in natural settings. Residents of retirement communities report that living within pleasant landscaped grounds is important (Browne, 1992), and office employees report that plants make them feel calmer and more relaxed (Larsen, Adams, Deal, Kweon, & Tyler, 1998; Randall, Shoemaker, Relf, & Geller, 1992). In urban settings, gardens and gardening have been linked to a range of social benefits, ranging from improved property values to greater conviviality (for example, Patel, 1992). A study of children with attention deficit hyperactivity disorder found that playing in natural settings reduced ADHD symptoms more than playing in built settings (Kuo & Taylor, 2004). It has been suggested that regular opportunities for nature contact is an essential—and diminishing—aspect of wholesome child development (Louv, 2005).

Contact with nature increasingly seems to offer health benefits, a principle that can be applied in many ways to building and community design.

Mental Health

The built environment may have an effect on mental health if people find some places to be soothing and restorative and other places irritating and depressing. Tradition and research in architecture, geography, landscape architecture, urban planning, and environmental psychology support this concept (Alexander et al., 1997; Frumkin, 2003; Gallagher, 1993; R. Kaplan, Kaplan, & Ryan, 1998; Tuan, 1977; Whyte, 1980). Some observers think that living in ugly or unpleasant places may adversely affect mental health. James Howard Kunstler (1993, 2005) suggests that sprawling suburban developments are isolating, disaggregated, and neurologically punishing and may contribute to obesity and depression.

Another set of links between the built environment and mental health pertains to the stressful effects of driving. Markers of this stress include increased heart rate and blood pressure and increased levels of stress hormones measured in urine. Driving-related stress is aggravated by certain personality traits, high levels of life stress in general, and situations such as crowded roads, unpredictability, and rude behavior by other drivers. It is therefore no surprise that automobile commuting—unavoidable, time-pressured driving performed ten times a week at crowded times of the day—has long been recognized as a stressor (Frumkin, 2004). Various studies have linked automobile commuting in congestion with increased blood pressure, back pain, cardiovascular disease, and self-reported stress (Belkic' et al., 1994; Koslowsky, Kluger, & Reich, 1995; Magnusson, Pope, Wilder, & Areskoug, 1996; Novaco, Stokols, Campbell, & Stokols, 1979; Pietri et al., 1992; Stokols, Novaco, Stokols, & Campbell, 1978). As people spend more time on more crowded roads, an increase in these health outcomes might be expected.

One possible indicator of such problems is aggressive driving. Substantial proportions of drivers report aggressive feelings while driving and confess to such behaviors as swearing out loud at other drivers, making threatening or hostile gestures, and even feeling that they "could gladly kill" other drivers (Hauber, 1980; Parry, 1968; Snow, 2000; Turner, Layton, & Simons, 1975). These aggressive thoughts can escalate into action, in episodes that have come to be called "road rage," episodes when "an angry or impatient driver tries to kill or injure another driver after a traffic dispute" (Rathbone & Huckabee, 1999). According to the American Automobile Association's Foundation for Traffic Safety, the interval from 1990 to 1996 saw a 51 percent increase in reported incidents of road rage. The foundation documented ten thousand reports of such incidents, resulting in 12,610 injuries and 218 deaths (Mizell, 1997). A variety of weapons were used, including guns, knives, clubs, fists, feet, and in some cases the vehicle itself.

Road rage is not well understood. Risk factors include male sex and psychological predispositions (Dahlen & Ragan, 2004; Smart, Stoduto, Mann, & Adlaf, 2004). Stress at home or work may combine with stress while driving to elicit anger (Hartley & el Hassani, 1994; Novaco, 1991). Data from Australia, Canada, and Europe suggest that traffic volume, travel distance, and the amount of time spent driving are risk factors (Harding, Morgan, Indermaur, Ferrante, & Blagg, 1998; Parker, Lajunen, & Summala, 2002; Smart et al., 2004). Long delays on crowded roads are likely to be a contributing factor.

It seems reasonable to hypothesize that anger and frustration among drivers are not restricted to their cars. When angry people arrive at work or at home, what are the implications for work and family relations? If the phenomenon known as "commuting stress" affects well-being and social relationships both on the roads and off, and if this set of problems is aggravated by increasingly long and difficult commutes on crowded roads, then the built environment may in this manner threaten mental health.

Social Capital

Social capital refers to the attitudes and behaviors that bind a community or a society together—attitudes such as trust and reciprocity and behaviors such as civic engagement and participation (Portes, 1998). A closely related concept is "sense of community." Social capital, especially more and better social relationships, is associated with health benefits (House, Landis, & Umberson, 1988; Kawachi, 1999). Conversely, conditions corresponding to low social capital—social isolation, social stratification, and income inequality—are associated with higher all-cause mortality, infant mortality, and mortality from a variety of specific causes, independent of income and poverty (G. A. Kaplan, Pamuk, Lynch, Cohen, &

Balfour, 1996; Kawachi & Kennedy, 1999; Kawachi, Kennedy, Lochner, & Pro-throw-Stith, 1997; Kennedy, Kawachi, & Prothrow-Stith, 1996; Lynch, Smith, Kaplan, & House, 2000; Lynch et al., 1998; Stanistreet, Scott-Samuel, & Bellis, 1999; Wilkinson, 1996).

Many factors, ranging from television and computer use to employment patterns, affect levels of social capital. The built environment may play a role (Calthorpe, 1993; Mo & Wilkie, 1997; Putnam, 2000). After the Second World War, many Americans flocked to newly developing suburbs, drawn in part by the promised sense of community. In Park Forest, Illinois, in the 1950s, William Whyte (1956) observed an almost frantic pace of socializing, a "hotbed of participation." Investigators in Levittown, on New York's Long Island, described many social organizations that formed during the 1950s, such as babysitting co-ops, Tupperware parties, Little League, and service on the school board and PTA (Baxandall & Ewen, 2000).

But other observers have noted adverse consequences of suburban design on social capital. For example, Ewing believes that "strong communities of place, where neighbors interact, have a sense of belonging, and have a feeling of responsibility for one another are harder to find" in suburbs than in traditional small towns or cities (1997, p. 117).

Several features of suburban community design may undermine social capital. First, urban sprawl and associated long commutes restrict the time and energy people have available for civic involvement. Putnam (2000) reports that commute time is one of the most important demographic variables in predicting civic involvement. He writes that "each ten additional minutes in daily commuting time cuts involvement in community affairs by 10 percent—fewer public meetings attended, fewer committees chaired, fewer petitions signed, fewer church services attended, and so on" (p. 213).

Second, the built environment may or may not provide opportunities for spontaneous, informal social interaction. Traditional towns and cities typically include "great good places"—the "cafés, coffee shops, bookstores, bars, hair salons, and other hangouts at the heart of a community" where people may gather to socialize (Oldenburg, 1989). In contrast, recently developed suburbs tend to lack such places.

Third, the built environment could affect social capital by either promoting or devaluing the public realm. People who use exercise machines at home or relax in their back yards rather than jog or picnic in parks may have little feeling for parks and other public assets. Recent voting trends suggest that suburban voters prefer limited government programs and place little emphasis on such social goals as eliminating discrimination and reducing poverty. They also tend to reject initiatives such as park acquisition and mass transit (Oliver, 2001; Putnam, 2000; Teaford & Kilpinen, 1997).

Fourth, relatively homogeneous communities, segregated by social class and race, may obviate the political discourse that is important to social capital. Oliver (2001) suggests that in homogeneous suburban communities, social conflicts between citizens are transformed into conflicts between political institutions. This removes incentives for people to become personally involved in the political process, reducing levels of civic participation.

Finally, many homogeneous suburban neighborhoods offer housing appropriate to only one stage in the life cycle, so that couples who wanted large houses and lots while raising children need to leave the neighborhood when they are ready to downsize to smaller lodging. The use of property taxes to fund schools may be a further incentive for empty-nesters to depart communities with young families. The systematic departure of families after living in a neighborhood for twenty years reduces social capital.

Such evidence suggests that features of the built environment may either promote or diminish social capital (Burchell et al., 1998; Frumkin, Frank, & Jackson, 2004). In general, evidence suggests that walkability, public spaces, and mixed uses are associated with improvements in social capital, while automobile dependence, absence of public spaces, and low density have a negative impact. In these ways, the built environment may indirectly but significantly affect health.

Populations at Special Risk

As with many environmental exposures, features of the built environment are likely to affect some groups more than others. Groups that deserve special attention in this regard include women, children, the elderly, poor people, people of color, and people with disabilities.

Women

In automobile-dependent areas, women play a disproportionate role as chauffeurs—taking children to school, play dates, or soccer games; taking elderly parents to the doctor; and running errands to the grocery store, post office, or bank. One study (Surface Transportation Policy Project, 2002) found that two-thirds of all chauffeur trips are made by women and that married women with school-aged children were averaging more than five automobile trips a day, 21 percent more than the average for men. Among women, 50.4 percent of trips were made for chauffeuring, compared with 41.1 percent among men. Time spent in the car per day averaged sixty-six minutes for married women with school-aged children and seventy-five minutes for single mothers. The image of the suburban "soccer mom" in a minivan turned out to reflect long hours at the wheel providing transportation and delivery services. For women in suburban and exurban areas, faced with a large burden of driving, the built environment must seem very much a women's health issue.

Children

Children are also a vulnerable population, in several ways. First, the burdens of air pollution fall heavily on children, since they breathe disproportionately more air than adults, have more outdoor exposure time, and have developing respiratory systems (Etzel & Balk, 2003). Asthma prevalence is high in children, and asthmatic children are especially susceptible to exposure to ozone and other respiratory irritants. Ozone increases acute respiratory symptoms in children in the short term and may impair lung growth (Künzli et al., 1997) and increase the probability of developing asthma (McConnell et al., 2002) following long-term exposure. This is an issue in densely trafficked areas, such as alongside busy roadways, and it is an issue on a regional scale when high levels of driving increase the air pollution burden.

Second, children have been hard hit by the physical inactivity associated with shifting travel patterns. The disappearance of walking and bicycling to school, discussed earlier, together with other changes in activity patterns and diet, have contributed to a rapid increase in childhood overweight and obesity (Hedley et al., 2004; Ogden, Flegal, Carroll, & Johnson, 2002). The consequences include low self-esteem; increased risk of diabetes, hyperlipidemia, and other diseases; and an increased risk of being overweight in adulthood (Dietz, 1998; Serdula et al., 1993). Third, children are especially susceptible to automobile-related injuries and fatalities, particularly when they are pedestrians or bicyclists (Schieber & Thompson, 1996). Fourth, children need certain cues and stimuli from their environment for normal development; these may include contact with nature and opportunities to navigate and learn wayfinding (Bronfenbrenner, 1979; Louv, 2005; R. C. Moore, 1997; Spencer & Woolley, 2000). Children in built environments that feature little nature contact or that require being driven everywhere instead of walking or bicycling (and exploring) may suffer as a result. Finally, the decline of social capital may be especially worrisome for children. The adage that "it takes a village to raise a child" reflects a traditional understanding, supported by both theory and empirical research, that children benefit from cohesive communities (Earls & Carlson, 2001; Morrow, 2002).

The Elderly

The elderly represent the fastest-growing age segment of the U.S. population. Aging inevitably includes declines in function such as impaired vision and mobility. Many elderly people become unable to drive. Accordingly, elderly persons are disfranchised in communities in which driving is the only practical means of transportation and in which walkable destinations are scarce. In contrast, walkable communities, where destinations such as stores, libraries, and churches are located close to where people live, offer ideal opportunities for elders to maintain their mobility and independence. Physical activity is a powerful protector of health in the elderly (Mazzeo, Cavanagh, & Evans, 1998).

Poor People and People of Color

Poor people and people of color are affected in many ways by the design of the built environment. John Kain (1968) identified a systematic spatial mismatch in which blacks were trapped in the inner city by housing discrimination, while the job base was increasingly moving outward. "Sprawl is related to poverty and inequality," Paul Jargowsky (2002, p. 51) observes, "mainly because sprawl creates a greater degree of separation between the income classes." For city dwellers without automobiles, public transit rarely provides affordable, efficient access to suburban jobs (Bullard & Johnson, 1997; Bullard, Johnson, & Torres, 2000). The health consequences of poverty, especially in urban centers, are widely recognized (Berkman & Kawachi, 2000; Marmot & Wilkinson, 1999).

Some specific health effects of the built environment fall disproportionately on poor people and people of color. For example, home injury risks are more common among disadvantaged populations, who frequently rent housing in poorly maintained buildings (Cubbin, LeClere, & Smith, 2000; Shenassa, Stubbendick, & Brown, 2004). Pedestrian fatalities follow a similar pattern. In suburban Orange County, California, Latinos comprise 28 percent of the population but account for 43 percent of pedestrian fatalities (Marosi, 1999). In the Virginia suburbs of Washington, D.C., Hispanics make up 8 percent of the population but account for 21 percent of pedestrian fatalities (Moreno & Sipress, 1999). The reasons for this disproportionate impact are complex and may involve the probability of being a pedestrian (perhaps related to low access to automobiles and public transportation), road design in areas where members of minority groups walk, and behavioral and cultural factors. Built environment interventions to reduce injuries should target such disadvantaged populations.

People with Disabilities

Finally, aspects of the built environment have a major impact on the health and well-being of people with disabilities. Transportation systems designed for cars rather than pedestrians are especially unfriendly to those with special transportation needs. People in wheelchairs need sidewalks and paths that are sufficiently wide and level to allow safe and convenient passage, with curb cuts at appropriate locations. People with visual impairments need audible pedestrian signals at intersections to facilitate safe crossings (Barlow et al., 2003). Crossing signals need to be timed to allow people with disabilities enough time to reach the other side. In some cases, traffic-calming measures designed to protect most pedestrians, such as roundabouts, pose special challenges for those who are blind. Careful planning is needed to provide safe and convenient mobility for all, and design guidelines are available (American Association of State Highway and Transportation Officials, 2001; Institute of Transportation Engineers, 1998). Undertaking such changes requires an awareness of the needs of people with disabilities, as well as a broader orientation to safe, nonmotorized travel.

Conclusion

The built environment may affect health and well-being on many spatial scales, from a piece of furniture to an entire metropolitan area, and in many ways, from cardiovascular to respiratory to mental health to sense of community. Recognizing these links, the health sciences have identified many opportunities to create built environments that prevent injury and illness and promote health. Ergonomists help design safe, comfortable furniture; industrial hygienists help assess and control indoor air problems; and sanitarians help control rodent infestations in buildings. Equally important, professionals in other fields also shape the health and safety of built environments. Architects design buildings, planners lay out neighborhoods, landscape architects create parks, and traffic engineers design roadways. All these professionals play a major, if sometimes unrecognized, role in public health.

A health impact assessment (HIA) is a new tool that offers promise for bringing attention prospectively to the health consequences of decisions in the design of the built environment (Dannenberg et al., 2006; Kemm, Parry, & Palmer, 2004). An HIA is defined as "a combination of procedures, methods, and tools by which a policy, program, or project may be judged as to its potential effects on the health of a population and the distribution of those effects within the population" (European Centre for Health Policy, 1999). An HIA can be used to improve communication between local health departments and community decision makers, enabling the latter to consider improved designs to favor health promotion or minimize adverse effects on health.

One example of a comprehensive approach to the built environment is known as "smart growth," a set of land use and transportation principles that include mixed land uses, higher density balanced by the preservation of green spaces, transportation alternatives including pedestrian infrastructure and transit, attractive communities with a strong sense of place, and effective, coordinated regional planning based on community and stakeholder participation (Bollier, 1998; Calthorpe, 1993; Calthorpe & Fulton, 2001; Congress for the New Urbanism, 2000; Langdon, 1994; Local Government Commission, 1991; Newman & Kenworthy, 1999). Smart growth has been recognized as offering a range of health benefits (Frumkin et al., 2004), and planners and health professionals are increasingly cooperating to implement and evaluate smart growth principles.

Most aspects of the built environment are designed and constructed to achieve many goals, of which health is only one; others include efficiency, profitability, environmental performance, and aesthetics. However, the health implications of the built environment are increasingly being recognized and documented by rigorous evidence.

Health professionals and other community leaders need to act on this evidence, contributing their perspective to planning and design of the built environment. Activities that can be used by local citizens to enhance community well-being include participating in public hearings with zoning and planning boards, writing letters to newspapers, and joining local groups that advocate for public health and environmental improvements. All citizens can benefit when places are designed to optimize community well-being.

References

Aiello, J. R., Nicosia, G., & Thompson, D. E. (1979). Physiological, social, and behavioral consequences of crowding on children and adolescents. *Child Development, 50,* 195–202.

Alexander, C., Ishikawa, S., Silverstein, M., Jacobson, M., Fiksdahl-King, I., & Angel, S. (1997). *A pattern language: Towns, buildings, construction.* New York: Oxford University Press.

American Academy of Pediatrics. (2001). Falls from heights: Windows, roofs, and balconies. *Pediatrics, 107,* 1188–1191.

American Association of State Highway and Transportation Officials. (2001). *A policy on geometric design of highways and streets* (4th ed.). Publ. No. GDHS-4. Washington, DC: Author.

Arnold, C. L., & Gibbons, C. J. (1996). Impervious surface coverage: The emergence of a key environmental indicator. *Journal of the American Planning Association, 62,* 243–258.

Bannerman, R. T., Owens, D. W., Dodds, R. B., & Hornewer, N. J. (1993). Sources of pollutants in Wisconsin stormwater. *Water Science and Technology, 28,* 241–259.

Barlow, J. M., Bentzen, B. L., Tabor, L. S., & Pedestrian and Bicycle Information Center. (2003, May). *Accessible pedestrian signals: Synthesis and guide to best practice.* Washington, DC: National Research Council. Retrieved October 17, 2006, from http://www.walkinginfo.org/aps/home.cfm

Bauman, A. E. (2004). Updating the evidence that physical activity is good for health: An epidemiological review, 2000–2003. *Journal of Science and Medicine in Sport, 7*(1 Suppl.), 6–19.

Baxandall, R., & Ewen, E. (2000). *Picture windows: How the suburbs happened.* New York: Basic Books.

Beauchemin, K. M., & Hays, P. (1996). Sunny hospital rooms expedite recovery from severe and refractory depression. *Journal of Affective Disorders, 40,* 49–51.

Belkic´, K., Savic´, C., Theorell, T., Rakic´, L., Ercegovac, D., & Djordjevic´, M. (1994). Mechanisms of cardiac risk among professional drivers. *Scandinavian Journal of Work and Environmental Health, 20,* 73–86.

Bell, M. L., & Samet, J. M. (2005). Air pollution. In H. Frumkin (Ed.), *Environmental health: From global to local* (pp. 331–361). San Francisco: Jossey-Bass.

Bergner, L., Mayer, S., & Harris, D. (1971). Falls from heights: A childhood epidemic in an urban area. *American Journal of Public Health, 61,* 90–96.

Berkman, L. F., & Kawachi, I. (2000). *Social epidemiology.* New York: Oxford University Press.

Bhaduri, B., Harbor, J., Engel, B., & Grove, M. (2000). Assessing watershed-scale long-term hydrologic impacts of land-use change using a GIS-NPS model. *Environmental Management, 26,* 643–658.

Blair, S. N., Kampert, J. B., Kohl, H. W., III, Barlow, C. E., Macera, C. A., Paffenbarger, R. S., Jr., et al. (1996). Influences of cardiorespiratory fitness and other precursors on cardiovascular disease and all-cause mortality in men and women. *Journal of the American Medical Association, 276,* 205–210.

Bollier, D. (1998). *How smart growth can stop sprawl.* Washington, DC: Essential Books.

Bronfenbrenner, U. (1979). *The ecology of human development.* Cambridge, MA: Harvard University Press.

Brook, R. D., Franklin, B., Cascio, W., Hong, Y., Howard, G., Lipsett, M., et al. (2004). Air pollution and cardiovascular disease: A statement for healthcare professionals from the Expert Panel on Population and Prevention Science of the American Heart Association. *Circulation, 109,* 2655–2671.

Browne, A. (1992). The role of nature for the promotion of well-being in the elderly. In D. Relf (Ed.), *The role of horticulture in human well-being and social development* (pp. 75–79). Portland, Ore.: Timber Press.

Bullard, R. D. (1990). *Dumping in Dixie: Race, class, and environmental quality.* Boulder, CO: Westview Press.

Bullard, R. D., & Johnson, G. S. (Eds.). (1997). *Just transportation: Dismantling race and class barriers to mobility.* Stony Creek, CT: New Society.

Bullard, R. D., Johnson, G. S., & Torres, A. O. (2000). *Sprawl city: Race, politics, and planning in Atlanta.* Washington, DC: Island Press.

Bunn, F., Collier, T., Frost, C., Ker, K., Roberts, I., & Wentz, R. (2003). Area-wide traffic calming for preventing traffic related injuries. *Cochrane Database of Systematic Reviews, 1,* art. CD003110.

Burchell, R. W., Shad, N. A., Listokin, D., Phillips, H., Downs, A., Seskin, S., et al. (1998). *The costs of sprawl—revisited.* Transportation Research Board Rep. No. 39. Washington, DC: National Academies Press.

Calle, E. E., Rodriguez, C., Walker-Thurmond, K., & Thun, M. J. (2003). Overweight, obesity, and mortality from cancer in a prospectively studied cohort of U.S. adults. *New England Journal of Medicine, 348,* 1625–1638.

Callender, E., & Rice, K. C. (2000). The urban environmental gradient: Anthropogenic influences on the spatial and temporal distributions of lead and zinc in sediments. *Environmental Science and Technology, 34,* 232–238.

Calthorpe, P. (1993). *The next American metropolis: Ecology, community, and the American dream.* Princeton, NJ: Princeton Architectural Press.

Calthorpe, P., & Fulton, W. (2001). *The regional city: Planning for the end of sprawl.* Washington, DC: Island Press.

Cayless, S. M. (2001). Slip, trip and fall accidents: Relationship to building features and use of coroners' reports in ascribing cause. *Applied Ergonomics, 32,* 155–162.

Centers for Disease Control and Prevention. (1999). Motor vehicle safety: A 20th-century public health achievement. *Morbidity and Mortality Weekly Report, 48,* 369–374.

Centers for Disease Control and Prevention, National Center for Injury Prevention and Control. (2005). *Falls and hip fractures among older adults.* Retrieved October 17, 2006, from http://www.cdc.gov/ncipc/factsheets/falls.htm

Cervero, R. (1989). *America's suburban centers: The land use–transportation link.* Boston: Unwin Hyman.

Cervero, R., & Gorham, R. (1995). Commuting in transit versus automobile neighborhoods. *Journal of the American Planning Association, 61,* 210–225.

Cervero, R., & Kockelman, K. (1997). Travel demand and the three Ds: Density, diversity, and design. *Transportation Research Record, 2,* 199–219.

Congress for the New Urbanism. (2000). *Charter for the new urbanism.* New York: McGraw-Hill.

Cote, A. (1984). Field test and evaluation of residential sprinkler system: Part III. *Fire Technology, 20,* 41–46.

Craig, C. L., Brownson, R. C., Cragg, S. E., & Dunn, A. L. (2002). Exploring the effect of the environment on physical activity: A study examining walking to work. *American Journal of Preventive Medicine, 23*(Suppl. 2), 36–43

Cubbin, C., LeClere, F. B., & Smith, G. S. (2000). Socioeconomic status and injury mortality: Individual and neighbourhood determinants. *Journal of Epidemiology and Community Health, 54,* 517–524.

Curriero, F. C., Patz, J. A., Rose, J. B., & Lele, S. D. (2001). The association between extreme precipitation and waterborne disease outbreaks in the United States, 1948–1994. *American Journal of Public Health, 91,* 1194–1199.

Dahlen, E. R., & Ragan, K. M. (2004). Validation of the propensity for angry driving scale. *Journal of Safety Research, 35,* 557–563.

Dannenberg, A. L., Bhatia, R., Cole, B. L., Dora, C., Fielding, J. E., Kraft, K., et al. (2006). Growing the field of health impact assessment in the United States: An agenda for research and practice. *American Journal of Public Health, 96,* 262–270.

Dellinger, A. M., & Staunton, C. E. (2002). Barriers to children walking and biking to school: United States, 1999. *Morbidity and Mortality Weekly Review, 51,* 701–704.

Dierberg, F. E. (1991). Non-point source loadings of nutrients and dissolved organic carbon from an agricultural-suburban watershed in east central Florida. *Water Research, 25,* 363–374.

Dietz, W. H. (1998). Health consequences of obesity in youth: Childhood predictors of adult disease. *Pediatrics, 101,* 518–525.

Dockery, D. W., Pope, C. A., III, Xu, X., Spengler, J. D., Ware, J. H., Fay, M. E., et al. (1993). An association between air pollution and mortality in six U.S. cities. *New England Journal of Medicine, 329,* 1753–1759.

Duffy, J. F., & Wright, K. P., Jr. (2005). Entrainment of the human circadian system by light. *Journal of Biological Rhythms, 20,* 326–338.

Duke, J., Huhman, M., & Heitzler, C. (2003). Physical activity levels among children aged 9–13 years: United States, 2002. *Morbidity and Mortality Weekly Report, 52,* 785–788.

Earls, F., & Carlson, M. (2001). The social ecology of child health and well-being. *Annual Review of Public Health, 22,* 143–166.

Ekman, L. (1996). *On the treatment of traffic safety analysis: A non-parametric approach applied on vulnerable road users* (Bulletin 136). Lund, Sweden: Department of Technology and Society, Lund Institute of Technology.

Elvik, R. (2001). Area-wide urban traffic calming schemes: A meta-analysis of safety effects. *Accident Analysis and Prevention, 33,* 327–336.

Environmental Protection Agency. (2001a). *Inventory of U.S. greenhouse gas emissions and sinks, 1990–1999* (EPA Publ. No. 236-R-01-001). Washington, DC: Author.

Environmental Protection Agency. (2001b). *Our built and natural environments: A technical review of the interactions between land use, transportation, and environmental quality* (EPA Publ. No. 231-R-01-002). Washington, D.C.: Author.

Environmental Protection Agency, Office of Transportation and Air Quality. (2006). *Mobile source emissions: Past, present, and future.* Retrieved October 17, 2006, from http://www.epa.gov/otaq/invntory/overview/pollutants/index.htm

Epstein, P. R. (2000). Is global warming harmful to health? *Scientific American, 283,* 50–57.

Erdmann, T. C., Feldman, K. W., Rivara, F. P., Heimbach, D. M., & Wall, H. A. (1991). Tap water burn prevention: The effect of legislation. *Pediatrics, 88,* 572–577.

Ernst, M., & McCann, B. (2002). *Mean streets, 2002.* Washington, DC: Surface Transportation Policy Project and Environmental Working Group. Retrieved October 17, 2006, from http://www.transact.org/PDFs/ms2002/MeanStreets2002.pdf

Etzel, R. A., & Balk, S. J. (Eds.). (2003). *Pediatric environmental health* (2nd ed.). Elk Grove Village, IL: American Academy of Pediatrics Committee on Environmental Health.

European Centre for Health Policy. (1999). *Health impact assessment: Main concepts and suggested approach.* Brussels, Belgium: World Health Organization Regional Office for Europe. Retrieved October 17, 2006, from http://www.who.dk/document/PAE/Gothenburg paper.pdf

Evans, G. W. (2003). The built environment and mental health. *Journal of Urban Health, 80,* 536–555.

Evans, G. W., Lepore, S. J., Shejwal, B. R., & Palsane, M. N. (1998). Chronic residential crowding and children's well-being: An ecological perspective. *Child Development, 69,* 1514–1523.

Evans, G. W., Saegert S., & Harris, R. (2001). Residential density and psychological health among children in low-income families. *Environment and Behavior, 33,* 165–180.

Ewing, R. (1997). Is Los Angeles–style sprawl desirable? *Journal of the American Planning Association, 63,* 107–126.

Ewing, R., Schieber, R. A., & Zegeer, C. V. (2003). Urban sprawl as a risk factor in motor vehicle occupant and pedestrian fatalities. *American Journal of Public Health, 93,* 1541–1545.

Feldman, K. W., Schaller, R. T., Feldman, J. A., & McMillon, M. (1978). Tap water scald burns in children. *Pediatrics, 62,* 1–7.

Fishman, R. (1987). *Bourgeois utopias: The rise and fall of suburbia.* New York: Basic Books.

Flegal, K. M., Carroll, M. D., Kuczmarski, R. J., & Johnson, C. L. (1998). Overweight and obesity in the United States: Prevalence and trends, 1960–1994. *International Journal of Obesity and Related Metabolic Disorders, 22,* 39–47.

Frank, L. D., Andresen, M. A., & Schmid, T. L. (2004). Obesity relationships with community design, physical activity, and time spent in cars. *American Journal of Preventive Medicine, 27,* 87–96.

Frank, L. D., & Pivo, G. (1995). Impacts of mixed use and density on utilization of three modes of travel: Single-occupant vehicle, transit, and walking. *Transportation Research Record, 1466,* 44–52.

French, S. A., Story, M., & Jeffery, R. W. (2001). Environmental influences on eating and physical activity. *Annual Review of Public Health, 22,* 309–335.

Frumkin, H. (2003). Healthy places: Exploring the evidence. *American Journal of Public Health, 93,* 1451–1455.

Frumkin, H. (2004). White coats, green plants: Clinical epidemiology meets horticulture. *Acta Horticulturae, 639,* 15–26,

Frumkin, H., Frank, L. D., & Jackson, R. J. (2004). *Urban sprawl and public health: Designing, planning, and building for healthy communities.* Washington, DC: Island Press.

Gallagher, W. (1993). *The power of place: How our surroundings shape our thoughts, emotions, and actions.* New York: Poseidon Press.

Gannon, J. J., & Musse, M. K. (1989). *E. coli* and enterococci levels in urban stormwater, river water, and chlorinated treatment plant effluent. *Water Research, 23,* 1167–1176.

Garreau, J. (1991). *Edge city: Life on the new frontier.* New York: Doubleday.

Gill, T. M., Williams, C. S., Robison, J. T., & Tinetti, M. E. (1999). A population-based study of environmental hazards in the homes of older persons. *American Journal of Public Health, 89,* 553–556.

Gillham, O. (2002). *The limitless city: A primer on the urban sprawl debate.* Washington, DC: Island Press.

Haines, A., & Patz, J. A. (2004). Health effects of climate change. *Journal of the American Medical Association, 291,* 99–103.

Hall, P. (1998). *Cities in civilization.* London: Weidenfeld & Nicolson.

Halperin, K. (1993). A comparative analysis of six methods for calculating travel fatality risk. *Risk: Health, Safety and Environment, 4,* 15–33.

Handy, S., Boarnet, M., Ewing, R., & Killingsworth, R. (2002). How the built environment affects physical activity: Views from urban planning. *American Journal of Preventive Medicine, 23*(Suppl. 2), 64–73.

Harding, R. W., Morgan, F. H., Indermaur, D., Ferrante, A. M., & Blagg, H. (1998). Road rage and the epidemiology of violence: Something old, something new. *Studies on Crime and Crime Prevention, 7,* 221–228.

Hartley, L., & el Hassani, J. (1994). Stress, violations, and accidents. *Applied Ergonomics, 25,* 221–230.

Hauber, A. R. (1980). The social psychology of driving behavior and the traffic environment: Research on aggressive behavior in traffic. *International Review of Applied Psychology, 29,* 461–474.

Hedley, A. A., Ogden, C. L., Johnson, C. L., Carroll, M. D., Lurtin, L. R., & Flegal, K. M. (2004). Prevalence of overweight and obesity among U.S. children, adolescents, and adults, 1999–2002. *Journal of the American Medical Association, 291,* 2847–2850.

Heschong, L. (2003a, October). Windows and Classrooms: A Study of Student Performance and the Indoor Environment. Attachment 7 to Public Interest Energy Research Program. *Integrated Energy Systems: Productivity and Building Science* (Publ. No, 500-03-082). Sacramento: California Energy Commission. Retrieved October 27, 2006, from http://www.energy.ca.gov/reports/2003-11-17_500-03-082_A-07.pdf

Heschong, L. (2003b, October). Windows and Offices: A Study of Office Worker Performance and the Indoor Environment. Attachment 9 to Public Interest Energy Research Program. *Integrated Energy Systems: Productivity and Building Science* (Publ. No. 500-03-082). Sacramento: California Energy Commission. Retrieved October 17, 2006, from http://www.energy.ca.gov/reports/2003-11-17_500-03-082_A-09.pdf

Horne, J. A., & Reyner, L. A. (1995). Sleep-related vehicle accidents. *British Medical Journal, 4,* 565–567.

House, J. S., Landis, K. R., & Umberson, D. (1988). Social relationships and health. *Science, 241,* 540–545.

Humpel, N., Owen, N., & Leslie, E. (2002). Environmental factors associated with adults' participation in physical activity: A review. *American Journal of Preventive Medicine, 22,* 188–199.

Institute of Transportation Engineers. (1998). *Design and safety of pedestrian facilities.* Washington, DC: Author.

Istre, G. R., McCoy, M. A., Stowe, M., Davies, K., Zane, D., Anderson, R. J., et al. (2003). Childhood injuries due to falls from apartment balconies and windows. *Injury Prevention, 9,* 349–352.

Jackson, K. T. (1985). *Crabgrass frontier: The suburbanization of the United States.* New York: Oxford University Press.

Jacobsen, P. L. (2003). Safety in numbers: More walkers and bicyclists, safer walking and bicycling. *Injury Prevention, 9,* 205–209.

Jargowsky, P. A. (2002). Sprawl, concentration of poverty, and urban inequality. In G. D. Squires (Ed.), *Urban sprawl: Causes, consequences, and policy responses.* Washington, DC: Urban Institute Press.

Kahn, P. H., Jr., & Kellert, S. R. (Eds.). (2002). *Children and nature: Psychological, sociocultural, and evolutionary investigations.* Cambridge, MA: MIT Press.

Kain, J. F. (1968). Housing segregation, Negro employment, and metropolitan decentralization. *Quarterly Journal of Economics, 82,* 175–197.

Kampert, J. B., Blair, S. N., Barlow, C. E., & Kohl, H. W., III. (1996). Physical activity, physical fitness, and all-cause and cancer mortality: A prospective study of men and women. *Annals of Epidemiology, 6,* 452–457.

Kaplan, G. A., Pamuk, E., Lynch, J. W., Cohen, R. D., & Balfour, J. L. (1996). Income inequality and mortality in the United States. *British Medical Journal, 312,* 999–1003.

Kaplan, R. (1992). The psychological benefits of nearby nature. In D. Relf (Ed.), *The role of horticulture in human well-being and social development.* Portland, Ore.: Timber Press.

Kaplan, R. (2001). The nature of the view from home: Psychological benefits. *Environment and Behavior, 33,* 507–542.

Kaplan, R., Kaplan, S., & Ryan, R. L. (1998). *With people in mind: Design and management of everyday nature.* Washington, DC: Island Press.

Kaplan, S., Talbot, J. F., & Kaplan, R. (1988). Coping with daily hassles: The impact of nearby nature on the work environment. Washington, DC: USDA Forest Service, North Central Forest Experiment Station.

Kawachi, I. (1999). Social capital and community effects on population and individual health. *Annals of the New York Academy of Science, 896,* 120–130.

Kawachi, I., & Kennedy, B. P. (1999). Income inequality and health: Pathways and mechanisms. *Health Services Research, 34,* 215–227.

Kawachi, I., Kennedy, B. P., Lochner, K., & Prothrow-Stith, D. (1997). Social capital, income inequality, and mortality. *American Journal of Public Health, 87,* 1491–1498.

Kemm, J., Parry, J., & Palmer, S. (2004). *Health impact assessment: Concepts, theory, techniques, and applications.* New York: Oxford University Press.

Kennedy, B. P., Kawachi, I., & Prothrow-Stith, D. (1996). Income distribution and mortality: Cross-sectional ecological study of the Robin Hood index in the United States. *British Medical Journal, 312,* 1004–1007.

Knauth, P., & Hornberger, S. (2003). Preventive and compensatory measures for shift workers. *Occupational Medicine (Oxford), 53,* 109–116.

Kockelman, K. M. (1997). Travel behavior as a function of accessibility, land use mixing, and land use balance: Evidence from San Francisco Bay Area. *Transportation Research Record, 1607,* 116–125.

Koplan, J. P., & Dietz, W. H. (1999). Caloric imbalance and public health policy. *Journal of the American Medical Association, 282,* 1579–1581.

Koslowsky, M., Kluger, A. N., & Reich, M. (1995). *Commuting stress: Causes, effects, and methods of coping.* New York: Plenum Press.

Kuczmarski, R. J., Flegal, K. M., Campbell, S. M., & Johnson, C. L. (1994). Increasing prevalence of overweight among U.S. adults: The National Health and Nutrition Examination Surveys, 1960 to 1991. *Journal of the American Medical Association, 272,* 205–211.

Kuller, R., & Lindsten, C. (1992). Health and behavior of children in classrooms with and without windows. *Journal of Environmental Psychology, 12,* 305–317.

Kunstler, J. H. (1993). *The geography of nowhere: The rise and decline of America's man-made landscape.* New York: Simon & Schuster.

Kunstler, J. H. (2005). *Big and blue in the USA.* Retrieved July 14, 2006, from http://www.oriononline.org/pages/oo/curmudgeon/index_BigAndBlue.html

Künzli, N., Lurmann, F., Segal, M., Ngo, L., Balmes, J., & Tager, I. B. (1997). Association between lifetime ambient ozone exposure and pulmonary function in college freshmen: Results of a pilot study. *Environmental Research, 72,* 8–23.

Kuo, F. E. (2001). Coping with poverty: Impacts of environment and attention in the inner city. *Environment and Behavior, 33,* 5–34.

Kuo, F. E., & Sullivan, W. C. (2001a). Aggression and violence in the inner city: Effects of environment via mental fatigue. *Environment and Behavior, 33,* 543–571.

Kuo, F. E., & Sullivan, W. C. (2001b). Environment and crime in the inner city: Does vegetation reduce crime? *Environment and Behavior, 33,* 343–367.

Kuo, F. E., & Taylor, A. F. (2004). A potential natural treatment for attention-deficit/hyperactivity disorder: Evidence from a national study. *American Journal of Public Health, 94,* 1580–1586.

Laberge-Nadeau, C., Maag, U., Bellavance, F., Lapierre, S. D., Desjardins, D., Messier, S., et al. (2003). Wireless telephones and the risk of road crashes. *Accident Analysis and Prevention, 35,* 649–660.

Lack L., & Wright, H. (1993). The effect of evening bright light in delaying the circadian rhythms and lengthening the sleep of early morning awakening insomniacs. *Sleep, 16,* 436–443.

Langdon, P. (1994). *A better place to live: Reshaping the American suburb.* Amherst: University of Massachusetts Press.

Larsen, L., Adams, J., Deal, B., Kweon, B. S., & Tyler, E. (1998). Plants in the workplace: The effects of plant density on productivity, attitudes, and perceptions. *Environment and Behavior, 30,* 261–282.

Leden, L. (2002). Pedestrian risk decreases with pedestrian flow: A case study based on data from signalized intersections in Hamilton, Ontario. *Accident Analysis and Prevention, 34,* 457–464.

Lee, I. M. (2003). Physical activity and cancer prevention: Data from epidemiologic studies. *Medicine and Science in Sports and Exercise, 35,* 1823–1827.

Lee, I. M., & Paffenbarger, R. S., Jr. (2000). Associations of light, moderate, and vigorous intensity physical activity with longevity. *American Journal of Epidemiology, 151,* 293–299.

Lewy, A. J., Kern, H. A., Rosenthal, N. E., & Wehr, T. A. (1982). Bright artificial light treatment of a manic-depressive patient with seasonal mood cycle. *American Journal of Psychiatry, 139,* 1496–1498.

Lienhardt, C. (2001). From exposure to disease: The role of environmental factors in susceptibility to and development of tuberculosis. *Epidemiologic Review, 23,* 288–301.

Local Government Commission. (1991). *Awhahnee principles.* Retrieved July 14, 2006, from http://www.lgc.org/ahwahnee/principles.html

Loo, C. M., & Smetana, J. (1978).The effects of crowding on the behavior and perception of 10-year-old boys. *Environmental Psychology and Nonverbal Behavior, 2,* 226–249.

Lourens, P. F., Vissers, J. A., & Jessurum, M. (1999). Annual mileage, driving violations, and accident involvement in relation to drivers' sex, age, and level of education. *Accident Analysis and Prevention, 31,* 593–597.

Louv, R. (2005). *Last child in the woods: Saving our children from nature-deficit disorder.* Chapel Hill, NC: Algonquin Press.

Lynch, J. W., Kaplan, G. A., Pamuk, E. R., Cohen, R. D., Heck, K. E., Balfour, J. L., et al. (1998). Income inequality and mortality in metropolitan areas of the United States. *American Journal of Public Health, 88,* 1074–1080.

Lynch, J. W., Smith, G. D., Kaplan, G. A., & House, J. S. (2000). Income inequality and mortality: Importance to health of individual income, psychosocial environment, or material conditions. *British Medical Journal, 320,* 1200–1204.

Macera, C. A., Jones, D. A., Yore, M. M., Jones, D. A., Ainsworth, B. E., Kimsey, C. D., et al. (2003). Prevalence of physical activity, including lifestyle activities among adults: United States, 2000–2001. *Morbidity and Mortality Weekly Review, 52,* 764–769.

Magnusson, M. L., Pope, M. H., Wilder, D. G., & Areskoug, B. (1996). Are occupational drivers at an increased risk for developing musculoskeletal disorders? *Spine, 21,* 710–717.

Marmot, M., & Wilkinson, R. G. (1999). *Social determinants of health.* New York: Oxford University Press.

Marosi, R. (1999, November 28). Pedestrian deaths reveal O.C.'s car culture clash. *Los Angeles Times,* p. A1.

Maxwell, L. E. (2003). Home and school density effects on elementary school children: The role of spatial density. *Environment and Behavior, 35,* 566–578.

Maxwell, L. E. (2006). Crowding. In H. Frumkin, R. Geller, & L. Rubin (with J. Nodvin) (Eds.), *Safe and healthy school environments* (pp. 13–19). New York: Oxford University Press.

Mazzeo, R., Cavanagh, P., & Evans, W. (1998). American College of Sports Medicine position stand: Exercise and physical activity for older adults. *Medicine and Science in Sports and Exercise, 30,* 992–1008.

McConnell, R., Berhane, K., Gilliland, F., London, S. J., Islam, T, Gauderman, W. J., et al. (2002). Asthma in exercising children exposed to ozone: A cohort study. *Lancet, 359,* 386–391.

Mizell, L. (1997, March). Aggressive driving. In *Aggressive driving: Three studies.* Washington, DC: AAA Foundation for Traffic Safety. Retrieved July 14, 2006, from http://www.aaafoundation.org/pdf/agdr3study.pdf

Mo, R., & Wilkie, C. (1997). *Changing places: Rebuilding community in the age of sprawl.* New York: Henry Holt.

Mokdad, A. H., Bowman, B. A., Ford, E. S., Vinicor, F., Marks, J. S., & Koplan, J. P. (2001). The continuing epidemics of obesity and diabetes in the United States. *Journal of the American Medical Association, 286,* 1195–1200.

Mokdad, A. H., Ford, E. S., Bowman, B. A., Dietz, W. H., Vinicor, F., Bales, V. S., et al. (2003). Prevalence of obesity, diabetes, and obesity-related health risk factors, 2001. *Journal of the American Medical Association, 289,* 76–79.

Mokdad, A. H., Serdula, M. K., Dietz, W. H., Bowman, B. A., Marks, J. M., & Koplan, J. P. (1999). The spread of the obesity epidemic in the United States, 1991–1998. *Journal of the American Medical Association, 282,* 1519–1522.

Moore, E. O. (1981). A prison environment's effect on health care service demands. *Journal of Environmental Systems, 11,* 17–34.

Moore, R. C. (1997). The need for nature: A childhood right. *Social Justice, 24,* 203–221.

Moreno, S., & Sipress, A. (1999, August 27). Fatalities higher for Latino pedestrians: Area's Hispanic immigrants apt to walk but unaccustomed to urban traffic. *The Washington Post,* p. A1.

Morrow, V. (2002). Children's experiences of "community": Implications of social capital discourses. In C. Swann & A. Morgan (Eds.), *Social capital for health: Insights from qualitative research* (pp. 9–28). London: National Health Service, Health Development Agency.

Mumford, L. (1961). *The city in history: Its origins, its transformations, and its prospects.* New York: Harcourt, Brace & World.

Must, A., Spadano, J., Coakley, E. H., Field, A. E., Colditz, G., & Dietz, W. H. (1999). The disease burden associated with overweight and obesity. *Journal of the American Medical Association, 282,* 1523–1529.

National Assessment Synthesis Team. (2000). *Climate change impacts on the United States: The potential consequences of climate variability and change.* New York: Cambridge University Press.

National Highway Traffic Safety Administration. (2004). *Traffic safety facts, 2004: A compilation of motor vehicle crash data from the Fatality Analysis Reporting System and the General Estimates System.* (DOT Publ. No. HS 809 919). Washington, DC: Author.

National Safety Council. (2004). *Injury facts* (2004 ed.). Itasca, IL: Author.

Newman, P., & Kenworthy, J. (1999). *Sustainability and cities: Overcoming automobile dependence.* Washington, DC: Island Press.

Noble, C. (1999). Lifeline for a landscape: Baltimore-Washington area. *American Forests, 105,* 37–39.

Novaco, R. (1991). Aggression on roadways. In R. Baenninger (Ed.), *Targets of violence and aggression* (pp. 253–326). Amsterdam: Elsevier.

Novaco, R., Stokols, D., Campbell, J., & Stokols, J. (1979). Transportation, stress, and community psychology. *American Journal of Community Psychology, 7,* 361–380.

Ogden, C. L., Flegal, K. M., Carroll, M. D., & Johnson, C. L. (2002). Prevalence and trends in overweight among U.S. children and adolescents, 1999–2000. *Journal of the American Medical Association, 288,* 728–732.

Oldenburg, R. (1989). *The great good place: Cafés, coffee shops, community centers, beauty parlors, general stores, bars, hangouts, and how they get you through the day.* New York: Paragon House.

Oliver, J. E. (2001). *Democracy in suburbia.* Princeton, NJ: Princeton University Press.

Ossenbruggen, P. J., Pendharkar, J., & Ivan, J. (2001). Roadway safety in rural and small urbanized areas. *Accident Analysis Prevention, 33,* 485–498.

Pack, A. M., Cucchiara, A., Schwab, C. W., Rodgman, E., & Pack, A. L. (1994). Characteristics of accidents attributed to the driver having fallen asleep. *Sleep Research, 23,* 141.

Parker, D., Lajunen, T., & Summala, H. (2002). Anger and aggression among drivers in three European countries. *Accident Analysis and Prevention, 34,* 229–235.

Parry, M. H. (1968). *Aggression on the road*. London: Tavistock.

Patel, I. C. (1992). *Community gardening fact sheet for Rutgers cooperative research and extension*. Retrieved November 15, 2006, from http://www.rcre.rutgers.edu/pubs/publication.asp?pid=FS624

Pietri, F., Leclerc, A., Boitel, L., Chastang, J. F., Morcet, J. F., & Blondet, M. (1992). Low-back pain in commercial travelers. *Scandinavian Journal of Work and Environmental Health, 18*, 52–58.

Pope, C. A., III, Thun, M. J., Namboodiri, M. M., Dockery, D. W., Evans, J. S., Speizer, F. E., et al. (1995). Particulate air pollution as a predictor of mortality in a prospective study of U.S. adults. *American Journal of Respiratory and Critical Care Medicine, 151*, 669–674.

Portes, A. (1998). Social capital: Its origins and applications in modern sociology. *Annual Review of Sociology, 24*, 1–24.

Powell, K. E., Martin, L. M., & Chowdhury, P. P. (2003). Places to walk: Convenience and regular physical activity. *American Journal of Public Health, 93*, 519–521.

Pucher, J., & Dijkstra, L. (2000). Making walking and cycling safer: Lessons from Europe. *Transportation Quarterly, 54*, 25–51.

Pucher, J., & Dijkstra, L. (2003). Promoting safe walking and cycling to improve public health: Lessons from the Netherlands and Germany. *American Journal of Public Health, 93*, 509–516.

Putnam, R. (2000). *Bowling alone: The collapse and revival of American community*. New York: Simon & Schuster.

Randall, K., Shoemaker, C. A., Relf, D., & Geller, E. S. (1992). Effects of plantscapes in an office environment on worker satisfaction. In D. Relf (Ed.), *The role of horticulture in human well-being and social development*. Portland, Ore.: Timber Press.

Rathbone, D. B., & Huckabee, J. C. (1999, June). *Controlling road rage: A literature review and pilot study*. Washington, DC: AAA Foundation for Traffic Safety.

Redelmeier, D. A., & Tibshirani, R. J. (1997). Association between cellular-telephone calls and motor vehicle collisions. *New England Journal of Medicine, 336*, 453–458.

Retting, R. A., Ferguson, S. A., & McCartt, A. T. (2003). A review of evidence-based traffic engineering measures designed to reduce pedestrian–motor vehicle crashes. *American Journal of Public Health, 93*, 1456–1463.

Roberts, I. (1993). Why have child pedestrian death rates fallen? *British Medical Journal, 306*, 1737–1739.

Roberts, I., Marshall, R., & Norton, R. (1992). Child pedestrian mortality and traffic volume in New Zealand. *British Medical Journal, 305*, 283.

Runyan, C. W., & Casteel, C. (Eds.). (2004). *The state of home safety in America* (2nd ed.). Washington, DC: Home Safety Council. Retrieved October 17, 2006, from http://www.homesafetycouncil.org/state_of_home_safety/stateofhomesafety.aspx

Runyan, C. W., Johnson, R. M., Yang, J., Waller, A. E., Perkis, D., Marshall, S. W., et al. (2005). Risk and protective factors for fires, burns, and carbon monoxide poisoning in U.S. households. *American Journal of Preventive Medicine, 28*, 102–108.

Saegert, S. (1982). Environment and children's mental health: Residential density and low-income children. In A. Baum & J. E. Singer (Eds.), *Handbook of psychology and health* (Vol. 2, pp. 247–271). Mahwah, NJ: Erlbaum.

Saelens, B. E., Sallis, J. F., Black, J. B., & Chen, D. (2003). Neighborhood-based differences in physical activity: An environment scale evaluation. *American Journal of Public Health, 93*, 1552–1558.

Saelens, B. E., Sallis, J. F., & Frank, L. D. (2003). Environmental correlates of walking and cycling: Findings from the transportation, urban design, and planning literatures. *Annals of Behavioral Medicine, 25,* 80–91.

Sallis, J. F., Bauman, A., & Pratt, M. (1998). Physical activity interventions: Environmental and policy interventions to promote physical activity. *American Journal of Preventive Medicine, 15,* 379–397.

Sarkar, S., Nederveen, A.A.J., & Pols, A. (1997). Renewed commitment to traffic calming for pedestrian safety. *Transportation Research Record, 1578,* 11–19.

Sattin, R. W., Rodriguez, J. G., DeVito, C. A., & Wingo, P. A. (1998). Home environmental hazards and the risk of fall injury events among community-dwelling older persons. *Journal of the American Geriatric Society, 46,* 669–676.

Schieber, R. A., & Thompson, N. J. (1996). Developmental risk factors for childhood pedestrian injuries. *Injury Prevention, 2,* 228–236.

Serdula, M. K., Ivery, D., Coates, R. J., Freedman, D. S., Williamson, D. F., & Byers, T. (1993). Do obese children become obese adults? A review of the literature. *Preventive Medicine, 22,* 167–177.

Sesso, H. D., Paffenbarger, R. S., Jr., & Lee, I. M. (1998). Physical activity and breast cancer risk in the College Alumni Health Study (United States). *Cancer Causes and Control, 9,* 433–439.

Shaper, A. G., Wannamethee, S. G., & Walker, M. (1997). Body weight: Implications for the prevention of coronary heart disease, stroke, and diabetes mellitus in a cohort study of middle-aged men. *British Medical Journal, 314,* 1311–1317.

Shaw, G. R. (1994, July). Impact of residential street standards on neo-traditional neighbourhood concepts. *Institute of Transportation Engineers Journal, 64,* 30–33.

Shenassa, E. D., Stubbendick, A., & Brown, M. J. (2004). Social disparities in housing and related pediatric injury: A multilevel study. *American Journal of Public Health, 94,* 633–639.

Smart, R., Stoduto, G., Mann, R., & Adlaf, E. (2004). Road rage experience and behavior: *Vehicle, exposure, and driver factors. Traffic Injury Prevention, 5,* 343–348.

Smith, N. A. (2000). *Lighting for health and safety.* Oxford: Butterworth-Heinemann.

Snow, R. W. (2000, January). *1999 National Highway Safety Survey: Monitoring American's attitudes, opinions, and behaviors.* Mississippi State: Social Science Research Center, Mississippi State University.

Spencer, C., & Woolley, H. (2000). Children and the city: A summary of recent environmental psychology research. *Child Care, Health, and Development, 26,* 181–198.

Stanistreet, D., Scott-Samuel, A., & Bellis, M. A. (1999). Income inequality and mortality in England. *Journal of Public Health Medicine, 21,* 205–207.

Staunton, C. E., Frumkin, H., & Dannenberg, A. L. (2006). Injury prevention through environmental design. In L. S. Doll, S. E. Bonzo, J. A. Mercy, & D. A. Sleet (Eds.), *Handbook of injury and violence prevention.* Secaucus, NJ: Springer.

Stokols, D., Novaco, R., Stokols, J., & Campbell, J. (1978). Traffic congestion, type A behavior, and stress. *Journal of Applied Psychology, 63,* 467–480.

Stunkard, A. J., Faith, M. S., & Allison, K. C. (2003). Depression and obesity. *Biological Psychiatry, 54,* 330–337.

Surface Transportation Policy Project. (2002). *High-mileage moms: The report.* Washington, DC: Author. Retrieved October 17, 2006, from http://www.transact.org/report.asp?id=184

Teaford, J. C., & Kilpinen, J. T. (1997). *Post-suburbia: Government and politics in the edge cities.* Baltimore: Johns Hopkins University Press.

Tennessen, C. M., & Cimprich, B. (1995). Views to nature: Effects on attention. *Journal of Environmental Psychology, 15,* 77–85.

Transportation Research Board, Committee on Physical Activity, Health, Transportation and Land Use. (2005). *Does the built environment influence physical activity? Examining the evidence* (TRB Special Report No. 282). Washington, DC: Author. Retrieved October 17, 2006, from http://trb.org/publications/sr/sr282.pdf

Trost, S. G., Owen, N., Bauman, A. E., Sallis, J. F., & Brown, W. (2002). Correlates of adults' participation in physical activity: Review and update. *Medicine and Science in Sports and Exercise, 34,* 1996–2001.

Tuan, Y.-F. (1977). *Space and place: The perspective of experience.* Minneapolis: University of Minnesota Press.

Turner, C. W., Layton, J. F., & Simons, L. S. (1975). Naturalistic studies of aggressive behavior: Aggressive stimuli, victim visibility, and horn honking. *Journal of Personality and Social Psychology, 31,* 1098–1107.

Ulrich, R. S. (1984). View through a window may influence recovery from surgery. *Science, 224,* 420–421.

Ulrich, R. S., Simons, R. F., Losito, B. D., & Fiorito, E. (1991). Stress recovery during exposure to natural and urban environments. *Journal of Environmental Psychology, 11,* 201–230.

U.S. Department of Health and Human Services. (1996). *Physical activity and health: A report of the surgeon general.* Atlanta: Author.

Van Metre, P. C., Mahler, B. J., & Furlong, E. T. (2000). Urban sprawl leaves its PAH signature. *Environmental Science and Technology, 34,* 64–70.

Van Someren, E.J.W., Kessler, A., Mirmirann, M., & Swaab, D. F. (1997). Indirect bright light improves circadian rest-activity rhythm disturbances in demented patients. *Biological Psychiatry, 41,* 955–963.

Wannamethee, S. G., Shaper, A. G., & Walker, M. (1998). Changes in physical activity, mortality, and incidence of coronary heart disease in older men. *Lancet, 351,* 1603–1608.

Wannamethee, S. G., Shaper, A. G., Walker, M., & Ebrahim, S. (1998). Lifestyle and 15-year survival free of heart attack, stroke, and diabetes in middle-aged British men. *Archives of Internal Medicine, 158,* 2433–2440.

Wei, M., Kampert, J. B., Barlow, C. E., Nichaman, M. Z., Gibbons, L. W., Paffenbarger, R. S., Jr., et al. (1999). Relationship between low cardiorespiratory fitness and mortality in normal-weight, overweight, and obese men. *Journal of the American Medical Association, 282,* 1547–1553.

Whyte, W. H. (1956). *The organization man.* New York: Simon & Schuster.

Whyte, W. H. (1958, January). Urban sprawl. *Fortune,* pp. 102–109.

Whyte, W. H. (1980). *The social life of small urban spaces.* Washington, DC: Conservation Foundation.

Wilkinson, R. G. (1996). *Unhealthy societies: The afflictions of inequality.* London: Routledge.

Willett, W. C., Dietz, W. H., & Colditz, G. A. (1999). Guidelines for healthy weight. *New England Journal of Medicine, 341,* 427–434.

Zielinski, J. (2000). The benefits of better site design in commercial development. In T. R. Schueler & H. K. Holland (Eds.), *The practice of watershed protection* (pp. 647–656). Ellicott City, MD: Center for Watershed Protection.

CHAPTER THIRTEEN

CREATING HEALTHY FOOD ENVIRONMENTS AND PREVENTING CHRONIC DISEASE

Leslie Mikkelsen, Catherine S. Erickson, Marion Nestle

Food is a unique component of life in that it provides the nutrition necessary for our health and survival while also playing a central role in the customs and traditions that add meaning to our lives. Although our need for food is fundamentally biological, we select our diets in the context of the social, economic, and cultural environments in which we live. In particular, what and where foods are available, the price of foods, and the advertising and promotion of foods each influence the choices we make. Taken together, these elements are often referred to as the *food environment*.

Ideally, the food environment would support biological needs, meaning that healthy, nutritious food would be readily available, affordable, and appealing to our palates. Unfortunately, the food environment in the United States today is characterized by a proliferation of heavily marketed snacks and sodas, doughnut shops and fast-food chains, and foods that are highly processed and "supersized."

This food environment has largely been shaped by the business practices of corporations that dominate the U.S. food industry and the ways in which these

Portions of this chapter are adapted from M. Nestle, Introduction: The food industry and "eat more" in M. Nestle, *Food politics: How the food industry influences nutrition and health*, © 2002 by Regents of the University of California.

practices interact with consumer preferences. Fierce competition for consumer food dollars has contributed to a proliferation of new foods and beverages formulated to tap into our biological preferences for foods high in calories, especially fat and sugars (Brownell & Horgen, 2004). Social trends, such as women entering the workforce and families moving to distant suburbs, creating longer commutes for parents, have contributed to a demand for quickly consumed convenience and take-out foods. As a result of this interplay between what people want to eat and what the food industry offers, people in the United States are eating more food, more often, in more places, and more frequently on the go—in automobiles, for example.

The impact of this food environment on health is of major concern as the United States faces an epidemic of caloric excess and its health consequences. Primary prevention activities supporting more healthful eating practices are urgently needed. By creating a food environment that encourages and supports diets rich in fruits, vegetables, legumes, and whole grains and balanced in calories, it should be possible to reduce risks in the overall population for high blood pressure, cardiovascular disease, type-2 diabetes, and certain types of cancer.

Although this chapter focuses primarily on the nutritional aspects of the food environment, other aspects of this environment are also important. The dominant industrialized agricultural system that produces cheap raw ingredients for processed food requires heavy use of synthetic pesticides, herbicides, and fertilizers; these kill wildlife and contribute to cancer, birth defects, neurological disorders, and asthma in humans. Concentrated animal feeding operations (CAFOs) are major sources of air and water pollution (International Society for Ecology and Culture, n.d.). The rising prevalence of antibiotic-resistant bacteria has been linked to the routine nontherapeutic use of antibiotics in animal husbandry, which constitutes 70 percent of all antibiotic use in the United States (Mellon, Benbrook, & Lutz-Benbrook, 2001). Further, transportation of produce for an average of 1,500 to 2,100 miles contributes to heavy truck traffic on our highway system and diesel exhausts linked to cancer, asthma, and other respiratory illnesses (Pirog, Van Pelt, Enshayan, & Cook, 2001). Concerns about these issues have increased interest in sustainable food systems and a new social movement focused on production methods that enhance environmental quality, protect natural resources, and provide a livable income and fair working conditions for growers and laborers.

For the past several decades, public health efforts to improve dietary intake have been primarily limited to disseminating educational messages about the importance of healthful eating and to building individual skills in food purchasing and preparation. Although nutrition education is always important, it is not sufficient to change eating habits in an environment that promotes consumption of heavily advertised and ever-available processed and fast foods. Given that the current food environment is shaped in large part by food industry practices and government policies, improving health behaviors requires focusing on the very practices and polices of these institutions. People need to know how to make healthful food choices, but it also needs to be easy for them to make such choices.

Transforming the food environment is a multistep process; some of its aspects, such as the busy lives of working families, are not readily altered. It is possible, however, to transform food products—what foods are offered, their availability, and the ways they are promoted. Creating food environments that motivate and support individuals to follow nutrition recommendations should make it easier to achieve long-term, broad-based improvements in eating trends. Furthermore, by adopting more ecologically sustainable production methods, the food system will support both good nutrition and a healthy natural environment.

Recently, public health advocates and practitioners have been working to achieve this type of transformation. They are developing and implementing comprehensive environmental approaches to community nutrition that make healthful foods more widely available in schools, workplaces, and neighborhoods. These strategies derive from those used in other health campaigns, such as those used in tobacco control, to change industry practices, government policies, and community norms.

This chapter describes the current status of nutrition and the food environment in the United States and highlights promising new public health strategies for improving the environment in order to make healthful food accessible, affordable, and attractive to all Americans.

The Status and Consequences of Current Eating Habits

What a Healthful Diet Looks Like Versus What We Really Eat

To promote health as effectively as possible, diets must achieve balance. They must provide enough energy (calories) and vitamins, minerals, and other essential nutrients to prevent deficiencies and support normal metabolism. At the same time, they must not include *excessive* amounts of calories and other nutritional factors that might promote the development of chronic diseases.

Fortunately, the optimal range of intake of most dietary components is quite broad. People throughout the world eat many different foods and follow many different dietary patterns that promote excellent health and longevity. As with other behavioral factors that affect health, diet interacts with individual genetic composition as well as with cultural, economic, and geographical factors. On a population basis, the balance between getting enough of the right kinds of nutrients and avoiding too much of the wrong kinds is best achieved by diets that include large proportions of energy from plant foods—fruits, vegetables, legumes, and grains, especially whole grains. Such diets tend to be relatively low in calories but high in vitamins, minerals, fiber, and other components of plants (phytochemicals) that act together to protect against disease.

Research tells us that the American diet is out of balance. On average, people in the United States today are consuming more calories and engaging in less physical activity than in previous decades, resulting in caloric imbalances that can lead to weight gain and chronic disease. They are also eating more highly processed, nutrient-poor foods in place of whole plant foods, resulting in nutritional imbalances that can lead to deficiencies.

The numbers tell the story. The calories provided by the U.S. food supply increased from 3,200 calories per capita per day in 1980 to 3,900 per capita per day in the late 1990s, an increase of 700 calories per day. These figures tend to overestimate the amounts actually consumed because they do not account for waste, but they give some indication of trends. During the decades from 1971 to 2000, the average daily energy intake for men increased from 2,450 to 2,618 calories and for women from 1,542 to 1,877 calories (Wright, Kennedy-Stephenson, Wang, McDowell, & Johnson, 2004). This suggests a trend toward caloric intakes that exceed the average estimated energy requirements for most adults as recommended by the Institute of Medicine's Food and Nutrition Board (2002).

In the United States, the increased calories come from eating more food in general but especially more of foods high in carbohydrates (grain dishes, soft drinks, juice drinks, desserts, and salty snack foods) (Wright et al., 2004). At least one-quarter of the calories in the U.S. diet are estimated to come from foods high in refined sugar or fat and containing few micronutrients (Block, 2004).

Despite consuming excess calories, most people in the United States are not meeting the nutritional recommendations established by the U.S. Department of Agriculture [USDA], the government agency responsible for developing the MyPyramid food guidance system (USDA, n.d.). The average consumption of whole-grain foods is just one serving per day, well below recommended levels. And although the number of vegetable servings appears close to recommendations of five to nine a day, half the servings come just from three foods: iceberg lettuce, potatoes (frozen, fresh, in the form of chips and fries), and canned tomatoes. When fried potatoes are excluded from the count, vegetable servings fall below three per day. Servings of added fats are at least one-third higher than recommended, and caloric sweeteners are half again as high (Kantor, 1999).

The Health Consequences of the Current U.S. Diet

Early in the twentieth century, when the principal causes of death and disability among people in the United States were infectious diseases related in part to the inadequate intake of calories and nutrients, the goals of health officials, nutritionists, and the food industry were identical—to encourage people to eat more of all kinds of food. Throughout that century, improvements in the economy affected the diets in important ways: people obtained access to foods of greater variety, their diets improved, and nutrient deficiencies gradually declined. The principal nutritional problems among people in the United States shifted to those of *overnutrition*—eating too much food or too much of certain kinds of food.

This trend has been observed across the globe. It is one of the great ironies of nutrition that the traditional plant-based diets consumed by the poor in many countries are ideally suited to meeting nutritional needs as long as caloric intake is adequate. Once people become more economically advantaged, they enter a nutrition transition in which they abandon traditional plant-based diets and begin eating more meat, fat, and processed foods. By replacing plant foods with nutritionally depleted snacks and treats, people may eat sufficient or excess calories and yet still not obtain the nutrients necessary for healthy body functioning.

The consequences of this shift are far-reaching. Health experts suggest that the combination of poor diet and sedentary lifestyle contributes to about 365,000 of the 2 million or so annual deaths in the United States, about the same number and proportion affected by cigarette smoking (McGinnis & Foege, 1993; Mokdad, Marks, Stroup, & Gerberding, 2005). The medical costs for just six diet-related health conditions—coronary heart disease, cancer, stroke, diabetes, hypertension, and obesity—exceeded $70 billion in 1995 (Frazão, 1999). The costs of obesity and its consequences were estimated at around $117 billion in 2000 (Office of the Surgeon General, 2001).

While reversing these trends presents a great challenge, it is worth the attempt; improving eating habits holds great promise for disease prevention. Research has shown that women who follow dietary recommendations display half the rates of coronary heart disease observed among those who eat poor diets, and women who are also active and do not smoke cigarettes have less than one-fifth the risk. Some authorities believe that just a 1 percent reduction in intake of saturated fat across the population would prevent more than thirty thousand cases of coronary heart disease annually and save more than $1 billion in health care costs. Such estimates indicate that even small dietary changes can produce large benefits when their effects are multiplied over an entire population (Stampfer, Hu, Manson, Rimm, & Willett, 2000).

The Food Environment

Every day, most people in the United States make numerous decisions about what to eat. These choices have an important impact on their health and functioning. Unfortunately, the environment in which individuals make food choices is one in which so-called junk foods are widely available, heavily advertised, and inexpensive and in which fresh foods are often difficult to find, of poor quality, or prohibitively expensive. The circumstances of work and place also affect individuals' decisions: when time is at a premium, concerns about convenience and cost often outweigh those about health.

Individuals have little direct control over the range of available food choices. Large food corporations are the dominant force that determines the foods we find on supermarket shelves, in convenience stores, and in schools and other institutions. Fast foods that are low in fiber and high in calories have been the primary response to consumers' demand for convenience. In a time of agricultural abundance, the corporate mandate is straightforward—encourage people to eat more food, more often. While health food remains a niche market, junk food and supersizing are the most effective options for generating profits for shareholders.

To develop comprehensive solutions to address the nation's epidemic of poor nutrition, it is important to understand the complexity and interaction of the many factors that influence not only the choices people make but also the choices available to them. This section describes food industry marketing imperatives, how these imperatives influence community food environments, and the context of food choices within the broader food system.

The U.S. Food Industry and Today's Food Supply

Here we use the term *food industry* to refer to companies that produce, process, manufacture, sell, and serve foods and beverages. The U.S. food industry is the remarkably successful result of twentieth-century trends that led from small farms to giant corporations, from a society that cooked at home to one that buys nearly half its meals prepared and consumed elsewhere, and from a diet based on "whole" foods grown locally to one based largely on foods that have been processed in some way and transported long distances. Designed for uniformity and long shelf life, many food products are made from highly processed ingredients that have lost their natural taste and nutritional value. Producers rely on added fat, salt, sweeteners, and (frequently) artificial flavors and colors to make these foods palatable.

The U.S. food industry is highly concentrated. In 2002, four companies accounted for 52 percent of the $32 billon total value of shipments in the soft drink industry. Similarly, the four largest snack food manufacturers took in 56 percent of the industry's $17 billion in total shipments (U.S. Census Bureau, 2006). In 2003, several U.S. companies, including Philip Morris (Kraft Foods), PepsiCo, and Tyson Foods, ranked among the ten largest food companies in the world (Higgins, 2004). Other U.S. companies, such as ConAgra and Sara Lee, ranked among the top one hundred worldwide companies. These corporations have adopted several techniques to attract customers and maximize profits.

Emphasize Highly Processed Foods and Sweetened Beverages. The food industry produces large numbers of sweet foods and ones that are "energy-dense," meaning high in calories, fat, and sugar. The human preference for such foods probably has biological origins. For thousands of years, humans had to work hard for their food. It was an evolutionary advantage to consume high-calorie foods during the rare times they were available (Brownell & Horgen, 2004). Such preferences drive the development of new food products, the menus in restaurants, and the allocation of food advertising dollars.

In the United States, food marketers introduce fifteen to twenty thousand new food products every year into a food system that already contains more than three hundred thousand food products. More than two-thirds of new products are condiments, candies and snacks, baked goods, soft drinks, and dairy products (cheese products and ice cream novelties). These products compete for shelf space in supermarkets that stock about fifty thousand products each. Processed, frozen, and baked goods accounted for more than 40 percent of supermarket sales in 2000, while produce represented only 9 percent (Harris, Kaufman, Martinez, & Price, 2002). Most fast-food restaurants follow a similar trend; they feature high-fat meals devoid of fruits and vegetables and whole grains. Instead, they serve oversized burgers with added cheese or sauces, fried chicken, and pizza.

Supersize It. Marketing methods that encourage people to eat more include substantial increases in the sizes of food packages and restaurant portions (Young & Nestle, 1995). From an industry standpoint, larger portions make good marketing sense. The cost of food is low relative to labor and other expenses, and large portions attract consumers. However, one of the dangers of the increased availability of enlarged portions is "portion distortion": as portion sizes grow, so do consumers' perceptions of what constitutes a single serving. For example, serving size standards defined by the USDA define a standard serving of grain as one slice of white bread, 1 ounce of ready-to-eat cereals or muffins, or half a cup of rice or pasta. A marketplace jumbo bakery muffin weighing 7 ounces would actually exceed a full day's grain allowances with some left over for the next day, yet a consumer might reasonably believe that a single muffin constitutes a single serving.

The practice of "bundling"—adding sides like fries and a soft drink to a fast-food sandwich—is responsible for some of the largest increases in calorie content. Fountain drinks cost the least to add; they provide excess calories along with high profit margins for retailers. Large portions may contribute to weight gain unless people compensate with diet and exercise, and the excess calories may crowd out healthier foods in the diet. Research reveals that adults consume more calories when served larger portion sizes and do not necessarily compensate by decreasing caloric intake at later meals (Diliberti, Bordi, Conklin, Roe, & Rolls, 2004; Roe, Rolls, Kral, Meengs, & Wall, 2004; Rolls, Morris, & Roe, 2002).

Offer Convenience. In the last quarter of the twentieth century, the proportion of women with children who entered the workforce greatly expanded, and many people began to work longer hours and commute longer distances to make ends meet. As a result, many of today's families have less time to shop for, prepare, and serve home-cooked meals (Bowers, 2000).

These societal changes at least partly explain why nearly half of all meals are prepared or consumed outside the home, why fast food is the fastest-growing segment of the food service industry, and why the practice of snacking nearly doubled from the mid-1980s to the mid-1990s (Zizza, Siega-Riz, & Popkin, 2001). The food industry has responded to the demand for convenience by producing heat-and-serve meals; prepackaged sandwiches, salads, entrees, and desserts; "power bars"; yogurt in tubes; prepackaged cereal in a bowl; hot food bars and take-out chicken; and foods designed to be eaten directly from the package. Many such products are high in calories, fat, sugar, or salt but marketed as nutritious because they contain added vitamins.

These food products, and the advertising that promotes them, relegate cooking to a low-priority chore. Even cookbook authors are scaling back their instructions in deference to the growing number of adults who simply do not know how to cook (Sagon, 2006). Nutritionists and traditionalists may lament such developments, but demand for convenience stimulates the food industry to create even more products that can be consumed quickly and with minimal preparation.

Promote Health Benefits. In 1990, the U.S. government passed the Nutrition Labeling and Education Act (NLEA) requiring "nutrition facts" labels on all packaged foods. In return for placing the label on their products, food companies induced Congress to allow them to make two kinds of health claims on product labels: nutrient content claims and claims of health benefits.

Food manufacturers knew that promotion of nutritional advantages with messages such as "low-fat," "no cholesterol," "high-fiber," or "contains calcium" increased sales, as did the use of health claims ("lowers cholesterol," "prevents cancer"). They knew that nutrition ranks second after taste as the factor most frequently influencing food purchases (Guthrie, Derby, & Levy, 1999). Because the NLEA allowed companies to say that their products were high in vitamins and minerals, the law encouraged the addition of such nutrients to food products.

Breakfast cereals, juice drinks, and even candy could bear labels proclaiming "contains 100% of 10 vitamins" or similar statements, even if most of their energy came from added sugars.

The NLEA allowed claims for health benefits, but Food and Drug Administration (FDA) efforts to hold such claims to a rigorous scientific standard were routinely challenged in court by food companies. Eventually, the FDA was forced to relinquish attempts to require much in the way of scientific substantiation for health claims. The result is evident in the marketplace, especially in the cereal section of supermarkets. It has long been possible to find cereals claiming to lower cholesterol levels or prevent heart disease or cancer; now you can also find cereals labeled as promoting a healthy immune system or as weight-loss products.

Perhaps more insidious is the emergence of manufacturers' self-endorsements with "health seals" based on their own criteria. For example, PepsiCo has launched the "Smart Spot" program, which features a label with a checkmark and the phrase "Smart Choices Made Easy." These include Baked Lays and some Cap'n Crunch cereals. Kraft has "Sensible Solution" labels on such products as CarbWell Oreos and certain Lunchables (University of California-Berkeley School of Public Health, 2005).

Invest in Marketing. Food and food service companies spend more than $12 billion annually on direct media advertising in magazines and newspapers and on radio, television, and billboards ("Domestic Advertising," 2006). In 2005, for example, McDonald's spent $742.3 million, Burger King $268.8 million, Taco Bell $231.7 million, and Coke and Diet Coke $317 million just on direct media advertising. Even small products have impressive advertising budgets, as illustrated by expenditures of $83 million for M&M candies ("Top 100 Megabrands," 2006).

Marketing techniques have expanded far beyond direct media to include product placement, character licensing, special events, in-school activities, books, and games. An estimated $10 billion is spent each year in the United States on food and beverage marketing aimed specifically at children (McGinnis, Grootman, & Kraak, 2006). In total, food companies spend more than $30 billion annually to advertise and promote their products to the public. Most of this astronomical sum is used to promote the most highly processed and elaborately packaged fast foods. Nearly 70 percent of food advertising is for convenience foods, candy and snacks, alcoholic beverages, soft drinks, and desserts, whereas just 2.2 percent is for fruits, vegetables, grains, or beans (Gallo, 1999).

Advertisers deliberately promote food brands to children, at home and at school, in an effort to influence food and beverage purchases and to encourage lifelong brand loyalty. Unfortunately, young children, especially those under the age of eight, have difficulty discerning the difference between television advertising and programming; it is not until around the age of eleven that most children are able to comprehend the purpose of advertising (McGinnis et al., 2006).

Despite protestations by marketers that advertising is a minor element in food choice, research shows that food sales increase with intensity, repetition, and visibility of advertising messages (Novelli, 1990). Successful campaigns are carefully researched, targeted to specific groups, and repeated frequently. In the report *Food Marketing to Children and Youth: Threat or Opportunity?* the Institute of Medicine concluded that advertising unquestionably influences children's food and beverage preferences, purchase requests, and dietary intake (McGinnis et al., 2006).

The Neighborhood Food Landscape

The U.S. food industry has been highly successful in making snack foods, fast foods, baked goods, and sweetened beverages available at every turn. Many urban areas and suburban malls are dominated by fast-food outlets, making it easy for customers to be attracted by the sights and smells of the latest fad in ice cream, baked goods, or high-calorie coffee drinks. Corporations set specific goals for expanding their presence in new geographical areas and ensuring easy access. For example, Starbucks often places outlets across the street from one another.

Fast-food restaurants deliberately open in areas easily accessed by children and adolescents. A Chicago study found fast-food restaurants to be significantly more clustered in areas close to schools than would be expected if they were randomly distributed throughout the city. The median distance from any school to the nearest fast-food restaurant was less than one-third of a mile, and the great majority of schools (78 percent) were located within a half mile of a fast-food place (Austin et al., 2005).

Fresh foods are not equally accessible to all neighborhoods. The lack of supermarkets, grocery stores, and farmer's markets in neighborhoods where the primary residents are low-income, people of color, or immigrants is well documented (Chung & Myers, 1999; Cotterill & Franklin, 1995; Kantor, 1999; Morland, Wing, Diez, & Poole, 2001; Shaffer, 2002). The phenomenon of supermarket flight—the gradual disappearance of supermarkets from inner cities and other low-income neighborhoods—over the past forty years has left the typical low-income neighborhood with 30 percent fewer supermarkets than higher-income areas (Cotterill & Franklin, 1995). This lack of access is compounded by lower household car ownership and nonexistent or cumbersome public transportation options. According to a 2002 study of more than ten thousand residents in 221 census tracts in Maryland, North Carolina, Mississippi, and Minnesota, ready access to supermarkets is associated with higher fruit and vegetable consumption (Morland, Wing, & Diez, 2002).

Although supermarkets are the largest purveyors of produce in any neighborhood, they provide far larger quantities of junk food. Many display junk foods and sodas in high-traffic areas at the ends of aisles or in special displays. Boxes of sweetened cereals featuring toys and popular cartoon characters are placed on low shelves where children can see them. Supermarket chains collect "slotting fees" from product manufacturers to place products in these prime locations.

Schools have not been immune to food industry forces. Formerly relegated to the faculty lounge, vending machines now line the walls of high schools. Branded fast food is available in school cafeterias. Those foods and others sold outside the federally funded school breakfast and lunch programs are known as "competitive foods." Such foods are a source of income for food service departments, school programs, and extracurricular activities. Unlike federally qualified meal programs, competitive foods are not required to meet specific nutritional standards, yet they can be sold in schools as à la carte cafeteria items or through vending machines or school stores and at events elsewhere on school grounds. The most common foods offered are candy, chips, desserts, ice cream, and soft drinks (Samuels & Associates, 2000). Companies, particularly soda companies, have targeted schools for exclusive marketing contracts that prominently feature their products. Most often the corporation provides donations of money or equipment in exchange for the exclusive right to sell its products in schools and to display marketing messages to students.

The Broader Food System Context

In recent decades, U.S. farm policy has driven down the price of a few farm commodities, including corn and soybeans, through subsidies. The low cost of corn and soybeans, which are used to produce high-fructose corn syrup (a sweetener) and hydrogenated vegetable oil (a fat), has contributed to a proliferation of inexpensive crackers, chips, soda, and candy, among other processed foods, on grocery store shelves. The low cost of corn used for animal feed has also reduced the price of beef and other meats. In the United States, the retail price of fruits and vegetables has increased nearly 40 percent since 1985, while the cost of fats and sugars has declined (Schnoover & Muller, 2006). In this sense, U.S. agricultural subsidy programs are incongruent with the government's nutritional guidelines.

Studies have shown that refined grains, added sugars, and added fats are among the lowest-cost sources of dietary energy in grocery stores, while lean meats, fish, and fresh fruit and vegetables generally cost more (Drewnowski & Darman, 2005; Jetter & Cassady, 2005). In restaurants, high-fat, high-sodium fast foods and sugary drinks are relatively inexpensive compared to salads and healthier options. This does not go unnoticed by consumers: in a California survey, about one-third of respondents cited expense as a barrier to eating low-fat foods and fresh fruits and vegetables (California Department of Health and Human Services, 1999). Researchers have shown that reducing the relative price of low-fat snacks and fruits and vegetables stimulates adolescents and adults to purchase healthier products from vending machines (French et al., 2001).

This system raises questions of "externalities," costs that are hidden from consumers. Cheap food has hidden nutritional costs. It stimulates the overconsumption of low-nutrient foods that contribute to chronic disease. Further, cheap food has ecological costs. Government price supports and subsidies for water, fertilizers, and other inputs benefit industrial farms that employ practices that deplete the soil, expose humans and animals to hazardous toxins, and adversely affect health in other ways (Jacobson, 2006).

Prevention Solutions

Although the crises of poor nutrition and caloric imbalance are daunting, there is optimism within the public health community that transformation of the food environment is possible and is indeed beginning to take hold. What is especially promising about the movement for change is that it involves leaders in many fields, including public health, city planning and urban design, sustainable agriculture, transportation, education, and public policy. Pooling expertise and resources, innovative leaders, policymakers, and foundations, as well as advocates, are researching and taking new approaches to address issues such as increased access to healthful and affordable food and decreased availability and marketing of less healthful foods. They are working to identify issues that capture the imagination of the public and methods that will most effectively influence nutrition and physical activity behaviors in a more healthful direction. The following examples describe strategies that hold promise for improving nutrition at the community level.

Create Model School Food Environment

To date, much of the energy dedicated to improving the food environment has centered on schools. As parents and policymakers began to understand the scope of childhood obesity and poor nutrition, they started actively pursuing solutions to protect students' short- and long-term health. Though institutional changes generally originated one school at a time through the activism of interested parents and students, early successes inspired broader efforts at the district and state levels. Much room for improvement remains within schools, but the progress in the past five years demonstrates that food environments can indeed be improved substantially.

In with the Healthy, Out with the Junk. Across the country, individual schools and state and local governments have enacted policies that emphasize offering fresh, nutritious food items to students. For example, changes to meal service in Flagstaff, Arizona, included adding salad bars in secondary schools and fruit and vegetable bars in all elementary schools. The New York City school system is committed to meet USDA guidelines for all foods sold at mealtimes and in vending machines by 2008 and is already serving more fruits and vegetables; limiting beverages to water, milk, and 100 percent juice; and reducing the amount of highly processed foods served (Center for Science in the Public Interest, 2003). To improve capabilities to prepare fresh meals in school cafeterias, communities are remodeling kitchens or passing ordinances stipulating that all new schools must be built with full kitchens (Vallianatos, 2005). In Healdsburg, California, remodeling the kitchen at the local high school was part of an effort to serve fewer branded, prepackaged meals and to prepare more fresh meals on site (California Food Policy Advocates, 2003). Providing adequate time and space for students to eat meals in an unhurried manner has also become a planning priority in some districts (Vallianatos, 2005).

Going hand in hand with efforts to increase the availability of healthy foods are efforts to decrease the availability of junk foods. Many school districts and several states have enacted policies restricting or eliminating the sale of soda and unhealthy snacks in vending machines and cafeterias or reducing the number of hours that vending machines are available. West Virginia was an early pioneer in this effort; it passed comprehensive nutrition standards in 1993 setting limits for the fat and sugar content of all foods sold during the school day (Stuhldreher, Koehler, Harrison, & Deel, 1998). More recently, California passed a bill with stronger standards for fat, sugar, and calorie content that apply to meals and snacks sold anywhere on campus during school hours. A second California law bans the sale of sodas during the school day at elementary, middle, and high schools (California Center for Public Health Advocacy, 2005).

Schools are also making efforts to reduce food marketing and commercialism on campus. The Los Angeles Unified School District, one of the largest districts in California, passed an Obesity Prevention Motion in 2003 establishing strict guidelines for the foods and beverages sold during school hours and calling for an elimination of contracts and relationships between the district and branded fast-food products. In Mercedes, Texas, the school board has banned all advertising for unhealthy food or beverages on school grounds. In San Francisco, schools are prohibited from using curriculum materials that feature food company brand names (Vallianatos, 2005). Such efforts demonstrate that school districts are finding ways to limit students' exposure to food marketing and to tailor approaches to the specific concerns of their communities.

Bringing the Farm to the Cafeteria Table. Schoolyard gardens and farm-to-school partnerships are emerging as effective strategies for including locally grown, fresh produce in student meals. In addition to introducing students to a variety of fruits and vegetables, many of these programs bridge the gap between cafeteria table and classroom by providing instruction about agriculture and nutrition.

Students participating in schoolyard gardens experience the rewards of watching foods grow and tasting the fruits and vegetables they have tended with their own hands. The "edible schoolyard" at King Middle School in Berkeley, California, provides opportunities for students to grow, harvest, prepare, cook, serve, and eat meals, as well as clean up afterward—all while engaging in conversation with peers and teachers. Teachers of all subject areas use the gardens as a springboard for student lessons in history, mathematics, or language, for example. Today, nearly all of Berkeley's schools have gardens, and a third of these produce vegetables that are included in the preparation of school meals (Heeter, 2006).

Farm-to-school partnerships expand the offerings available to school cafeterias and enable local farmers to develop an additional source of revenue. As with schoolyard gardens, the programs provide opportunities to teach students about the sources of the foods they eat. Inspired by the actions of local school districts, Connecticut and Massachusetts have passed bills requiring schools to give preference to locally produced foods for school meals (Heeter, 2006).

Schoolyard gardens and farm-to-school partnerships can be as varied as the climates and environments in which they take place and can be successfully initiated top-down at the school district level or bottom-up from parents or local farmers.

Ensure That Workplaces Support Healthy Food Norms

Just as students need nutritious foods to thrive at school, adults also benefit from the availability of healthy foods and beverages in the workplace. It has long been demonstrated that the physical and social environment of the workplace influences health-related behaviors (Stokols, Pelletier, & Fielding, 1996). As with the enactment of restrictions on smoking, government agencies and health care institutions have taken the lead in improving workplace food environments in the hope that such actions will have a ripple effect, influencing food norms across the community as a whole.

The types of food available in employee cafeterias, in vending machines, and at work-sponsored events frequently determine what people eat throughout the day. Typically, one meal a day is consumed at work, and snacks are often eaten to relieve pressure or during breaks throughout the workday. Applying nutrition standards to all cafeteria meals and vending machine items can provide employees with healthier food options and promote overall well-being. Regulations vary from standards that follow the USDA's nutrition guidelines to those that restrict or completely eliminate junk food.

In San Antonio's Bexar County, Texas, for example, the Fit City initiative established nutrition guidelines for vending machines. These require the machines to be stocked primarily with low-fat foods and milk, water and juices, and low-fat, low-sugar snacks. Many employers in the city, including several hospitals, have voluntarily joined this effort (Kulick, 2005). Although vending machines are a logical starting place for many companies, a focus on healthy options in cafeterias is equally important. The Cleveland Clinic, one of the nation's top cardiac hospitals, recently revamped its cafeteria menu to include more healthy options and to offer nutritional information to guide purchasing choices.

However, one food source in the workplace is often overlooked for nutritional quality: food provided by an employer at meetings and other gatherings. Often food is used to entice employees to participate in a company event or meeting. Employers can provide healthful, nutritious snacks while still engaging employee participation by substituting healthier food options for high-fat, calorie-dense foods; providing a fruit basket with special, seasonal items; or using nonfood incentives.

Ensure the Availability of Healthful Food in All Neighborhoods

Several aspects of the neighborhood food environment can ultimately influence dietary behavior, including the types of retail outlets present, the product mix offered, the quality and cultural appropriateness of available foods, and the affordability of foods. Community-based efforts to improve neighborhood food environments have traditionally focused on increasing access to healthy foods while also decreasing the prevalence of unhealthy foods. In today's market economy, doing so requires the involvement of multiple stakeholders and a long-term outlook.

Attracting Supermarkets to Underserved Areas. Returning supermarkets and mid-sized grocery stores to underserved neighborhoods is one avenue for increasing access to healthful food. The increased availability of fresh fruits and vegetables is a major factor in increasing consumption, as shown by a landmark study in 2002, based on more than ten thousand residents in 221 census tracts, which found that black residents increased fruit and vegetable intake by an average of 32 percent for each supermarket located in their census tract (Morland et al., 2002). In the United Kingdom, a preliminary before-and-after comparison demonstrated improvements in dietary behavior following the introduction of a large chain supermarket (Wrigley, Warm, Margetts, & Whelan, 2002).

Many cities are exploring public-private partnerships as a way to meet the public's need for community infrastructure, facilities, and services. Public-private partnerships are agreements between government and private sector organizations that feature shared investments, risks, responsibilities, and rewards. Such arrangements often involve the financing, design, construction, operation, and maintenance of public infrastructure and services (British Columbia Ministry of Municipal Affairs, 1999). Cities such as Philadelphia, Boston, and New York have used public-private partnerships to bring supermarkets into underserved areas (Pothukuchi, 2000).

Although supermarkets and mid-sized stores usually provide quality and variety of foods at affordable prices, they are not a viable solution for all underserved communities. These stores are extremely costly and time-consuming investments, requiring government subsidies or allowances as well as a suitable building site.

Establishing Accessible Farmers' Markets or Farm Stands. Farmers' markets and farm stands are increasingly popular and serve as a valuable source of fresh produce and other goods. Underserved areas particularly benefit from the presence of convenient sources of fresh fruits and vegetables (Conrey, Frongillo, Dollahite, & Griffin, 2003). In addition to supplying fresh produce, farmers' markets and farm stands may offer job training and professional development opportunities as well as a community space for meetings and entertainment.

Several elements emerge as key to the success of farmers' markets in reaching low-income consumers: price and availability of familiar products, community ownership, transportation to markets, flexible market hours, employment of sales staff from the neighborhood, use of a community organizing approach for outreach, and promotions or sales tailored to the economic level of the community. By supporting small and mid-range farmers, these farmers' markets help preserve farm lands and promote more sustainable production methods. They do not, however, carry other staples and have limited hours and must be supplemented with other retail outlets. Farmers' markets also require a strong customer base in order to survive. Successful markets depend on customers' being able to use food stamps as well as WIC and Senior Farmers' Market Nutrition Program vouchers to pay for produce (Fisher, 1999).

Assisting Small Store Owners in Carrying and Selling Fresh Foods. Families living in underserved communities often rely on small neighborhood stores for much of their daily food. These stores often do not have the space, staff expertise, or equipment to carry fresh produce. As a result, the quality and selection of fresh food offered in small neighborhood stores is often poor. Providing training and in-

Promoting Supermarket Investment: The Pennsylvania Fresh Food Financing Initiative

Recognizing that residents of low-income communities in Philadelphia were experiencing high rates of diet-related chronic disease, the nonprofit Philadelphia Food Trust (PFT) launched an effort to bring supermarkets into low-income areas where access to fresh food and produce was poor. The PFT documented the communities' health disparities in the report *Food for Every Child* and concluded that the highest-income neighborhoods of Philadelphia had 156 percent more supermarkets than the lowest-income neighborhoods and that the low-income areas of the greater Philadelphia region fell seventy supermarkets short of the number needed. *Food for Every Child* galvanized political support and inspired the development of the Food Marketing Task Force.

The leadership taskforce released another report, *Stimulating Supermarket Development: A New Day for Philadelphia,* with ten recommendations to increase the number of supermarkets in the city's underserved communities by creating a more positive environment for supermarket development. Leaders of the task force, along with two state representatives, pushed for the development of the Pennsylvania Fresh Food Financing Initiative in the fall of 2004. The initiative serves the financing needs of supermarket operators that plan to operate in these underserved communities, where infrastructure costs and credit needs cannot be accommodated solely by conventional financial institutions.

The first supermarket to be funded under the initiative opened its doors in September 2004. To date, the Pennsylvania Fresh Food Financing Initiative has committed resources to five supermarket projects and devoted $6 million in grants and loans to leverage this investment. These five projects will result in the creation of 740 new jobs and represents $22,378,000 in total project costs. In addition, there are currently over twenty projects in the financing pipeline, ranging from 6,000-square-foot corner stores to 60,000-square-foot full-service supermarkets.

Additional information is available at http://www.thefoodtrust.org.

Source: Prevention Institute, with the assistance of Hannah Burton, formerly of The Food Trust.

centives to store owners can improve their ability to offer a greater variety of products and therefore influence consumption patterns.

Strategies have involved training store owners to purchase and handle produce, assisting store owners to increase shelf space for healthier items, and expanding dairy sections to include low-fat and nonfat milk. Training and grants for stores to upgrade storage equipment and enhance store layout and signage and to market changes to neighborhood residents enhance the success of these efforts.

San Francisco high school students participating in a program sponsored by Literacy for Environmental Justice (LEJ), a nonprofit youth organization, launched an effort to improve the availability of fresh foods in the low-income Bayview–Hunters Point neighborhood. After helping one store improve its produce selection to account for 30 percent of overall sales, students and the youth and LEJ staff recruited public and private support for an incentive program for area merchants. The resulting Good Neighbor Project offers benefits to qualifying store owners in energy efficiency, local advertising, business training, cooperative buying, in-store promotions, and participation in branding campaigns. In return, the merchants must agree to stock certain minimum amounts of produce, remove most tobacco and alcohol advertising, and maintain a clean appearance.

The advantages of such programs are that they support small business owners within a neighborhood community. They are also less time-intensive and less costly than programs designed to develop supermarkets. But they require genuine commitments from the store owners to make changes and must address several challenges: it is difficult for small stores to match the low prices, high quality, and selection of larger stores; changing product selection means risking losing profits; and smaller stores are not always valued by community residents.

Addressing Restaurant Menus and Locations. As more and more families consume a greater proportion of their calories away from home, the variety and quality of prepared restaurant menu items increasingly influence consumption patterns. Restaurants are an important element of the neighborhood food environment and have been shown to be potential mediators in patterns of vegetable consumption (Glanz & Hoelscher, 2004). Encouraging restaurants and carry-out dining establishments to make nutritional information available; to offer more selections lower in fat, sugar, and sodium; and to feature more fresh produce should expand the ability of families to make healthful food choices.

In addition to improving access to more healthful foods, advocates and community residents have also sought ways to limit the presence of less healthful junk foods. Land use and zoning regulations hold particular promise for improving neighborhood environments for nutrition and activity. A few examples from around the country include efforts in Concord, Massachusetts, and Calistoga, California, to prohibit fast-food outlets and drive-through service restaurants; in Warner, New Hampshire, to regulate the density of fast-food restaurants by requiring a specific spacing distance between restaurants in its commercial district; and in Detroit, Michigan, where fast-food restaurants must be located a minimum of 500 feet away from any school site (Mair, Pierce, & Teret, 2005).

The legal basis for these actions may be more to protect the character of historic neighborhoods or to reduce traffic in commercial or residential areas than to improve health, although health improvement may be the underlying goal.

Eliminate Advertising of Less Healthful Foods to Children

The serious nature of nutrition-related chronic disease warrants action to prevent the advertising of less healthful junk foods and beverages directly to children. Restrictive actions require federal legislation or regulation by the Federal Trade Commission (FTC).

Currently, there are few restrictions or standards in the United States for food advertising and marketing aimed at children. In the late 1970s, the FTC attempted to institute restrictions on advertising to children and to require nutrition information in certain food advertisements. These efforts met with strong opposition from the food industry and eventually failed (Valkenburg, 2000). However, in recent years, consumer, public health, and parent advocates have taken up this issue with renewed interest.

Strong policies do exist in other countries. According to a Consumers International report on television advertising aimed at children (Dibb, 1996), Denmark, Norway, Sweden, and Finland do not permit commercial sponsorship of children's programs. Sweden and Norway do not permit television advertising to children under age twelve and do not allow advertisements during children's programming. Australia does not allow advertisements during programming for preschoolers, and the Flemish region of Belgium prohibits advertising in the five minutes immediately preceding and following children's programs.

The Institute of Medicine has called on food and beverage manufacturers to shift their marketing resources toward significantly healthier items. Historically, voluntary action by industry has not made a meaningful difference. The Children's Advertising Review Unit (CARU), operated by the Better Business Bureau, was established in 1974 to ensure that marketing aimed at children is "truthful, accurate, and sensitive to the special nature of children" (CARU, 2003). Under CARU's watch, during the 1990s, there was a twentyfold increase in expenditures on advertising that targeted children. Furthermore, between 1994 and 2004, more than 4,400 new food and beverage products were targeted to children and youth, the majority of which were high in calories, sugar, or fat and low in nutrients (McGinnis et al., 2006). Perhaps with this perspective in mind, the Institute of Medicine recommends that if improvements are not implemented on a voluntary basis, they should be mandated through legislation.

Align Agricultural Policy with Public Health Goals

Although arguments about how best to improve the farm system and the food supply are complex, there is a need for advocates in agriculture, environmental health, and public health to explore ways to align government agriculture policies to support more healthful eating patterns and sustainable production methods. Careful policy analysis is needed as the basis for developing agricultural policies that meet the economic and health needs of farmers, agricultural workers, and consumers. The U.S. Farm Bill, which Congress must reauthorize every several years, presents an opportunity for broad advocacy for health goals. The Farm Bill must address commodity supports as well as nutrition (for example, the food stamp program). Shifts in subsidies for agricultural commodities may be one area of focus, but other changes in federal and state regulations or tax policies might help transform the food environment to make healthier foods more affordable and available. The Farm Bill also provides an opportunity to create incentives to conserve soil, prevent air and water pollution, preserve farmland surrounding urban areas, and take other actions to reduce environmental hazards associated with industrial agriculture.

Health Care Without Harm

The public health and health care sectors are partnering to bring attention to the links between human health and sustainable food systems. An example of these links can be found in hospital food use. Hospitals and agriculture are not often thought as being connected, but hospitals feed thousands of patients, staff, and visitors every day, millions every year. It is therefore conceivable that hospital food purchasing practices and policies could influence agricultural practices in some of the same ways that restaurant practices do. In fact, hospitals can become ongoing and reliable partners in advocating for sustainable agriculture.

Founded in 1996, Health Care Without Harm (HCWH) is a global coalition of more than four hundred organizations in fifty-two countries working to transform the health care industry so that it is no longer a source of harm to people and the environment. In the United States, HCWH has worked to eliminate the use of thermometers and other medical devices containing mercury and to ensure safer practices for handling medical waste by encouraging hospitals to switch from waste incinerators to safer nonburning waste technologies. HCWH is now applying its success working collaboratively with hospitals to a campaign focused on sustainable food systems. HCWH members encourage hospitals to provide nutritionally improved food for patients, staff, and the general public by adopting food procurement policies that are ecologically sound, economically viable, and socially responsible. By using their buying power to change the ways in which food is produced, health care institutions can demonstrate an understanding of the inextricable links between human, public, and ecosystem health.

There are steps health care institutions can take, both small and large, to change their practices and support sustainable agriculture. Many facilities have already switched to purchasing milk produced without using recombinant bovine growth hormone. Hospitals may also consider purchasing foods produced without synthetic chemicals and antibiotics. For example, hospitals can purchase USDA-certified organic foods, which are approved by a government-endorsed certifier to ensure that the food has been developed without the use of antibiotics, growth hormones, or most conventional pesticides and synthetic chemicals (USDA, 2002). Saint Luke's Hospital in Duluth, Minnesota, offers certified organic produce at the cafeteria salad bar, serves certified fair-trade coffee, and is in the process of securing antibiotic-free poultry (Marie Kulick, senior associate, Institute for Agriculture and Trade Policy, personal communication, July 27, 2006). Buying locally can also become a priority for some facilities: hospitals can work with local farmers or growers' collaboratives to include seasonal and local options on hospital menus. Fletcher Allen Health Care in Burlington, Vermont, purchases milk, cheese, and organic produce from area farmers (Kulick, 2005). Other hospitals bring fresh produce to their facilities by hosting regular farmers' markets or creating on-site gardens. For example, Kaiser Permanente's Oakland Medical Center in California instituted the facility's first farmers' market in 2003, providing locally grown organic food as a service to workers and the community. Kaiser now has twenty-nine on-site farmers' markets at medical facilities across the country (Roosevelt, 2006). Dominican Hospital in Santa Cruz, California, has its own on-site organic garden that supplies produce for the cafeteria (Kulick, 2005).

By adopting food purchasing policies and practices that support health and sustainable food systems, health care can lead the way in redefining healthy food and shifting U.S. demand for sustainable food products.

More information is available at http://www.noharm.org.

Conclusion

The movement to transform the food environment is in its early stages. A variety of leaders—from public health practitioners to investigative journalists, from researchers to policymakers—have been making the case that eating habits cannot be changed by information and promotional messages alone. The environment must be changed to facilitate more healthful eating and activity patterns. Many school districts, work sites, government agencies, and health care institutions are making environmental changes to improve access to healthful, sustainably produced food and to decrease the promotion and presence of junk foods. Such local actions constitute the core of a movement to create new social norms in the United States, norms that favor the consumption of fruits, vegetables, whole grains, and legumes, all of which are currently lacking in the American diet. Government regulations as well as voluntary institutional efforts will be needed to propel changes in the food environment that are significant enough to reverse current trends in chronic disease rates related to poor nutrition.

References

Austin, S. B., Melly, S. J., Sanchez, B. N., Patel, A., Buka, S., & Gortmaker, S. L. (2005). Clustering of fast food restaurants around schools: A novel application of spatial statistics to the study of food environments. *American Journal of Public Health, 95*, 1575–1581.

Block, G. (2004). Foods contributing to energy intake in the U.S.: Data from NHANES III and NHANES 1999–2000. *Journal of Food Composition and Analysis, 17*, 439–447.

Bowers, D. E. (2000). Cooking trends echo changing roles of women. *FoodReview, 23*(1), 23–29.

British Columbia Ministry of Municipal Affairs. (1999, May). *Public-private partnership: A guide for local government.* Vancouver: British Columbia Ministry of Municipal Affairs. Retrieved July 11, 2006, from http://www.mcaws.gov.bc.ca/lgd/pol_research/mar/PPP

Brownell, K. D., & Horgen, K. B. (2004). *Food fight: The inside story of the food industry, America's obesity crisis, and what we can do about it.* New York: McGraw-Hill.

California Center for Public Health Advocacy. (2005). *California SB 12 (Escutia): School nutrition standards—summary* and *California SB 695 (Escutia) healthy beverage bill.* Davis: Author. Retrieved October 18, 2006, from http://www.publichealthadvocacy.org

California Department of Health and Human Services. (1999). *California Dietary Practices Survey: Overall trends in healthy eating among adults, 1989–1997,* Pt. 2. (1999). Sacramento: Author.

California Food Policy Advocates. (2003). *Improving meal quality in California's schools: A best practices guide for school meal service.* San Francisco: Author. Retrieved October 18, 2006, from http://www.cfpa.net/obesity/MealQualityReport_May2003.pdf

Center for Science in the Public Interest. (2003, September). *School foods tool kit: A guide to improving school foods and beverages,* Pt. 2: *Case studies.* Washington, DC: Author. Retrieved May 24, 2006, from http://www.cspinet.org/schoolfoodkit/school_foods_kit_part3.pdf

Children's Advertising Review Unit. (2003). *Self-regulatory guidelines for children's advertising.* New York: Council of the Better Business Bureau's Children's Advertising Review Unit. Retrieved June 25, 2006, from http://www.caru.org/index.asp

Chung, C., & Myers, S. L. (Eds.). (1999). Do the poor pay more for food? An analysis of grocery store availability and food price disparities. *Journal of Consumer Affairs, 33*, 276–296.

Conrey, E. J., Frongillo, E. A., Dollahite, J. S., & Griffin, M. R. (2003). Integrated program enhancements increased utilization of farmers' market nutrition program. *Journal of Nutrition, 133*, 1841–1844.

Cotterill, R., & Franklin, A. (Eds.). (1995). *The urban grocery store gap.* Storrs: Food Marketing Policy Center, University of Connecticut.

Dibb, S. (1996). *A spoonful of sugar: Television food advertising aimed at children—an international comparative study.* London: Consumers International.

Diliberti, N., Bordi, P. L., Conklin, M. T., Roe, L. S., & Rolls, B. J. (2004). Increased portion size leads to increased energy intake in a restaurant meal. *Obesity Research, 12*, 562–568.

Domestic advertising spending by category. (2006, June 26). *Advertising Age,* p. 6.

Drewnowski, A., & Darman, N. (2005). The economics of obesity: Dietary energy density and energy cost. *American Journal of Clinical Nutrition, 82*(Suppl.), 265S–273S.

Fisher, A. (1999). *Hot peppers and parking lot peaches: Evaluating farmers' markets in low-income communities.* Venice, CA: Community Food Security Coalition.

Food and Nutrition Board, Institute of Medicine. (2002). *Dietary reference intakes for energy, carbohydrate, fiber, fat, fatty acids, cholesterol, protein, and amino acids.* Washington, DC: National Academies Press.

Frazão, E. (1999). High costs of poor eating patterns in the United States. In E. Frazão (Ed.), *America's eating habits: Changes and consequences* (pp. 5–32). Washington, DC: U.S. Department of Agriculture.

French, S. A., Jeffrey, R. W., Story, M., Breitlow, K. K., Baxter, J. S., Hannan, P., et al. (2001). Pricing and promotion effects on low-fat vending snack purchases: The CHIPS study. *American Journal of Public Health, 91,* 112–117.

Gallo, A. E. (1999). Food advertising in the U.S. In E. Frazão (Ed.), *America's eating habits: Changes and consequences* (pp. 173–180). Washington, DC: U.S. Department of Agriculture.

Glanz, K., & Hoelscher, D. (2004). Increasing fruit and vegetable intake by changing environments, policy, and pricing: Restaurant-based research, strategies, and recommendations. *Preventive Medicine, 39*(Suppl. 2), 88–93.

Guthrie, J. F., Derby, B. M., & Levy, A. S. (1999). What people know and do not know about nutrition. In E. Frazão (Ed.), *America's eating habits: Changes and consequences* (pp. 243–280). Washington, DC: U.S. Department of Agriculture.

Harris, J. M., Kaufman, P. R., Martinez, S. W., & Price, C. (2002). *The U.S. food marketing system: Competition, coordination, and technological innovations into the 21st century* (Publ. No. AER-811). Washington, DC: U.S. Department of Agriculture. Retrieved July 12, 2006, from http://www.ers.usda.gov/publications/aer811

Heeter, C. (2006, March 9). In Berkeley, Calif., lunch has become a learning experience. *Christian Science Monitor,* p. 14. Retrieved June 28, 2006, from http://www.csmonitor.com/2006/0309/p14s03-legn.html

Higgins, K. (2004, October 4). The world's top 100 food and beverage companies: Diets define profit and loss. *Food Engineering, 76*(10), 58.

International Society for Ecology and Culture. (n.d.). *Local food toolkit: Factsheet.* Retrieved July 20, 2006, from http://www.isec.org.uk/toolkit/factsheet.html

Jacobson, M. (2006). *Six arguments for a greener diet.* Washington, DC: Center for Science in the Public Interest.

Jetter, K. M., & Cassady, D. L. (2005, March). *The availability and cost of healthier food items* (Issue Brief No. 29). Davis: University of California Agricultural Issues Center.

Kantor, L. S. (1999). A dietary assessment of the U.S. food supply. *Family Economics and Nutrition Review, 12,* 51–54.

Kulick, M. (2005, May). *Healthy food, healthy hospitals, healthy communities: Stories of health care leaders bringing fresher, healthier food choices to their patients, staff, and communities.* Minneapolis, MN: Institute for Agriculture and Trade Policy. Retrieved July 27, 2006, from http://www.environmentalobservatory.org/library.cfm?refid=72927

Mair, J. S., Pierce, M. W., & Teret, S. P. (2005). *The use of zoning to restrict fast-food outlets: A potential strategy to combat obesity* [Monograph]. Johns Hopkins and Georgetown Universities. Retrieved June 28, 2006, from http://www.publichealthlaw.net/Research/Affprojects.htm#Zoning

McGinnis, J. M., & Foege, W. H. (1993). Actual causes of death in the United States. *Journal of the American Medical Association, 270,* 2207–2212.

McGinnis, J. M., Gootman, A. J., & Kraak, V. I. (Eds.). (2006). *Food marketing to children and youth: Threat or opportunity?* Washington, DC: National Academies Press. Retrieved June 15, 2006, from http://www.nap.edu/catalog/11514.html#toc

Mellon, M., Benbrook, C., & Lutz-Benbrook, K. (2001). *Hogging it: Estimates of antimicrobial abuse in livestock.* Cambridge, MA: Union of Concerned Scientists. Retrieved July 11, 2006, from http://www.ucsusa.org/index.html

Mokdad, A. H., Marks, J. S., Stroup, D. F., & Gerberding, J. L. (2005). Correction: Actual causes of death in the United States, 2000. *Journal of the American Medical Association, 293,* 293–294.

Morland, K., Wing, S., & Diez, R. A. (2002). The contextual effect of the local food environment on residents' diets: The Atherosclerosis Risk in Communities study. *American Journal of Public Health, 92,* 176–177.

Morland, K., Wing, S., Diez, R. A., & Poole, C. (2001). Neighborhood characteristics associated with the location of food stores and food service places. *American Journal of Preventive Health, 22,* 23–29.

Novelli, W. D. (1990). Applying social marketing to health promotion and disease prevention. In K. Glanz, F. M. Lewis, & B. K. Rimer (Eds.), *Health behavior and health education: Theory, research, and practice* (pp. 342–349). San Francisco: Jossey-Bass.

Office of the Surgeon General. (2001). *The Surgeon General's call to action to prevent and decrease overweight and obesity.* Rockville, MD: U.S. Department of Health and Human Services.

Pirog, R., Van Pelt, T., Enshayan, K., & Cook, E. (2001). *Food, fuel, and freeways: An Iowa perspective on how far food travels, fuel usage, and greenhouse gas emissions.* Ames: Leopold Center for Sustainable Agriculture, Iowa State University.

Pothukuchi, K. (2000). *Attracting grocery retail investment to inner-city neighborhoods: Planning outside the box.* Detroit, MI: Wayne State University.

Roe, L. S., Rolls, B. J., Kral, T. V., Meengs, J. S., & Wall, D. E. (2004). Increasing the portion size of a packaged snack increases energy intake in men and women. *Appetite, 42,* 63–69.

Rolls, B. J., Morris, E. L., & Roe, L. S. (2002). Portion size of food affects energy intake in normal-weight and overweight men and women. *American Journal of Clinical Nutrition, 76,* 1207–1213.

Roosevelt, M. (2006, May). Healthier hospital food [Electronic version]. *Time Magazine, 167*(21). Retrieved November 14, 2006, from http://www.time.com/time/magazine/article/0,9171,1194018,00.html

Sagon, C. (2006, March 18). Cooking 101: Add 1 cup of simplicity: Cookbooks simplify terms as kitchen skills dwindle. *Washington Post,* p. A1.

Samuels & Associates. (2000). *2000 California High School Fast Food Survey: Findings and recommendations.* Sacramento, CA: Public Health Institute.

Schnoover, H., & Muller, M. (2006). *Food without thought: How U.S. farm policy contributes to obesity.* Minneapolis, MN: Institute for Agricultural and Trade Policy.

Shaffer, A. (2002). *The persistence of Los Angeles' grocery store gap.* Los Angeles: Urban and Environmental Policy Institute.

Stampfer, M. J., Hu, M. F., Manson, J. E., Rimm, E. B., & Willett, W. C. (2000). Primary prevention of coronary heart disease in women through diet and lifestyle. *New England Journal of Medicine, 343,* 16–22.

Stokols, D., Pelletier, K. R., & Fielding, J. E. (1996). The ecology of work and health: Research and policy directions for the promotion of employee health. *Health Education Quarterly, 23,* 137–158.

Stuhldreher, W. L., Koehler, A. N., Harrison, M. K., & Deel, H. (1998). The West Virginia standards for school nutrition. *Journal of Child Nutrition and Management, 22,* 79–86.

Top 100 megabrands. (2006, June 26). *Advertising Age,* pp. 23, 29, 62, 64, 102.

U.S. Census Bureau. (2006). *Concentration ratios, 2002: 2002 economic census: Manufacturing, subject series.* Washington, DC: U.S. Department of Commerce. Retrieved October 18, 2006, from http://www.census.gov/prod/ec02/ec0231sr1.pdf

U.S. Department of Agriculture. (2002, April). *Organic food labels and standards: The facts.* Washington, DC: Author. Retrieved July 31, 2006, from http://www.ams.usda.gov/nop/Consumers/brochure.html

U.S. Department of Agriculture. (n.d.). *Steps to a healthier you.* Washington, DC: Author. Retrieved June 13, 2006, from http://www.mypyramid.gov

University of California-Berkeley School of Public Health. (2005, November). Health pitches on packages. *UC-Berkeley Wellness Letter, 22*(2), 6.

Valkenburg, P. M. (2000). Media and youth consumerism. *Journal of Adolescent Health, 27*(Suppl.), 52–56.

Vallianatos, M. (2005, June). *Healthy school food policies: A checklist.* Los Angeles: Center for Food and Justice, Urban and Environmental Policy Institute, Occidental College. Retrieved June 28, 2006, from http://departments.oxy.edu/uepi/cfj/publications/healthy_school_food_policies_05.pdf

Wright, J. D., Kennedy-Stephenson, J., Wang, C. Y., McDowell, M. A., & Johnson, C. L. (2004). Trends in intake of energy and macronutrients: United States, 1971–2000. *Morbidity and Mortality Weekly Report, 53,* 80–82.

Wrigley, N., Warm, D., Margetts, B., & Whelan, A. (2002). Assessing the impact of improved retail access on diet in a "food desert": A preliminary report. *Urban Studies, 92,* 2061–2082.

Young, L. R., & Nestle, M. (1995). Portion sizes in dietary assessment: Issues and policy implications. *Nutrition Review, 53,* 149–158.

Zizza, C., Siega-Riz, A. M., & Popkin, B. M. (2001). Significant increase in young adults' snacking between 1977–1978 and 1994–1996 represents a cause for concern! *Preventive Medicine, 32,* 303–310.

CHAPTER FOURTEEN

STRENGTHENING THE COLLABORATION BETWEEN PUBLIC HEALTH AND CRIMINAL JUSTICE TO PREVENT VIOLENCE

Deborah Prothrow-Stith

Over the last two decades in the United States, public health practitioners, policy makers, and researchers have charted new territory by increasingly using public health strategies to understand and prevent youth violence, which has traditionally been considered a criminal justice problem. The utilization of public health approaches has generated several contributions to the understanding and prevention of violence, including new and expanded knowledge in surveillance, delineation of risk factors, and program design, including implementation and evaluation strategies.

While public health activities generally complement those of criminal justice, confrontations, challenges and turf issues within this cross-disciplinary enterprise remain inevitable. Continued progress is dependent upon expanded efforts and greater collaboration within both disciplines. This chapter addresses two objectives that have implications for future research and prevention activities:

- Review the history and implications of addressing violence as a public health problem
- Compare and contrast public health and criminal justice approaches to violence

This article originally appeared in the *Journal of Law, Medicine, and Ethics.* Copyright © 2004 by the American Society of Law, Medicine, and Ethics. Reprinted with permission.

Violence as a Public Health Problem

Understanding Public Health

Before discussing the role of public health in violence prevention, it is important to explain what is meant by public health because polling data show that there is not widespread familiarity with the profession ("Public opinion about public health," 1998). Contrasting medicine with public health is illustrative and provides a context for understanding the basic tenets and approaches within public health.

Harvey Fineberg, former Dean of the Harvard School of Public Health and current President of the Institutes of Medicine, highlights several important distinctions in his momentous comparison of the two disciplines as shown in Table 14.1. Medicine responds to the health problems (diseases) of individuals with efforts to treat, cure, reduce harm, and prevent further complications. In contrast, public health addresses the health problems of populations (neighborhoods, cities, states, age cohorts, employee groups) using epidemiology to identify the major problems; understand risk factors; follow rates of morbidity and mortality; design, implement, and evaluate programmatic and policy oriented prevention strategies.

In addition, the basic sciences of medicine (physiology, pathology, anatomy, histology, etc.) are substantially different from those within public health (epidemiology, economics, sociology, political science, behavioral sciences, etc.). Also, public health in the United States is a much younger discipline than medicine with a less well-funded and developed infrastructure (Institute of Medicine, 1988, 2003). However, despite its relative youth, public health is responsible for many of the contemporary contributions to increased longevity and holds substantial promise for similar impact on violence prevention.

The Case for Addressing Interpersonal Violence Using Public Health Strategies

There are at least four reasons why interpersonal violence became an important concern for public health professionals in the United States: (1) the contact health professionals have with victims and perpetrators of violence, (2) the magnitude of the problem, (3) the characteristics of violence, and (4) the application of public health strategies to both understanding and preventing violence which has yielded significant positive findings and offers further promise.

Contact with Victims and Perpetrators. In 1978, in a fairly common emergency room experience, a patient threatening to go out and seek revenge after being

TABLE 14.1. PUBLIC HEALTH VERSUS MEDICINE.

Public Health	Medicine
Primary Focus on Population	**Primary Focus on Individual**
Public service ethic, tempered by concerns for the individual	Personal service ethic, conditioned by awareness of social responsibilities
Emphasis on prevention, health promotion for the whole community	Emphasis on diagnosis and treatment, care for the whole patient
Public health paradigm employs a spectrum of interventions aimed at the environment, human behavior and lifestyle, and medical care	Medical paradigm places predominant emphasis on medical care
Multiple professional identities with diffuse public image	Well-established profession with sharp public image
Variable certification of specialists beyond professional public health degree	Uniform system for certifying specialists beyond professional medical degree
Lines of specialization organized, for example, by: • analytical method (epidemiology) • setting and population (occupational health) • substantive health problem (nutrition) • skills in assessment, policy development, and assurance	Lines of specialization organized, for example, by: • organ system (cardiology) • patient group (pediatrics) • etiology, pathophysiology (oncology, infectious disease) • technical skill (radiology)
Biologic sciences central, stimulated by major threats to health of populations; move between laboratory and field	Biologic sciences central, stimulated by needs of patients; move between laboratory and bedside
Numeric sciences an essential feature of analysis and training	Numeric sciences increasing in prominence, though still a relatively minor part of training
Social sciences an integral part of public health education	Social sciences tend to be an elective part of medical education
Clinical sciences peripheral to professional training	Clinical sciences an essential part of professional training

Source: Courtesy of Harvey Fineberg.

treated for injuries received during a fight precipitated a physician's search for prevention strategies (Prothrow-Stith & Weissman, 1991). "Stitch them up and send them out" was the standard of care at that time. Nevertheless, the predictable and regular contact physicians and nurses have had with victims and perpetrators of violence, particularly in emergency departments, has caused many to begin to address this problem.

To this day, emergency room recidivism and the high mortality rates associated with violent injury continue to compel medical personnel toward violence prevention efforts. The American College of Emergency Physicians has included violence prevention on the agenda of their annual meetings since the late 1980s. The *Journal of the American Medical Association* has annually published a special issue of its journal dedicated to violence since 1998. The American Medical Association has published protocols and manuals for health providers on domestic violence, youth violence, child abuse, and rape and sexual assault.

New strategies, materials, and protocols for clinical intervention and prevention are regularly introduced and evaluated, reflecting the responsiveness of health care providers to the repeated contact they have with the tragedy of violence.

Magnitude of Violence. Homicide rates in the United States are mind-boggling when compared to those of other industrialized nations not at war. Not only is the United States' homicide rate 10 to 25 times higher than that of most industrialized nations, but the homicide rates actually rival some less developed countries facing war or considerable social, political, and economic turmoil (Krug, Powell, & Dalhberg, 1998; Wolfgang, 1986). The only good news in the disproportionately large rates of homicides in the United States is that it validates the preventable nature of violence.

Nonfatal episodes of violence are also a significant part of America's tragedy. The United States Federal Bureau of Investigation (2001) estimates that 1.8 million Americans are victims of violence each year, with adolescents at the greatest risk for victimization. Homicide is the leading cause of death for African Americans ages 15–24 and the second leading cause of death for all adolescents 15–19 (National Center for Injury Prevention and Control, 2001). A complete representation of the magnitude of violence is not available, however, because there are not reliable and consistent measures of nonfatal episodes of violence. In a biannual national survey of 13,000 adolescents, the Youth Risk Behavioral Surveillance System (YRBSS), 33 percent of respondents reported being in at least one physical fight in the previous year (boys 43 percent and girls 24 percent) and 4 percent reported being medically treated for injuries sustained in a fight during that same time period (Centers for Disease Control and Prevention, 2002).

Unreported and poorly reported episodes of violence (including intimate partner violence, child abuse, school assaults, etc.) represent an even larger part of the burden of injury requiring public health attention.

Characteristics of Violence in the United States. Public health strategies are required for violence prevention because criminal justice strategies primarily target stranger violence committed during another crime, not the significant problem of acquaintance, family, and intimate violence. Contrary to the stereotype, much of the violence experienced in the United States occurs among people who know each other. A typical homicide in the United States involves two people who know each other, are under the influence of alcohol, get into an argument, and have a handgun. In homicides of children and adolescents (0–17) in the U.S., 22 percent are killed by a parent, 5 percent by another family member, 36 percent by an acquaintance and 11 percent by a stranger (Snyder & Sickmund, 1999, p. 19). Even in the unlikely situation where all of 25 percent classified as an unknown relationship were all committed by strangers, the majority are committed by family, friends, and acquaintances.

In the cases of homicides and violence against women, the acquaintance nature of violent injury is even more compelling. According to the 2000 National Crime Victimization Survey, 62 percent of rape and sexual assaults came at the hands of a person the female victim called a friend or acquaintance, with 18 percent identified as intimate partners (National Institute of Justice, 2000). In the National Violence Against Women Survey, 25 percent of the women said that current or former spouses, cohabiting partner, or a date had raped or physically assaulted them during their lifetime (Tjaden & Thoennes, 2000).

The stability of the significant presence of acquaintances, friends, and family among the perpetrators of violent injury (rape, assaults, and homicides) begs for prevention strategies beyond aggressive criminal justice efforts of blame and punish. Prevention in the setting where a victim and perpetrator know each other requires the policy, public awareness and education, and change in social norms that fall under the purview of public health.

Application of Public Health Strategies. Over the last two decades, public health professionals have applied traditional public health strategies to violence prevention. They have brought a different perspective and orientation to bear on the problem by applying public health techniques and strategies which complement and strengthen the criminal justice approach. Public health brings an analytic approach that identifies risk factors and important causes that could become the focus of preventive interventions.

Major risk factors for youth violence have been identified as outlined in Exhibit 14.1. These factors operate at different levels as illustrated in Figure 14.1. The individual and family levels have not only been the primary focus of research on violence, but also have dictated the public policy responses to violence. These risk factors, understood through the population-based approach of public health, highlight the importance of the macro influences such as poverty at the neighborhood level, gun availability, and social norms. The larger circles of community, society, and world influences come into greater focus through a public health lens.

EXHIBIT 14.1. RISK FACTORS FOR YOUTH VIOLENCE.

- Poverty and income inequality
- Access to guns
- Alcohol and other drug use
- Witnessing violence and victimization
- Biological or organic abnormalities
- Social and cultural factors, culture of violence

Source: Adapted from Prothrow-Stith & Spivak (2004).

FIGURE 14.1. LEVELS OF INTERACTION BETWEEN RISK FACTORS AND INDIVIDUALS.

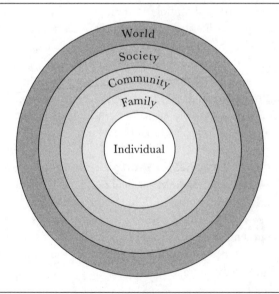

Public Health Defines Violence. A prevailing definition of violence within the public health profession was offered by the National Center for Injury Prevention and Control (2001) at the United States' Centers for Disease Control and Prevention (CDC). The CDC classifies both unintentional injuries (accidents) and intentional injuries (violence) as public health problems, as illustrated in Figure 14.2. Intentional injuries are divided into self-directed violence (suicides and suicide attempts) and interpersonal violence (assaults and homicides) (see Figure 14.3). Violence is defined by the CDC as "the threatened or actual use of physical force or power against another person, against oneself, or against a group or community that either results or is likely to result in injury, death, or deprivation."

This definition highlights the breadth of behaviors involved and does not limit it to physical violence. Also, the labels "perpetrator" and "victim" are often assigned based on the outcome of a fight (the person more injured is often labeled as the victim) with very little regard to the events leading up to the event and the roles of participants. Because public health is concerned with prevention and reduction of risk factors, the labels "victim" and "perpetrator," particularly with youth violence, are less helpful. Behaviors like spanking children, tackling on the football field, and rough play among peers all illustrate the important role of the receiver's interpretation.

FIGURE 14.2. CLASSIFICATION OF INJURY IN PUBLIC HEALTH.

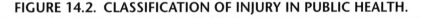

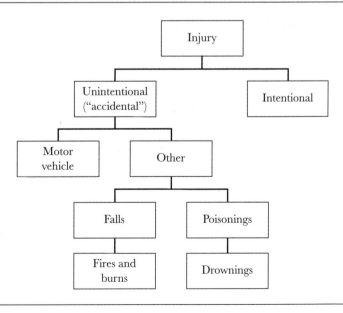

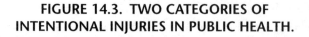

FIGURE 14.3. TWO CATEGORIES OF INTENTIONAL INJURIES IN PUBLIC HEALTH.

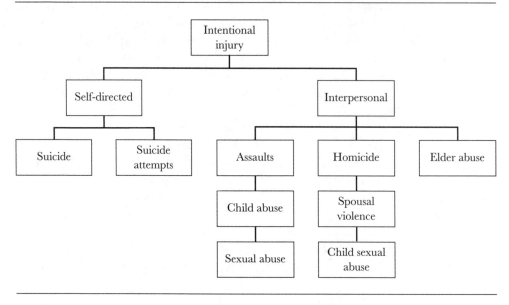

Public Health and Youth Violence Prevention in the United States

Over the last two decades, violence has been increasingly accepted within mainstream public health as a problem for its consideration. The major contribution resulting from designating violence as a public health problem is the acknowledgment that violence is preventable, not inevitable. Violence prevention leadership within public health has emerged from the Centers for Disease Control and Prevention, the Surgeon General's office, and many state and local health departments.

The Centers for Disease Control established its Violence Epidemiology Branch in 1983, for the study of homicide and suicide. This application of basic epidemiology and reporting techniques became part of the impetus for public health professionals across the country to confront the issue. In October 1985, then Surgeon General C. Everett Koop convened an invitational meeting, the Surgeon General's Workshop on Violence and Public Health, in Leesburg, Virginia. The professionally interdisciplinary meeting focused on assault and homicide, child abuse, rape and sexual assault, domestic violence, elder abuse, and suicide. The workshop and its proceedings, published in a special 1986 issue of *Public Health Reports,* were instrumental toward mainstreaming the issue of violence prevention for public health professionals. In 1994, the Centers for Disease Control established the National Center for Injury Prevention and Control, and every Surgeon General after Dr. Koop has encouraged the public health community to use its strategies to understand better and prevent violence.

In summary, the public health efforts to understand and prevent violence utilize standard methods and strategies including epidemiology, community outreach, screening, community-based programs, health education, behavior modification, public awareness, and education campaigns. Prevention strategies resemble efforts taken to prevent smoking, increase seat belt use, and promote child car seats. Though only two decades old and mostly comprised of relatively isolated initiatives scattered across the country, public health efforts to violence prevention demonstrate the potential for the same level of success the public health approach has had with reducing smoking and deaths from car crashes in the United States.

The analogy between violence prevention and other public health problems is not flawless, yet experience to date employing comparable techniques and strategies suggests that these efforts will continue and expand. The public health approaches to violence prevention that have evolved over the last two decades are described in many resources available through the National Center for Injury Prevention and Control at the Centers for Disease Control and Prevention and its Web site, http://www.cdc.gov/ncipc.

Public Health and Criminal Justice

Public health's venture into violence prevention has not always been well received. Many issues divide public health and criminal justice, including fundamental principles, core approaches, proactive vs. reactive strategies, prevention efforts vs. a punitive response to violence in addition to the usual issues arising out of cross-disciplinary collaboration such as different jargons, efforts to protect one's turf, and competition for funding. In many ways the differences between public health and medicine discussed earlier are analogous to the difference between public health and criminal justice.

The public health and criminal justice systems have been historically separate in their conceptualization of approaches to violence and the development of activities to reduce or prevent violence. The public health field has approached the issue through efforts to identify the risk factors related to violent behavior. The criminal justice system has approached the issue through efforts to identify and assign blame for criminal behavior, maintain public safety, and remove violent offenders from the community.

Historically, society has relied almost exclusively on the criminal justice system to respond to violence well rooted in a few assumptions: (1) violence is an individual's criminal choice, (2) punishment or the threat of punishment is a deterrent to violent acts, and (3) violence is an inevitable aspect of the behaviors of some people. Police, prosecutors, public defenders, judges, probation officers, and prison guards are part of a sophisticated system designed to respond to crimes after they have been committed by identifying, apprehending, prosecuting, punishing, and controlling the violent offender. Their primary function is not prevention. The prevention efforts that are a part of the criminal justice system are found in the passage of laws and the deterrence resulting from enforcement.

Viewed from the perspective of those interested in reducing violence, the criminal justice system's responses have had only limited success. Inherent limitations in the reactive nature of the criminal justice system are partly responsible. Deterrence, the mainstay prevention strategy, has limited prevention capacity (particularly in the context of violence among acquaintances and family). Rehabilitation, a form of prevention, is offered after a conviction and at variable levels of implementation from state to state.

Despite the fact that the juvenile justice system was created with a fundamental belief in the potential for prevention and rehabilitation among children, its major responsibility is punishment, particularly in this political climate. Many states are eliminating specialized juvenile justice systems for criminal offenses and incorporating youth into the adult criminal process.

Police and many of the laws they enforce are geared toward predatory violence that occurs among strangers on the street. As a result, the many episodes of violence among family, friends, and acquaintances that emerge from insults, frustrations, and festering disputes and that take place in intimate settings are less well addressed. Both the family and acquaintance characteristics of violence in the United States and the need for a more comprehensive set of prevention activities create the context for cooperation between public health and criminal justice. The two disciplines could offer complementary approaches.

Interdisciplinary Challenges

While there are examples of effective collaboration between public health and criminal justice, the professional associations, conferences, programmatic efforts, and academic publications remain distinct, for the most part. More effective collaboration beyond the existing silos of activity and competitive strategies would greatly improve society's capacity to save children from the devastating impact of interpersonal violence. Currently, both disciplines are defensive: criminal justice for its failure to meet societal expectations to control youth violence and public health for the slowness with which it has recognized and taken on the problem. However, considerable tension emerges from the divergent perspectives of the two disciplines and the fact that there are inadequate resources directed to addressing violence, which fosters competition rather than collaboration.

Public health is primarily focused on identifying causality (or its approximation) and intervening to control or reduce the risk factors; it has little interest in assigning blame or ensuring appropriate punishment and does not discriminate between victim and offender. The public health community may agree that justice must be done, but it is not professionally committed to the process. The criminal justice system, on the other hand, is deeply and morally rooted in "justice" and in criminal offenders being properly identified and punished. In this field there is less emphasis on the precursors or factors that may have led to the violent event. The criminal justice system is likely to consider external factors that might have motivated the offender to engage in violence as less important as they are largely irrelevant to judgment of guilt and innocence. Often public health efforts to understand and identify risk factors, particularly those associated with a specific episode of violence, are characterized as a search for excuses or a rationalization (read defense) for what is understood within criminal justice as an individual's malicious choice, a crime.

The more public health embraces multilevel socioecological models for understanding human behavior, the greater the threat to the principles of individual choice and responsibility. This tension between public health and criminal justice is unproductive. It threatens effective collaboration and frustrates the opportunity to pool resources and expertise at a time when resources are seriously inadequate and the problem is increasing. Healing this rift requires a more collaborative spirit from both disciplines. Public health "purists" must get beyond a religious dependence upon science and recognize the invaluable contributions and practical experiences of the criminal justice professionals. The criminal justice "moralists" must, in turn, recognize the limitations of a largely reactive agenda that focuses on blame and punishment.

Moving beyond these obstacles and successfully exploiting the complementary qualities of public health and criminal justice approaches requires following the examples of those who have put aside professional jealousies and utilized the expertise that both disciplines bring to the issue. This not only leads to a more creative process but also enhances productive working relationships.

Delineating Disciplinary Responsibilities: Primary, Secondary, and Tertiary Prevention

Devising conceptual frameworks that can alleviate interprofessional tension, facilitate definitions of roles in addressing the problem, and assist in developing a broader perspective on programmatic strategies involves breaking the spectrum of violence into levels that reflect different points of intervention (see Figure 14.4). This framework, used frequently in public health circles, structures approaches to problems into three stages: primary prevention, secondary prevention (or early intervention), and tertiary prevention (or treatment/rehabilitation). These distinctions have proved valuable in thinking about intervention efforts even though their boundaries are not discrete. In this discussion, it might be best to think of these distinctions in terms of concentric circles that widen out in space and time from a central point which is the occurrence of some violent event.

Primary prevention, which by definition addresses the broadest level of the general public, might seek to reduce the level of violence that is shown on television or to promote gun control. This would be an effort directed toward dealing with the public values and attitudes that may promote or encourage the use of violence.

Secondary prevention is distinguished from primary prevention in that it identifies narrowly defined subgroups or circumstances that are at high risk of being involved in or occasioning violence and focuses its attention on them. Thus, secondary prevention efforts might focus on urban poor, young men and women who are at particularly high risk of engaging in or being victimized by violence, and educating them in nonviolent methods of resolving disputes or displaying competence and power.

Tertiary prevention is distinguished from secondary and primary prevention in that it is a response to a violent event, not purely a preventive measure. Its focus

FIGURE 14.4. THE IDEAL RELATIONSHIP BETWEEN PUBLIC HEALTH AND CRIMINAL JUSTICE IN PREVENTING VIOLENCE.

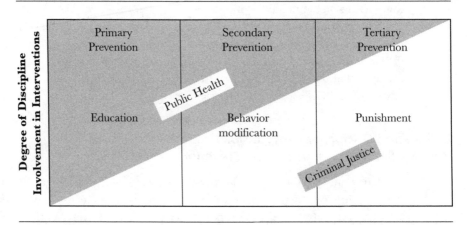

is on trying to reduce the negative consequences of a particular event after it has occurred, or on trying to find ways to use the event to reduce the likelihood of similar incidents occurring in the future. Thus, one might think of improved trauma care, on the one hand, and increased efforts to rehabilitate or incapacitate violent offenders, on the other hand, as tertiary prevention instruments in the control of or the response to violence.

Primary prevention instruments are those that can affect larger and larger populations, ideally at relatively low cost. Thus, primary prevention instruments tend to be those providing information and education on the problem of violence through the popular media—for example, the recruitment of Bill Cosby to the cause of using the media to prevent adolescent violence, or Sarah Brady's efforts to advocate for gun control laws and educate the public about the risks of handguns, rather than providing nonviolence training to the entire population. There are, of course, the ultimate long-term primary prevention goals, which have to do with eliminating some of the root causes of violence, such as social injustice and discrimination.

Tertiary prevention has generally involved incarceration. The major activities of the criminal justice system have historically involved the roles of the police, the courts, and the prison system in responding to criminal or violent events. Most resources have been directed to investigating and punishing criminal behavior. In the area of secondary prevention, the police have focused efforts on "situated" crime prevention and the juvenile justice system has made attempts at early intervention with youthful offenders, although the courts and probation system frequently ignored youth until their criminal behavior reached a relatively high level of concern. Primary prevention efforts have focused on elementary school drug and violence prevention education by the police, as well as on controlling commodities such as drugs, guns, and alcohol.

This model of three levels of prevention can be very useful when applied specifically to the issue of interpersonal violence. In the past, the criminal justice system has addressed each of the three points of intervention to varying degrees as represented, yet the bulk of the efforts have focused on the response to serious violent behavior with moderate attention to early identification and intervention and limited efforts in the area of primary prevention. The role and activities of the public health system are newer, less extensive, and therefore less evolved than those of the criminal justice system.

Traditionally, public health responded by treating violence-related injury in the emergency setting. Today, a new generation of committed health practitioners, community violence prevention practitioners, social workers, and community activists have devised numerous intervention programs to serve medium- to high-risk adolescents. At the primary prevention level, efforts have focused on gun control and safety and enhanced public awareness of risk factors and the true characteristics of most violence to dispel myths and modify societal values around the use of violence. Additionally, some educational interventions (for example, violence prevention curricula) have been applied to broader, less high-risk settings. Again, much of this work is relatively recent and therefore has not yet established a long track record to assess fully its effects. Finally, public health has applied its analytical expertise to enhance greatly the understanding of risk factors, allowing for a broader vision in the planning and development of preventive approaches (National Center, 2001; Prothrow-Stith & Weissman, 1991). In the area of secondary prevention, public health has been involved in the development of educational interventions specifically focused on behavior modification of high-risk individuals, particularly children and youth. Programs and curricula are currently in place across the country, addressing many of the risk factors for violence, including nonviolent problem solving and conflict resolution techniques (National Center, 2001).

Over the last three decades, the criminal justice system has increased its involvement in primary and secondary prevention efforts, highlighting and funding school-based and community-based initiatives to reduce children's access to guns, teach conflict resolution, provide needed social services, and evaluate best practices in prevention. In 1974, with the passage of the Juvenile Justice and Delinquency Prevention Act, the U.S. Department of Justice assumed primary responsibility for delinquency prevention programs, creating the Office of Juvenile Justice and Delinquency Prevention (OJJDP). The OJJDP encourages the development of model delinquency prevention programs and engages a multidisciplinary audience in violence prevention activities. It has been responsible for designating and highlighting "blueprint" programs as models and funding their replication.

One such program is the Boys and Girls Clubs of America's Gang Prevention Through Targeted Outreach. Other community groups refer at-risk boys to the program, who are then recruited. Early evaluations of these programs showed promise: data indicated that 39 percent of the boys did better at school and 93 percent of those who completed the program had not been further involved with the juvenile justice system (Arbreton & McClanahan, n.d.). These types of interventions reflect an important interface between the criminal justice and public health professions. With further attention and the dedication of resources of the public health system to this issue and the broadening vision of criminal justice, a more reasonable balance between prevention and treatment can be achieved in the future.

Boston, Massachusetts, with its dramatic and sustained decline in youth violence, serves as a model of multilevel programmatic activity with exemplary integration between public health and policing strategies (Prothrow-Stith & Spivak, 2004). Two decades of activities within public health and criminal justice and most importantly within the broader community of parents, teens, and survivors of violence resulted in the creation of an extensive set of programs for youth throughout the city. Boston's efforts reflect the range needed both to reduce the extent of violent behavior and to respond to the violence that does occur. It is not only an example for elected officials and community activists; it is also a model for professionals within public health and criminal justice.

Conclusion

Public health professionals began over two decades ago addressing the problem of violence because of their witness to its tragic toll on American children and understanding the limitation of the existing practice within criminal justice. The contributions made by public health professionals toward efforts to prevent violence have been tremendous. The continued application of public health strategies to the understanding and prevention of violence is essential to further progress.

Also, the interface between public health and criminal justice must be continually explored to ensure complementary strategies and activities. While examples of collaboration between the two disciplines exist, more effort must be placed on overcoming some of the inherent obstacles in order to create and fund a joint research and action agenda.

Recently, our national rates of violent crime have fallen; however, in smaller towns, among girls, and in younger children, the rates appear to be on the rise. Also, even with our lower national rates, there is far too much preventable injury daily. The emphasis of the public health system will always be on prevention, and the criminal justice system must place priority on aggressive responses to violence, but much possibility lies in enhancing the collaborative effort between both disciplines.

References

Arbreton, A.J.A., & McClanahan, W. S. *Targeted outreach: Boys & Girls Club of America's approach to gang prevention and intervention.* Retrieved November 15, 2006, from http://www.ppv.org/ppv/publications/assets/148_publication.pdf

Centers for Disease Control and Prevention. (2002, June 28). Youth risk behavior surveillance—United States, 2001. *Morbidity and Mortality Weekly Report, 51*(SS-4).

Federal Bureau of Investigation. (2001). *Uniform crime report: Crime in the United States.* Washington, DC: U.S. Department of Justice.

Institute of Medicine. (1988). *The future of public health.* Washington, DC: National Academies Press.

Institute of Medicine. (2003). *Who will keep the public healthy?* Washington, DC: National Academies Press.

Krug, E. G., Powell, K. E., & Dalhberg, L. L. (1998). Firearm-related deaths in the United States and 35 other high- and upper-middle-income countries. *International Journal of Epidemiology, 27,* 214–221.

National Center for Injury Prevention and Control. (2001). *Injury fact book, 2001–2002.* Atlanta: Centers for Disease Control and Prevention.

National Institute of Justice. (2000). *Criminal victimization 2000: Changes, 1999–2000, with Trends, 1993–2000.* Washington, DC: U.S. Department of Justice.

Prothrow-Stith, D., & Spivak, H. R. (2004). *Murder is no accident: Understanding and preventing youth violence in America.* San Francisco: Jossey-Bass.

Prothrow-Stith, D., & Weissman, M. (1991). *Deadly consequences: How violence is destroying our teenage population and a plan to begin solving the problem.* New York: HarperCollins.

Public opinion about public health—California and the United States 1996, 1998. (1998, February 6). *MMWR, 47*(4), 69–73. Retrieved November 15, 2006, from http://www.cdc.gov/mmwr/preview/mmwrhtml/00051341.htm

Snyder, H., & Sickmund, M. (1999). *Juvenile offenders and victims: 1999 national report.* Washington, DC: Office of Juvenile Justice and Delinquency Prevention.

Tjaden, P., & Thoennes, N. (2000). *Full report of the prevalence, incidence and consequences of violence against women: Findings from the National Violence Against Women Survey.* Washington, DC: National Institute of Justice.

Wolfgang, M. E. (1986). Homicide in other industrialized countries. *Bulletin of the New York Academy of Medicine, 62,* 400–412.

CHAPTER FIFTEEN

THE LIMITS OF BEHAVIORAL INTERVENTIONS FOR HIV PREVENTION

Dan Wohlfeiler, Jonathan M. Ellen

For the past twenty-five years, prevention of HIV has relied heavily on be-havioral interventions aimed at reducing individual risk behaviors, including unprotected sex and sharing contaminated needles, which have been found to lead to infection. Whereas numerous studies have been conducted that demonstrate the effectiveness of behavioral interventions in increasing knowledge, changing attitudes, and reducing risky behaviors, fewer studies have demonstrated the im-pact of behavioral interventions on reducing HIV infections. This is significant since reducing infections is ultimately the goal of primary prevention efforts.

Behavioral interventions are a necessary but insufficient component of HIV prevention. This is due to their moderate success in reducing risky behaviors, their lesser success at decreasing infections, and sadly, their lack of demonstrated ef-fectiveness at altering the course of HIV epidemics. Structural factors, such as economic and racial disparities, fuel the HIV epidemic. Often they act by affect-ing sexual networks—the web of sexual partnerships.

In this chapter, we argue that reducing HIV infections requires more than re-lying on individual behavior change. We suggest two new directions for HIV pre-vention practitioners to take. The first is to take cues from other fields of public health, most notably injury prevention and tobacco control, which have used pol-icy as an integral part of the strategy to achieve desired outcomes. These fields, with more years of experience than HIV's quarter-century, have achieved greater success at developing economic, policy, environmental, and technological strategies that allow their prevention efforts to be more self-sustaining and less reliant on a constant infusion of public health resources, whether these are staff or financial support. This requires public health professionals to be facilitators of change in addition to service providers. Second, as part of a strategy that relies more heavily on structural interventions and policies, we suggest developing interventions that will directly affect the sexual networks that facilitate viral transmission.

Most of this chapter will rely on examples from the United States. This is not meant to diminish the importance of interventions in other countries. The relatively high level of resources available for behavioral interventions in the United States, the rich diversity of behavioral interventions, and the epidemiologic and sociopolitical context of the HIV epidemics in the United States make many aspects of the U.S. epidemic unique.

Epidemiology of HIV in the United States

By the end of 2004, more than 944,000 people had been diagnosed with AIDS in the United States, of whom 529,000 (56 percent) had died (Centers for Disease Control and Prevention [CDC], 2005a). Gay men and African Americans are the two communities most profoundly affected by HIV in the United States, which found fertile ground in these marginalized populations (Valleroy et al., 2000). However, the experiences of the gay and African American communities in confronting HIV are very different from each other.

Gay men and men who have sex with men (MSM) continue to make up the largest segment of infections (65 percent among adult males), even though the percentage of men who have sexual contact with other males is estimated at between 3 and 9 percent of the general population (Anderson & Stall, 2002; Laumann, Gagnon, Michael, & Michaels, 1994; Sell, Wells, & Wypij, 1995).

The AIDS epidemic, similar to other diseases and to other sexually transmitted diseases (STDs), is also increasingly marked by profound racial disparities. The CDC (2005a) reported that non-Hispanic African Americans, who represent 12.3 percent of the U.S. population, accounted for half of the HIV/AIDS cases diagnosed in 2004. Hispanics, who represent 19 percent of the adult population, account for 18 percent of the infections. Among adolescents diagnosed during 2003, 66 percent of those infected are African American; 21 percent are Hispanic. These disparities in infection rates cannot be explained by differences in risk behaviors. Numerous studies have concluded that individuals of different ethnicities report very similar rates of condom usage. Possible explanations and strategies to address these marked disparities will be addressed later in this chapter.

The HIV epidemic among the gay population is the only one in the world that is not correlated with poverty. The high STD and HIV rates among African Americans are often correlated with high levels of poverty, depletion of social capital, neighborhood disintegration, and community fragmentation (Fullilove, 1998; Fullilove, Green, & Fullilove, 2000). The gay community has fewer needs (for example, for improved jobs and housing) and fewer competing priorities (existence of high crime rates) that can affect a community's interest and ability to participate individually and collectively in HIV-specific interventions.

Roots of HIV Prevention

Shortly after the first cases were reported in the United States in 1981, HIV quickly spread through gay communities and through networks of injection drug users. By the mid-1980s, approximately one-half of the gay men in San Francisco and one-half of injection drug users in New York City were infected. Many of these people began developing illnesses rarely seen in young, otherwise healthy adults. By studying the characteristics of those who were first affected by these illnesses, epidemiologists were quickly able to determine that the disease was being transmitted sexually (Auerbach, Darrow, Jaffe, & Curran, 1984) and through injecting needles (CDC, 1982).

Many gay men quickly reduced their high-risk behavior. Most notably, they reduced the number of partners with whom they had unprotected sex (McCusick et al., 1985; Winkelstein et al., 1987). This was demonstrated both by numerous survey studies and through epidemiologic surveillance and modeling. In fact, the rates of infection plummeted almost as quickly as they had increased initially, largely as a result of the reduction in the number of partners.

A careful examination of the history of HIV/AIDS, particularly among gay men, reveals that profound behavior changes took place before any governmental support and funding became available. Early organizers used grassroots mobilizing and information distribution through the press, brochures, and posters to provide people at risk with the information they lacked about this new disease. For example, in San Francisco, reductions in risk behavior occurred as the gay community formed organizations and later engaged in more formal education efforts. Although many contemporary community-based interventions attempt to replicate the strategies used in these early community mobilizations, it is unlikely that they will ever have the impact or reach the scale of the early mobilizations, primarily because it is impossible to replicate the social context in which they occurred. In particular, it is unrealistic to hope to mobilize communities to the same extent as when HIV first took hold, when it had no known etiology or treatment.

Types of Behavioral Interventions and Their Success

Individual-Level Interventions

HIV testing to date has for the most part been accompanied by brief pretest and posttest counseling sessions that aim to inform an individual as to what the HIV test will and will not reveal, what strategies can reduce risk, and what sources of medical and social support are available in case of a positive result. This ambitious scope for brief sessions has long served as a mainstay of HIV prevention. Meta-analyses of multiple studies have demonstrated that the impact of counseling and testing is greatest for HIV-positive individuals, most of whom will take significant measures not to expose anyone else to the virus. The impact on HIV-negative individuals, however, is less pronounced (Weinhardt, Carey, Johnson, & Bickham, 1999).

Client-centered counseling offered by well-trained staff has been shown to help reduce STD transmission. A key study, Project Respect, demonstrated that client-centered counseling was more effective than either interactive counseling or didactic messages in reducing new STD infections (Kamb et al., 1998).

One of the most intensive and broad-based individual-level interventions, Project Explore, recruited more than four thousand high-risk gay and bisexual men to ten onetime counseling sessions. The intervention also included quarterly sessions aimed at maintaining the effect of the counseling sessions (Koblin, Chesney, & Coates, 2004). This is a level of intensity and scale that is much higher than the vast majority of HIV interventions are able to offer. Nevertheless, although the infection rate was lower in the intervention group than in the standard comparison group, the difference was not statistically significant.

Group-Level Interventions

Group workshops have long been used in public health to promote healthy behaviors and provide social support for them. AIDS prevention programs have relied on group-level interventions to reduce participants' risk in gay men and MSM of all ethnicities (Carballo-Dieguez et al., 2005; Peterson et al., 1996; Valdiserri et al., 1989), women (Kelly et al., 1994), injection drug users (el-Bassel & Schilling, 1992), and adolescents (Jemmott, Jemmott, & Fong, 1992; Rotheram-Borus et al., 2003). These have been used to convey information, to promote norms favoring risk reduction, and to recruit volunteers for further educational efforts. Both professional and volunteer facilitators have led these sessions. Studies have demonstrated that group workshops have been effective at reducing both sexual and drug-related risk behavior. Some group interventions convene only once; others may continue for weeks or months. Many of these interventions have recruited individuals who did not know each other previously and are unlikely to meet again except by chance after the intervention. Others recruit members of social networks, with the hope that the conversations and dynamics that emerge during the formal intervention will be more easily sustained afterward.

One example of a group-level intervention provided four group sessions lasting four hours each to sexually experienced African American girls aged fourteen to eighteen. Compared to a control group, participants reported more condom use and fewer new vaginal sex partners. The study also found small but promising declines in chlamydia infections and self-reported pregnancies (DiClemente et al., 2004).

Although many interventions have succeeded in reducing risk, there is less evidence of their effectiveness in reducing the incidence of HIV infections.

Community-Level Interventions

Community-level interventions often include both individual- and group-level interventions and aim to support the effectiveness of these interventions by supporting communitywide norms favoring risk reduction even among individuals who do not participate in the most intensive one-on-one and group-level interventions. These have relied heavily on diffusion models. Diffusion describes the processes whereby messages and norms are conveyed throughout a community. Rather than having to reach every individual, practitioners aim to reach a segment of the population, often popular opinion leaders who can then diffuse the message or norm throughout the rest of the community (Rogers, 1962). In some cases, these programs have been generated by the community itself (Wohlfeiler, 1997). Other programs, such as Mpowerment, have been launched by university researchers (Kegeles, Hays, & Coates, 1996). This project organized gay men, aged eighteen to twenty-nine, to conduct small group workshops, formal and informal outreach, and media and social events. Participants decreased rates of unprotected anal intercourse. No biological outcomes were measured, however.

Forces Promoting One-on-One Interventions

Multiple forces working together have pushed the field of HIV prevention to emphasize one-on-one interventions. As the importance of care and treatment increased, it became harder to mobilize volunteers for prevention. Pressures to be accountable to funders also resulted in the creation of programs that were easier to plan, implement, and measure. Finally, the need to constantly seek additional funding has driven many organizations, both governmental and nongovernmental, to choosing interventions that did not conflict with economic or political interests (Wohlfeiler, 2002).

The Limits of Behavioral Interventions

Behavioral interventions often require substantial resources to decrease the odds of risk behavior by approximately 25 percent (Herbst et al., 2005), which is the level reached by the more successful interventions (Johnson et al., 2002). As the Institute of Medicine (IOM) observes, "A program that achieves statistically significant social and behavioral changes still may not avert large numbers of new infections" (2001, p. 26). For behavioral interventions to succeed in reducing infections across a population, they need to reach a broad sector of the population, be of sufficient intensity, and reach the right individuals. In addition, interventions need to occur in supportive social environments and contexts.

Some of the largest-scale interventions do, in fact, reach significant percentages of their populations. However, most of these interventions are relatively low-intensity, such as one-on-one outreach interventions. These may be as simple as handing out information and condoms or as in-depth as conducting risk assessments, recruiting to more in-depth interventions, and testing for STDs or HIV (or both). These interventions may reach individuals at highest risk, often referred to as the "core group." Even if these individuals are reached, it is unlikely that a brief intervention will make an impact on their risk behavior, since many of these people have psychosocial needs that are not easily addressed by a workshop or counseling session or even ongoing counseling.

A further limitation of many interventions, particularly at the community level, is that they often offer the same "dose" of prevention regardless of the level of an individual's risk. For example, outreach workers may be as likely to offer the same messages, condoms, and invitations to workshops to an individual who has occasional unprotected sex with one partner that they would offer to an individual who has a new unprotected partner every week.

One of the largest-scale community-level interventions carried out targeting the entire gay community, the STOP AIDS Project, has been very successful in recruiting large numbers of men. However, the numbers have decreased over the years. In the mid-1980s, STOP AIDS was able to mobilize three hundred volunteers and recruit some seven thousand men (approximately 15 percent of the gay community) annually to workshops. This was a period marked by widespread fear and large numbers of individuals getting sick, visibly deteriorating—and dying. By the early 1990s, when the infection rate had fallen—but still before new treatments had become available—STOP AIDS was able to mobilize only half that many volunteers and recruit only twelve hundred men to workshops (Wohlfeiler, 2002).

As the lethality of the threat of HIV infection and its sequelae diminishes, thanks to more effective treatment, it becomes less likely that individuals will be motivated to take an active role in community-level interventions. Furthermore, behavioral interventions typically do not directly address the social contexts in which behavior occurs. Behavioral interventions typically recruit individuals to interventions, increase their knowledge, and in many cases, identify triggers to risk behavior, including situations where risk behavior is the most likely to occur. Such triggers may include going to a bar or socializing with peers who engage in high-risk behavior. Many of these contexts are difficult to alter, since they may require a change in social environments, including peer groups. In addition, individuals may have to overcome corporate practices that lead to environments that promote high-risk behaviors.

Corporate practices, including the products sold and promoted in particular neighborhoods, play an important role in shaping the context in which behavioral interventions occur. These practices often overwhelm and contradict behavioral interventions. For example, alcohol abuse and overconsumption are associated with STD acquisition (Cook & Clark, 2005), yet promotion of alcohol is a multi-million-dollar industry, and bars and other purveyors of alcohol are widespread. Considerable variation also exists in the commitment of the adult film industry (CDC, 2005b) and businesses that facilitate partners meeting one another (Internet companies, bathhouses and sex clubs, and large circuit parties) to support risk reduction (Wohlfeiler & Potterat, 2005).

Beyond legitimate questions regarding their effectiveness, behavioral interventions also have faced numerous obstacles related to infrastructure, political barriers, and network- and social-level contextual issues that further hamper their efficacy. Investment in public health and STD prevention has always been insufficient. According to the IOM (1997, p. 2), "Effective STD prevention efforts are hampered by biological characteristics of STDs, societal problems, unbalanced mass media messages, lack of awareness, fragmentation of STD-related services, inadequate training of health care professionals, inadequate health insurance coverage and access to services, and insufficient investment in STD prevention." In HIV prevention, government agencies have relied heavily on community-based organizations, on the principle that these organizations may be more appropriate than the government itself to reach communities with culturally appropriate interventions, mobilize community support, and gain access to communities that may distrust government agencies. However, with few exceptions, most of these agencies pay prevention management and line staff low salaries. This in turn creates high turnover rates among staff, which consequently creates a constant need to train new staff in both the theory and the skills necessary to design and implement effective interventions.

Political forces have also hampered scientifically based behavioral interventions. Support for abstinence-only education has increased, although these programs have been found to contain numerous inaccuracies and have little, if any, benefit in reducing incidence of STDs and HIV (Bruckner & Bearman, 2005). Meanwhile, prevention advocates spend considerable time and energy defending behavioral interventions from conservative forces, which means they have less time to spend on prevention efforts themselves.

New Treatments

Biomedical advances, in particular the discovery and widespread use of new treatments, far extend the lives of HIV-infected individuals. Many in the HIV prevention field have feared that "treatment optimism" has so substantially decreased the threat of HIV as to make prevention even more difficult. However, the relationship between optimism about treatment effectiveness and risk behavior is more complex and may not be unidirectional; risk behavior may both predict and be predicted by such treatment optimism (Huebner, 2005). Regardless of the individual perceptions of new treatment options, it is harder to mobilize community members around a "chronic," if still ultimately fatal, disease.

New treatments reduce individuals' infectiousness and, if widely used, can do so on a population level (Porco et al., 2004). HIV virulence (ease of infection) in a newly infected individual is high, and treatment can significantly decrease infectivity. In an effort to increase the number of individuals who know their HIV status and can then seek treatment, the CDC launched the Advancing HIV Prevention Initiative in 2003, which also aims to increase the integration of prevention and medical care (CDC, 2003).

Structural-Level Solutions to Preventing HIV

Structural interventions aim to modify the social, economic, and political structures and systems in which we live. These may affect legislation, media, health care, and the marketplace. They may include policy, technology, environmental, and economic interventions. Ideally, structural interventions should rely as little as possible on continued support from the public health sector's scarce resources. Thus rather than solely relying on outreach workers to surf the Web to answer questions, public health may be better served by working with Internet providers to provide links to factually correct information and resources. Many HIV behavioral practitioners are aware of the numerous contextual factors that contribute to HIV infection. However, similar to practitioners in other fields of public health, they often continue to pursue individual-level interventions (Millett, Peterson, Wolitski, & Stall, 2006; Wohlfeiler, 2002). As Trostle (2004) points out, behavioral interventions often accept the status quo of existing social dynamics and structures.

Structural interventions often take longer and may not yield immediately measurable benefits in the short term and perhaps not even in the generation in which they are implemented (Fenton & Imrie, 2005). However, given their effectiveness in other areas of public health, they represent a promising area for innovative efforts in HIV prevention.

Structural interventions have a longer history in areas of public health such as violence prevention, tobacco control, and regulation of alcohol consumption than in the prevention of HIV. While many structural interventions have yet to be evaluated in HIV prevention, some have proved effective.

Examples of Structural Interventions in HIV Prevention

Legalizing syringe exchange programs (SEPs), through which injection drug users (IDUs) may exchange used syringes for sterile ones, is one example of a structural intervention. A study of eighty-one cities around the world compared HIV infection rates among IDUs in cities that had SEPs with cities that did not have SEPs. HIV infection rates increased by 5.9 percent per year on average in the fifty-two cities without SEPs but decreased by 5.8 percent per year in the twenty-nine cities with SEPs. The study concluded that SEPs appear to lead to lower levels of HIV infection among IDUs (Hurley, Jolley, & Kaldor, 1997).

Preventing HIV Through Needle Exchange

The nation's first needle exchange program began as a form of civil disobedience in 1986. Incensed by a professor's comment that addicts should not be the focus of HIV prevention efforts because their behaviors could not be changed, Jon Parker, a public health student at Yale University and former heroin addict, began distributing and later exchanging needles and syringes on the streets of New Haven, Connecticut, and Boston, Massachusetts (Lane, 1993).

Parker's belief that addicts' behaviors could and must be changed was particularly relevant in New York City, where as early as 1983 as many as 50 percent of the city's two hundred thousand drug users were infected with HIV (Susman, 2001). New York City

---

(Continued)

was infamous for its "shooting galleries," where large groups of people shared needles, meaning that preventing the spread of HIV was intrinsically linked to the behavior of a large population of intravenous drug users (Drucker, n.d.). New York City's health department attempted to institute a needle exchange program as early as 1985, but the idea was met with immediate protest from law enforcement and from some prominent members of the African American community (Drucker, n.d.).

Many people believed that such a program would encourage drug use in the midst of a "war on drugs," and others expressed concern about the location of needle exchange facilities. That is, even many of the people who agreed with the concept of needle exchange did and still do not want needle exchanges taking place in their own back yards. To address both concerns, the New York City Department of Health opened an experimental exchange program in 1988 (Lane, 1993).

Injection drug users were accepted into the program only if they agreed to enter treatment and could participate only until a treatment slot became available (Lane, 1993). Each received one syringe imprinted with a health department logo and a photo identification card that exempted them from a law prohibiting the possession of drug paraphernalia. They were allowed to exchange only one syringe on each visit. Because there were difficulties housing the exchange program, it was located in the health department headquarters, far from most clients' neighborhoods and near the court house and police department (Lane, 1993).

These adaptations to earlier proposals won the support of the current mayor, Edward Koch, but not of his successor, David Dinkins, who in response to vocal community leaders closed the program in 1990, shortly after his election (Lane, 1993).

Subsequently, activists concerned about rising rates of HIV infection attempted to build community consensus for needle exchange programs. Their efforts were aided by Yale Professor Edward Kaplan's evaluation of the exchange program, which concluded that it had succeeded in reducing HIV transmission and in linking needle exchange with drug treatment and housing. Prevention policy shifted toward needle exchange and won the cautious support of the Dinkins administration (Lane, 1993).

According to Dr. Don Des Jarlais of the Beth Israel Medical Center, before the initiation of the needle exchange program, about 4 to 5 percent of drug users were becoming infected each year (Susman, 2001). The rate was reduced to about 1 percent per year after the exchange program started (Des Jarlais et al., 2000). Though still controversial, needle exchange programs in several cities now receive local, state, and even federal funding (Lane, 1993) because of ample evidence that they are effective in preventing the spread of HIV among intravenous drug users and thus preventing the spread of HIV in the greater community (Satcher, 2000). According to Des Jarlais, "Large-scale syringe exchange and voluntary HIV counseling and testing programs appear to have 'reversed' the HIV epidemic among injecting drug users in New York City." (p. 358).

Source: Prevention Institute.

Bathhouses and sex clubs have long been important institutions in the gay community, providing gay men and MSM an opportunity to meet sexual partners in a venue free from harassment. Considerable debates have taken place within the gay community and even within public health as to what role these institutions may play in facilitating HIV or STD transmission. Bathhouses and sex clubs also provide a good way to compare and contrast two approaches. Individual-level outreach happens in many bathhouses and sex clubs across the country. Structural changes have been attempted in some jurisdictions by instituting policies prohibiting unprotected sex and removing private rooms to enforce these policies. While there are no data to compare effects on infection rates, researchers at the University of California in San Francisco (UCSF) found that men who went to bathhouses and sex clubs in four cities—San Francisco, Chicago, Los Angeles, and New York—all had the same level of unprotected sex overall. But men in San Francisco, where owners have removed the private rooms and enforce rules regarding unprotected sex, reported having less of it in the clubs themselves (Woods et al., 2003). As will be discussed later, this may have important implications for transmission of STDs and HIV through a community's sexual networks. This is an example of how public health practitioners may gain more ground by modifying environments and policies rather than seeking to modify individuals' behavior.

In the Dominican Republic, researchers randomized brothels to two different arms of a study. In one arm, they encouraged voluntary strategies—group workshops and education—to promote condom usage. In another arm, they used those strategies as well as the threat of enforcement through legal strategies. Rather than relying exclusively on reports of changes in rates of condom use, they were able to document changes in the incidence of sexually transmitted infections. These researchers found that the two-pronged approach that used voluntary and policy strategies through mobilizing community and governmental will had a bigger impact than voluntary strategies alone (Kerrigan et al, 2006).

The Structure of Sexual Networks

Many behavioral interventions assume that an individual's risk is the result of his or her individual psychosocial factors. This is partially true. However, the risk to an individual is also determined by his or her sexual partners' levels of risk. Thus an individual's total risk is determined by the patterns and networks of sexual relationships among lower- and higher-risk individuals (Ellen, 2003; Klovdahl, Potterat, Woodhouse, Muth, & Muth, 1992; Morris, 1997; Morris & Kretzschmar, 1997). This has been documented in both young gay males and young African American females (Harawa et al., 2004). For example, young gay men who have partners older than thirty are at even greater risk than those who report having multiple younger partners or inject drugs, simply by virtue of the fact that their older partners are more likely to be infected (Blower & Service, 1997).

There is even stronger evidence among heterosexual adolescents that individual sexual behaviors are not associated with HIV in the United States. Adolescents at greatest risk for HIV are young men who have sex with men, and young minority women who have sex with men (Wilson et al., 2001). Studies comparing HIV-infected adolescent women to uninfected young women from the same community and similar household structure found no differences in number of recent sex partners (Ellen, Aral, & Madger, 1998). In fact, consistent condom use was higher among HIV-infected girls. Studies of acquisition of other STDs also suggest that individual factors have a limited impact on infection among adolescent women. STDs such as chlamydia and gonorrhea show a similar racial and sex distribution as HIV. A national study of adolescents found that risk factors such as consistency of condom use and alcohol use with sex do not mitigate the risk correlated with ethnicity, age, or gender, which are in turn each associated with sexual norms and sexual networks (Ellen et al., 1998). Interventions that focus on individuals, therefore, are unlikely to alter substantially the relationship between high- and lower-risk individuals or the structure of risk-taking networks.

As we have already explained, racial disparities in infection rates cannot be explained by differences in risk behavior between different races alone. Differences do exist, however, in the patterns and network structure of relationships, with higher rates of mixing between high- and lower-risk individuals taking place among African Americans, for example, than among other ethnicities (Laumann & Youm, 1999). This may be related, in part, to both mixing patterns among ethnicities and a shortage of African American males relative to females, due to disproportionate involvement in the criminal justice system and higher rates of mortality (Thomas & Sampson, 2005). AIDS rates have been found to be correlated with incarceration rates (Johnson & Raphael, 2005). Behavioral interventions that attempt to change individual behaviors while ignoring these factors are unlikely to succeed in reducing such disparities. Differences in network structure have been hypothesized to account for racial differences in both heterosexuals and gay men and MSM (Millett et al., 2006).

Focusing a new generation of structural interventions on sexual networks may hold substantial promise. One area of structural interventions that is likely to be the most promising is to focus on sexual network-level interventions in terms of both feasibility and impact (Johnson & Raphael, 2005; Laumann & Youm, 1999; Millett et al., 2006; Thomas & Sampson, 2005). Network-level interventions may be more cost-effective for a variety of populations, including injection drug users

(Neaigus, 1998). The following five principles of sexual network-level interventions may help guide practitioners (Wohlfeiler, 2005).

1. *Consider altering sexual network structures.* Many interventions promote social norms and facilitate communication of risk reduction messages (see, for example, Kelly, 1992; Latkin, Sherman, & Knowlton, 2003; Valente & Saba, 2001) while leaving networks intact. However, given that network structure itself confers risk (Klovdahl et al., 1992; Potterat, Rothenberg, & Muth, 1999; Rothenberg et al., 1998), practitioners should consider altering network structures themselves to gain an epidemiologic advantage. For example, providing "safe sex only" Internet sites or commercial sex venues may help reduce contact between high- and low-risk individuals.

2. *Focus on institutions that either facilitate partner mixing or disrupt ecologies of communities.* Institutions that facilitate mixing between high- and low-risk individuals and that also link different networks together (De, Singh, Wong, Yacoub, & Jolly, 2004) are particularly important for HIV prevention efforts. These include bars, Internet sites, bathhouses, and circuit parties. While a number of behavioral interventions exist within these settings, these have not been evaluated and are likely to be subject to the same limitations as described earlier in this chapter.

As noted previously, the criminal justice system also has a profound impact on the natural ecology of the African American community. By removing such a high percentage of African American men from communities, they leave in their wake a lower number of men than women, which may significantly contribute to the higher rates of concurrency among African Americans (Adimora & Schoenbach, 2005). Concurrency, which is defined as having multiple sexual partners at one time (Morris, 1997), increases the likelihood of HIV infection because earlier sexual partners can be infected through later encounters with the same sexual partners (Wohlfeiler & Potterat, 2003). (Serial monogamy, in contrast, implies no risk for an individual who ends a relationship with a partner before that partner gets infected.) These patterns of concurrency facilitate HIV transmission more efficiently than monogamy or even serial monogamy. Thus programs that focus on prisoners' transition to outside communities, conjugal visits, and efforts to further diminish the impact of prisons on communities may be particularly important in reducing transmission.

3. *Fragment networks by pulling low- and high-risk individuals apart.* Networks connect high- and low-risk individuals. By fragmenting networks, the potential exists to reduce transmission throughout the entire community. Creating Web sites and venues that attract specific segments may help. The marketplace is already doing this to some extent; for example: separate Internet sites exist for high- and low-risk gay men (Wohlfeiler & Potterat, 2005). Furthermore, the creation of sites that

cater to HIV-positive individuals is an example of a "pulling" strategy that violates no individual rights, gives HIV-positive individuals an opportunity to meet partners without having to risk stigma from disclosing status, and may help reduce transmission to HIV-negative individuals.

4. *Help people make informed choices about their sexual partners.* The Internet may be making it easier for people to find sexual partners, but it also provides public health with a unique opportunity. Disclosing HIV status is often an awkward process, and HIV-positive individuals often risk rejection from prospective partners. On the Internet, profile screens enable individuals to reveal their HIV-status once without having to disclose to a prospective partner each and every time. Web site profiles may also help individuals with low and high risk be more explicit about expressing their risk preferences, even at a site where high- and low-risk individuals mix. Encouraging more Web sites to adopt such practices is likely to become increasingly effective as the Internet becomes a more important means for people to meet partners.

5. *Maintain basic human rights and freedom of choice.* Risk behavior is ultimately a matter of individual choice, regardless of how it affects other people in a community. All of us may choose to smoke in our own homes and eat foods that jeopardize our health. As other chapters in this book attest, public health has sought to protect these individual rights while reducing the likelihood of harm to others (by restricting smoking in public places) and increasing informed choices (through menu labeling). These same principles may help public health practitioners as they seek to complement their behavioral interventions with network- and other structural-level interventions as they apply to HIV prevention.

Conclusion

Behavioral interventions will continue to play a strong and necessary role in the prevention of HIV. As new generations become sexually active and consider drug use and other high-risk behaviors, it is imperative that they have access to scientifically accurate and correct medical information that encourage risk reduction.

However, practitioners must also realize the inherent limitations of behavioral interventions in their depth, breadth, sustainability, and effectiveness. HIV practitioners will need to balance behavioral interventions with biomedical interventions, as well as to understand the complex relationship among these types of interventions. Practitioners would do well to attempt to achieve a balance across the spectrum of interventions, including biomedical interventions that seek to reduce the virulence of HIV-infected individuals. Although many tools exist to help practitioners understand the effectiveness of different interventions, few tools exist to help practitioners in allocating adequate resources to different interventions (Cohen, Wu, & Farley, 2004). There also remains a lack of understanding as to which of these interventions may have greater or lesser effectiveness in different populations or at different phases of the epidemic (Wasserheit & Aral, 1996).

Public health practitioners should look for new ways of reducing transmission that are cost-effective, promote truly informed choice, and maintain a respect for basic human rights. We contend that structural-level interventions, particularly those that affect the structure of sexual networks, hold particular promise for HIV prevention efforts.

References

Adimora, A. A., & Schoenbach, V. J. (2005). Social context, sexual networks, and racial disparities in rates of sexually transmitted infections. *Journal of Infectious Diseases, 191*(Suppl. 1), S115–S122.

Anderson, J. E., & Stall, R. (2002). Increased reporting of male-to-male sexual activity in a national survey. *Sexually Transmitted Diseases, 29,* 643–646.

Auerbach, D. M., Darrow, W. W., Jaffe, H. W., & Curran, J. W. (1984). Cluster of cases of the acquired immune deficiency syndrome: Patients linked by sexual contact. *American Journal of Medicine, 76,* 487–492.

Blower, S., & Service, S. (1997). Calculating the odds of HIV infection due to sexual partner selection. *AIDS and Behavior, 1,* 273–274.

Bruckner, H., & Bearman, P. (2005). After the promise: The STD consequences of adolescent virginity pledges. *Journal of Adolescent Health, 36,* 271–278.

Carballo-Dieguez, A., Dolezal C., Leu, C. S., Nieves, L., Diaz, F., Decena, C., et al. (2005). A randomized controlled trial to test an HIV-prevention intervention for Latino gay and bisexual men: Lessons learned. *AIDS Care, 17,* 314–328.

Centers for Disease Control. (1982). Pneumocystis pneumonia. *Morbidity and Mortality Weekly Report, 30,* 250–252.

Centers for Disease Control and Prevention. (2003). Advancing HIV prevention: New strategies for a changing epidemic, United States, 2003. *Morbidity and Mortality Weekly Report, 52,* 329–332.

Centers for Disease Control and Prevention. (2005a). *HIV/AIDS surveillance report, 2004.* Atlanta: U.S. Department of Health and Human Services.

Centers for Disease Control and Prevention. (2005b). HIV transmission in the adult film industry—Los Angeles, California, 2004. *Morbidity and Mortality Weekly Report, 54,* 923–926.

Cohen, D. A., Wu, S. Y., & Farley, T. A. (2004). Comparing the cost-effectiveness of HIV prevention interventions. *Journal of Acquired Immune Deficiency Syndrome, 37,* 1404–1414.

Cook, R. L., & Clark, D. B. (2005). Is there an association between alcohol consumption and sexually transmitted diseases? A systematic review. *Sexually Transmitted Diseases, 32,* 156–164.

De, P., Singh, A. E., Wong, T., Yacoub, W., & Jolly, A. M. (2004). Sexual network analysis of a gonorrhoea outbreak. *Sexually Transmitted Infections, 80,* 280–285.

Des Jarlais, D. C., Marmor, M., Friedmann, P., Titus, S., Aviles, E., Deren, S., et al. (2000). HIV incidence among injection drug users in New York City, 1992–1997: Evidence for a declining epidemic. *American Journal of Public Health, 3,* 352–359.

DiClemente, R. J., Wingood, G. M., Harrington, K. F., Lang, D. L., Davies, S. L., Hook, E. W., III, et al. (2004). Efficacy of an HIV prevention intervention for African American adolescent girls: A randomized controlled trial. *Journal of the American Medical Association, 292,* 171–179.

Drucker, E. (n.d.). New York, through the eye of the needle: Notes from the drug wars. Retrieved July 25, 2006, from http://www.drugtext.org/library/articles/89112.htm

el-Bassel, N., & Schilling, R. F. (1992). Fifteen-month follow-up of women methadone patients taught skills to reduce heterosexual HIV transmission. *Public Health Report, 107,* 500–504.

Ellen, J. M. (2003). The next generation of HIV prevention for adolescent females in the United States: Linking behavioral and epidemiologic sciences to reduce incidence of HIV. *Journal of Urban Health, 80*(4 Suppl. 3), iii40–iii49.

Ellen, J. M., Aral, S. O., & Madger, L. S. (1998). Do differences in sexual behaviors account for the racial/ethnic differences in adolescents' self-reported history of a sexually transmitted disease? *Sexually Transmitted Diseases, 25,* 125–129.

Fenton, K. A., & Imrie, J. (2005). Increasing rates of sexually transmitted diseases in homosexual men in western Europe and the United States: Why? *Infectious Disease Clinics of North America, 19,* 311–331.

Fullilove, R. E. (1998). Race and sexually transmitted diseases. *Sexually Transmitted Diseases, 25,* 130–131.

Fullilove, R. E., Green, L., & Fullilove, M. T. (2000). The Family-to-Family program: A structural intervention with implications for the prevention of HIV/AIDS and other community epidemics. *AIDS, 14*(Suppl. 1), S63–S67.

Harawa, N. T., Greenland, S., Bingham, T. A., Johnson, D. F., Cochran, S. D., Cunningham, W. E., et al. (2004). Associations of race/ethnicity with HIV prevalence and HIV-related behaviors among young men who have sex with men in 7 urban centers in the United States. *Journal of Acquired Immune Deficiency Syndrome, 35,* 526–536.

Herbst, J. H., Sherba, R. T., Crepaz, N., Deluca, J. B., Zohrabyan, L., Stall, R. D., et al. (2005). A meta-analytic review of HIV behavioral interventions for reducing sexual risk behavior of men who have sex with men. *Journal of Acquired Immune Deficiency Syndrome, 39,* 228–241.

Huebner, D. M. (2005). Is optimism really the enemy? New research on treatment optimism. *Focus, 20*(7), 5–6.

Hurley, S. F., Jolley, D. J., & Kaldor, J. M. (1997). Effectiveness of needle-exchange programmes for prevention of HIV infection. *Lancet, 349,* 1797–1800.

Institute of Medicine. (1997). *The hidden epidemic: Confronting sexually transmitted diseases.* Washington, DC: National Academies Press.

Institute of Medicine. (2001). *No time to lose: Getting more from HIV prevention.* Washington, DC: National Academies Press.

Jemmott, J. B., III, Jemmott, L. S., & Fong, G. T. (1992). Reductions in HIV risk-associated sexual behaviors among black male adolescents: Effects of an AIDS prevention intervention. *American Journal of Public Health, 82,* 372–377.

Johnson, R. C., & Raphael, S. (2005). *The effects of male incarceration dynamics on AIDS infection rates among African-American women and men.* Unpublished manuscript.

Johnson, W. D., Hedges, L. V., Ramirez, G., Semaan, S., Norman. L. R., Sogolow, E., et al. (2002). HIV prevention research for men who have sex with men: A systematic review and meta-analysis. *Journal of Acquired Immune Deficiency Syndrome, 30*(Suppl. 1), S118–S129.

Kamb, M. L., Fishbein, M., Douglas, J. M., Jr., Rhodes, F., Rogers, J., Bolan, G., et al. (1998). Efficacy of risk-reduction counseling to prevent human immunodeficiency virus and sexually transmitted diseases: A randomized controlled trial. *Journal of the American Medical Association, 280,* 1161–1167.

Kegeles, S. M., Hays, R. B., & Coates, T. J. (1996). The Mpowerment Project: A community-level HIV prevention intervention for young gay men. *American Journal of Public Health, 86,* 1129–1136.

Kelly, J. A. (1992). HIV risk behavior reduction following intervention with key opinion leaders of population: An experimental analysis. *American Journal of Public Health, 82,* 1483–1489.

Kelly, J. A., Murphy, D. A., Washington, C. D., Wilson, T. S., Koob, J. J., Davis, D. R., et al. (1994). The effects of HIV/AIDS intervention groups for high-risk women in urban clinics. *American Journal of Public Health, 84,* 1918–1922.

Kerrigan, D., Moreno, L., Rosario, S., Gomez, B., Jerez, H., Barrington, C., et al. (2006). Environmental-structural interventions to reduce HIV/STI risk among female sex workers in the Dominican Republic. *American Journal of Public Health, 96,* 120–125.

Klovdahl, A. S., Potterat J. J., Woodhouse, D. E., Muth, J., & Muth, S. Q. (1992). HIV infection in an urban social network: A progress report. *Bulletin de Methodologie Sociologique, 36,* 24–33.

Koblin, B., Chesney, M., & Coates, T. J. (2004). Effects of a behavioural intervention to reduce acquisition of HIV infection among men who have sex with men: The EXPLORE randomised controlled study. *Lancet, 364,* 41–50.

Lane, S. D. (1993). *Needle exchange: A brief history.* Menlo Park, CA: Henry J. Kaiser Family Foundation. Retrieved July 25, 2006, from http://www.aegis.com/law/journals/1993/HKFNE009.html

Latkin, C. A., Sherman, S., & Knowlton, A. (2003). HIV prevention among drug users: Outcome of a network-oriented peer outreach intervention. *Health Psychology, 22,* 332–339.

Laumann, E. O., Gagnon, J. H., Michael, R. T., & Michaels, S. (1994). *The social organization of sexuality.* Chicago: University of Chicago Press.

Laumann, E. O., & Youm, Y. (1999). Racial/ethnic group differences in the prevalence of sexually transmitted diseases in the United States: A network explanation. *Sexually Transmitted Diseases, 26,* 250–261.

McCusick, L., Wiley, J. A., Coates, T. J., Stall, R., Saika, G., Morin, S., et al. (1985). Reported changes in the sexual behavior of men at risk for AIDS, San Francisco, 1982–84: The AIDS Behavioral Research Project. *Public Health Reports, 100,* 622–629.

Millett, G. A., Peterson, J. L., Wolitski, R. J., & Stall, R. D. (2006). Greater risk for HIV infection of black men who have sex with men: A critical literature review. *American Journal of Public Health, 96,* 1007–1019.

Morris, M. (1997). Sexual networks and HIV. *AIDS, 11*(Suppl. A), S209–S216.

Morris, M., & Kretzschmar, M. (1997). Concurrent partnerships and the spread of HIV. *AIDS, 11,* 641–648.

Neaigus, A. (1998). The network approach and interventions to prevent HIV among injection drug users. *Public Health Reports, 113*(Suppl. 1), 140–150.

Peterson, J. L., Coates, T. J., Catania, J. A., Hauck, W. W., Acree, M., Daigle, D., et al. (1996). Evaluation of an HIV risk reduction intervention among African-American homosexual and bisexual men, *AIDS, 10,* 319–325.

Porco, T. C., Martin, J. N., Page-Shafer, K. A., Cheng, A., Charlebois, E., Grant, R. M., et al. (2004). Decline in HIV infectivity following the introduction of highly active anti-retroviral therapy. *AIDS, 18,* 81–88.

Potterat, J. J., Rothenberg, R. B., & Muth, S. Q. (1999). Network structural dynamics and infectious disease propagation. *International Journal of Sexually Transmitted Diseases and AIDS, 10,* 182–185.

Rogers, E. M. (1962). *Diffusion of innovations.* New York: Free Press.

Rothenberg, R. B., Potterat, J. J., Woodhouse, D. E., Muth, S. Q., Darrow, W. W., & Klovdahl, A. S. (1998). Social network dynamics and HIV transmission. *AIDS, 12,* 1529–1536.

Rotheram-Borus, M. J., Song, J., Gwadz, M., Lee, M., Van Rossem, R., & Koopman, C. (2003). Reductions in HIV risk among runaway youth. *Prevention Science, 4,* 173–187.

Satcher, D. (2000). *Evidence-based findings on the efficacy of syringe exchange programs: An analysis of the scientific research completed since April 1998.* Washington, DC: U.S. Department of Health and Human Services.

Sell, R. L., Wells, J. A., & Wypij, D. (1995). The prevalence of homosexual behavior and attraction in the United States, the United Kingdom, and France: Results of national population-based samples. *Archives of Sexual Behavior, 24,* 235–248.

Susman, E. (2001, August 13). New York needle exchange "reverses" AIDS. *United Press International Science News.* Retrieved July 25, 2006, from http://www.aegis.com/news/upi/2001/UP010805.html

Thomas, J. C., & Sampson, L. A. (2005). High rates of incarceration as a social force associated with community rates of sexually transmitted infection. *Journal of Infectious Diseases, 191*(Suppl. 1), S55–S60.

Trostle, J. A. (2004). *Cambridge studies in medical anthropology: Vol. 13. Epidemiology and culture.* New York: Cambridge University Press.

Valdiserri, R. O., Lyter, D. W., Leviton, L. C., Callahan, C. M., Kingsley, L. A., & Rinaldo, C. R. (1989). AIDS prevention in homosexual and bisexual men: Results of a randomized trial evaluating two risk reduction interventions. *AIDS, 3,* 21–26.

Valente, T. W., & Saba, W. P. (2001). Campaign exposure and interpersonal communication as factors in contraceptive use in Bolivia. *Journal of Health Communication, 6,* 303–322.

Valleroy, L. A., MacKellar, D. A., Karon, J. M., Rosen, D. H., McFarland, W., Shehan, D. A., et al. (2000). HIV prevalence and associated risks in young men who have sex with men. *Journal of the American Medical Association, 284,* 198–204.

Wasserheit, J. N., & Aral, S. O. (1996). The dynamic topology of sexually transmitted disease epidemics: Implications for prevention strategies. *The Journal of Infectious Diseases, 174*(Suppl. 2), 201–213.

Weinhardt, L. S., Carey, M. P., Johnson, B. T., & Bickham, N. L. (1999). Effects of HIV counseling and testing on sexual risk behavior. *American Journal of Public Health, 89,* 1397–1405.

Wilson, C. M., Houser, J., Partlow, C., Rudy, B. J., Futterman, D. C., & Friedman, L. B. (2001). The REACH (Reaching for Excellence in Adolescent Care and Health) project: Study design, methods, and population profile. *Journal of Adolescent Health, 29*(3 Suppl.), 8–18.

Winkelstein, W., Jr., Samuel, M., Padian, N. S., Wiley, J. A., Lang, W., Anderson, R. E., et al. (1987). The San Francisco Men's Health Study: III. Reduction in human immunodeficiency virus transmission among homosexual/bisexual men, 1982–86. *American Journal of Public Health, 76*, 685–689.

Wohlfeiler, D. (1997). Community organizing and community building among gay and bisexual men. In M. Minkler (Ed.), *Community organizing and community building for health* (pp. 230–243). New Brunswick, NJ: Rutgers University Press.

Wohlfeiler, D. (2002). From community to clients: The professionalisation of HIV prevention among gay men and its implications for intervention selection. *Sexually Transmitted Infections, 78*(Suppl. 1), i176–i182.

Wohlfeiler, D. (2005). Network-level interventions as feasible structural-level interventions with potentially high impact. In *Prevention strategies for STD and HIV prevention: What, where and when.* Amsterdam: International Society for Sexually Transmitted Diseases Research.

Wohlfeiler, D., & Potterat, J. J. (2003, April). *How do sexual networks affect HIV/STD prevention?* Center for AIDS Prevention Studies Fact Sheet No. 50E. Retrieved July 28, 2006, from http://www.caps.ucsf.edu/pubs/FS/networks.php

Wohlfeiler, D., & Potterat, J. J. (2005). Using gay men's sexual networks to reduce sexually transmitted disease (STD)/human immunodeficiency virus (HIV) transmission. *Sexually Transmitted Diseases, 32*(10 Suppl.), S48–S52.

Woods, W. J., Binson, D., Pollack, L. M., Wohlfeiler, D., Stall, R. D., & Catania, J. A. (2003). Public policy regulating private and public space in gay bathhouses. *Journal of Acquired Immune Deficiency Syndrome, 32*, 417–423.

NAME INDEX

A

Abbey, M., 50
Abelson, R., 10
Aboelata, M. J., 53
Abrams, B., 81
Ackerman, F., 247
Adams, J., 268
Adams, P. F., 50
Addis, M. E., 42
Adimora, A. A., 341
Adloaf, E., 269
Agron, P., 132
Aiello, J. R., 259
Airhihenbuwa, C. O., 34
Ajzen, I., 51
Akili, G., 174
Albee, G., 4, 5, 11
Alexander, C., 268
Alfano, M. S., 55
Alinsky, S., 99, 103, 104, 112
Allison, K. C., 262
Anda, R. F., 28, 30
Anderson, G. F., 10
Anderson, J. E., 330
Andresen, M. A., 262
Annadale, E., 43

Anthony, E. J., 66
Apelberg, B. J., 242
Aral, S. O., 340
Arbreton, A.J.A., 326
Ardell, D. B., 4
Areskoug, B., 268
Arias, E., 32
Ariel, E., 83
Armstrong, L., 46
Arnold, C. L., 266
Ashton, C., 224
Astbury, J., 54
Atkinson, A. J., 224
Atkinson, E. S., 42
Auerbach, D. M., 331
Auerbach, E., 111, 114
Austin, S. B., 296
Avila, M. M., 110

B

Bachar, J. J., 34
Bachmann, J., 6
Baer, N., 16
Bagwell, D. A., 223
Baker, Q. E., 110
Baldwin, G. T., 145, 214

Balfour, J. L., 270
Balk, S. J., 272
Baltodano, M., 114
Bandeh, J. G., 155
Bannerman, R. T., 267
Bardy, S., 325
Barlett, D. L., 10
Barlow, C. E., 261
Barlow, J. M., 274
Barnes, H. V., 67
Barnes, P. M., 50
Barnett, B., 103
Barocas, R., 74
Barrera, M., 83
Barrett, L. T., 217
Barrett-Connor, E., 51
Bauman, A. E., 261, 262
Baumeister, R., 70
Bautista, D. E., 82
Baxandall, R., 270
Beardslee, W., 67
Bearman, P., 336
Beauchamp, D. E., 122, 123, 124, 139
Beauchemin, K. M., 258
Becker, J., 211
Beckwith, D., 96, 112

348

SUBJECT INDEX

A

Access strategy: definition of, 182; developing, 191–195. *See also* Media advocacy

Access to care, as health disparity determinant, 29–30

Accident Prevention Committee of the American Academy of Pediatrics (Tennessee chapter), 163

Action for Healthy Kids, 148, 151, 157

Activist, 98

Ad Council, 15

Adolescents: prevention programs for depression and, 55–56; prevention of youth violence by, 320–321; risk factors for violence and, 318*e*; violence and, 316–317. *See also* Children

Advertising: eliminating less healthful food, 305; "health seals" self-endorsements by food industry, 295; media strategy using paid, 194; U.S. food industry expenditures on, 295–296

Advocates, 98

African Americans: environmental exposure outcomes for, 240, 244–245; HIV/AIDS rate among, 330, 331, 340; lack of health insurance by, 241; life expectancy of, 43. *See also* Racial/ethnic differences

After-school programs, 75

Agency for Healthcare Research and Quality, 11

Aggregate Exposures to Phthalates in Humans study (2002), 239

AIDS. *See* HIV/AIDS

Air pollution: built environment and, 263; concentrated animal feeding operations (CAFOs) source of, 288; Toxics Resolution in Multnomah County to reduce, 247–248

Alcohol: Friday Night Live (FNL) to prevent driving mixed with, 48–49; traffic injuries related to, 48

Alliance for Justice, 199

American Academy of Pediatrics, 259

American Association of State Highway and Transportation Officials, 274

American Automobile Association's Foundation for Traffic Safety, 269

American College of Emergency Physicians, 10, 316

American Dental Association, 8

American Heart Association, 52–53

American Medical Association, 316

Annie E. Casey Foundation, 78, 79

Antismoking legislation, 8

Asian Americans, 177–178

Asian and Pacific Islander American Health Forum, 178

Asian Pacific Islander Tobacco Control Network, 177

Asthma, 240

At-risk populations: built environment and, 271–274; Institute of Medicine on prevention and, 11

Australian Department of Transport and Regional Services, 47

Authentic voice stories, 196–197

B

Baby Milk Action, 15

Baby-Friendly Hospital Initiative, 17

Bathhouses, 339

BBC News, 15

Bean v. Southwestern Waste Management, 244

Behavioral interventions: as HIV prevention component, 329–330; HIV/AIDS and limits of, 334–336; HIV/AIDS and types of, 332–336; for sexual behavior, 332–334, 339–342. *See also* Prevention programs; Social change

Behavioral Risk Factor Surveillance System (CDC), 262

Belmont Report (National Commission), 224

Berkeley Public Health Services, 15

Best Start Social Marketing, 16

BMI (body mass index), 262

Boston Women's Health Book Collective, 103

Boys Clubs of America's Targeting Programs for Delinquency Intervention, 326

Breastfeeding, 13–15, 17–18

BREATH advocates, 177–178

British Columbia Ministry of Municipal Affairs, 302

Bronx Health REACH initiative, 35

Building Community (Gardner), 85

Built environment: buildings: crowding, 258–259; injury risk, 259–260; lighting, 258

Built environment: concept of, 257; health impact assessment (HIA) tool for evaluating, 274–275; intermediate scale: buildings, 258–260; large scale: from neighborhood to metropolis, 260–271; populations at special risk in, 271–274; small scale, 258. *See also* Community; Environmental health; Neighborhoods

Burger King, 295

Burns (residential), 260

C

CAFOs (concentrated animal feeding operations), 288

California Adolescent Health Collaborative, 56

California Center for Health Improvement, 190

California Center for Public Health Advocacy, 299

California Chamber of Commerce, 126

California Department of Health Services, 136, 206–207, 223, 298

California Department of Health Services' Tobacco Control Section (TCS), 220

California High School Fast Food Survey report (2000), 136

California Project LEAN (Leaders Encouraging Activity and Nutrition), 136

California Proposition 99, 8, 206

California Safe Cosmetics Act (2005), 239

California Smoke-Free Workplace Law (LA County), 223

California Tobacco Control Program (CTCP), 206

California Wellness Foundation, 79

California's Obesity Prevention Motion (2003), 299

Calorie intake, 290

Campaign for Safe Cosmetics, 238–239

Cancer Society, 144

Canvassing operations, 168, 171

Cardiovascular disease (CVD): described, 49; gender patterns of risks and outcomes, 49–52; implications for prevention, 52–54

Carnegie Task Force, 72

CBPR (community-based participatory research): environmental health application of, 249–251; evaluation using approach of, 209–210; as vital primary prevention strategy, 231–232

Center for Health, Environment and Justice, 246

Center for Science in the Public Interest, 299

Center for Third World Organizing, 100

Centers for Disease Control and Prevention (CDC): Behavioral Risk Factor Surveillance System of, 262; on cardiovascular disease-related deaths, 49; on environmental exposure impact, 237–238; environmental monitoring by, 247; on evaluating prevention programs, 206; evaluation framework developed by, 208*fig*–210; on HIV/AIDS in the U.S., 330; on impact of pollution policies, 6; on improving home safety, 260; injury classification by, 319; National Center for Injury Prevention and Control of, 316, 319, 321; on prevention efforts, 10; on prevention and health disparities, 11; Racial and Ethnic Approaches to Community Health program of, 34; on socializing men for health awareness, 53; on traffic injuries, 264; VERB Youth Media Campaign of, 213–214*t*; Violence Epidemiology Branch of, 320; website of, 321

"Challenging Corporate Abuses" (1993), 17

Change. *See* Behavioral interventions; Social change

Changing organizational practices, 17

Character Strengths and Virtues: A Handbook and Classification (Peterson and Seligman), 70

Chicago Neighborhood project, 75

Children: built environment risks for, 272; driven to school instead of walking, 265; food industry advertising directed toward, 295–296; impact of crowded environment on, 259. *See also* Adolescents; Schools

Children's Advertising Review Unit (CARU), 305

Cholera outbreak (England, 1854), 7

Citywide Liquor Coalition (Baltimore), 176